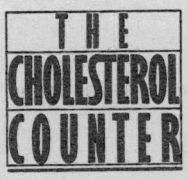

THE
CHOLESTEROL
COUNTER

ANNETTE B. NATOW, Ph.D., R.D., and JO-ANN HESLIN, M.A., R.D., are the authors of seven books on nutrition, including *The Pocket Encyclopedia of Nutrition, No-Nonsense Nutrition for Kids* and *Megadoses: Vitamins as Drugs* (all available from Pocket Books). They are faculty members of Adelphi University and previously taught at Downstate Medical Center and New York University. They have held editorial positions at the *Journal of Nutrition for the Elderly, American Baby* and *Prevention* magazines, and are regular contributors to health magazines and journals.

Books by Annette B. Natow and Jo-Ann Heslin

The Cholesterol Counter
Megadoses
No-Nonsense Nutrition for Kids
The Pocket Encyclopedia of Nutrition

Published by POCKET BOOKS

THE
CHOLESTEROL
COUNTER

Expanded and Updated

Annette Natow, Ph.D., R.D., and Jo-Ann Heslin, M.A., R.D.

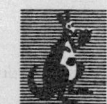

POCKET BOOKS

New York London Toronto Sydney Tokyo Singapore

An *Original* Publication of POCKET BOOKS

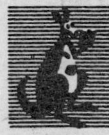

POCKET BOOKS, a division of Simon & Schuster Inc.
1230 Avenue of the Americas, New York, NY 10020

ISBN: 0-671-72762-1

First Pocket Books revised printing March 1989

10 9 8 7 6 5 4 3

POCKET and colophon are registered trademarks of
Simon & Schuster Inc.

Printed in the U.S.A.

———————

To our families, who support us through every project:
Harry, Allen, Irene, Sarah, Laura, Marty, George, Emily,
Steven, Joseph, Kristen and Karen

———————

ACKNOWLEDGMENTS

Without the tireless cooperation of Steven and Laura, *Cholesterol Counter* would never have been completed. A special thanks to Abe and Lillie Lefkowitz, who were there when we really needed them.

Our thanks also go to all the food manufacturers who graciously shared their data.

AUTHORS' NOTE

Sources of Data

Values in this counter have been obtained from the Composition of Foods, United States Department of Agriculture: Dairy and Egg Products, Agricultural Handbook No. 8-1; Spices and Herbs, Agricultural Handbook No. 8-2; Fats and Oils, Agricultural Handbook No. 8-4; Poultry, Agricultural Handbook No. 8-5; Soups, Sauces and Gravies, Agricultural Handbook No. 8-6; Sausages and Luncheon Meats, Agricultural Handbook No. 8-7; Fruit and Fruit Juices, Agricultural Handbook No. 8-9; Pork Products, Agricultural Handbook No. 8-10; Vegetables and Vegetable Products, Agricultural Handbook No. 8-11; Nut and Seed Products, Agricultural Handbook No. 8-12; Beef Products, Agricultural Handbook No. 8-13; Beverages, Agricultural Handbook No. 8-14; Finfish and Shellfish Products, Agricultural Handbook No. 8-15; Legumes and Legume Products, Agricultural Handbook No. 8-16.

Nutritive values of foods, United States Department of Agriculture, Home and Garden Bulletin No. 72.

Bowes & Church's Food Values of Portions Commonly Used (Philadelphia, PA: J.B. Lippincott Co., 1985).

Nutrients in Foods (Cambridge, MA: Nutrition Guild, 1983).

Information from food labels, manufacturers and processors. The values are based on research conducted prior to October 1988. Manufacturer's ingredients are subject to change, so current values may vary from those listed in the book.

"If only half a dozen foods were available the matter would be quickly settled."

MARY SWARTZ ROSE, PH.D.
Feeding the Family
The MacMillan Company
1919

CONTENTS

PART I
Brand Name and Generic Foods

CONTENTS xvii

xx CONTENTS

PART II
Restaurant, Take-Out and Fast-Food Chains

APPENDIX
Baby Foods

WHAT IS CHOLESTEROL?

High Cholesterol is a major risk factor for heart disease.
High Cholesterol is a major risk factor for stroke.
High Cholesterol increases your risk of colon and rectal cancer.
High Cholesterol plus high blood pressure may cause hearing loss.
High Cholesterol, fat-rich diets may cause gallstones.

Did you know that every year more than half a million Americans die from coronary heart disease—heart attack and stroke? That's more than the number of people who die from all forms of cancer! Heart attack and stroke disable even more people than they kill. Coronary heart disease is a disease not only of the old. One out of five men has a heart attack before he is fifty. Often, the heart attack or stroke that causes death or disability is the first sign you get that something is wrong.

Research shows that high cholesterol levels are one of the most important risk factors for heart disease. Lowering your cholesterol lowers your risk.

What is cholesterol?

Cholesterol is a white, waxy, fatlike substance that is part of every cell in your body. Cholesterol is important to body function. Hormones, nerve coverings, vitamin D, bile (used for digestion), and the fat that keeps your skin soft (sebum) are all made from cholesterol. Cholesterol makes up a major part of your brain. Cholesterol is needed by the body, but when the blood level of cholesterol in your blood gets too high, it's not healthy. Some of that extra cholesterol can be deposited on the artery wall, narrowing it and interfering with normal blood flow.

Where does cholesterol come from?

We get some cholesterol every time we eat any animal foods. Meat, poultry, fish, eggs, milk, yogurt, cheese and butter are all animal foods and contain cholesterol. Egg yolk is a major source of cholesterol. An average yolk contains about 270 milligrams. The egg white does not have any cholesterol. Caviar and organ meats like liver, heart and brains are very high in cholesterol.

There is no cholesterol in any food that grows in the ground. Vegetable oils, peanut butter, vegetables, fruits, cereals and grains contain no cholesterol.

Cholesterol is also made in the body. In fact most people make three times as much cholesterol as they get in the food they eat.

How do I know if my blood cholesterol is too high?

It is estimated that only ten percent of all American adults know their cholesterol level. The National Cholesterol Education Program recommends that all adults over age twenty find out their total cholesterol level. A blood test can tell you. Below are average blood cholesterol levels of Americans, but they are not the most healthy levels.

AVERAGE BLOOD CHOLESTEROL LEVELS*

AGE	MALES	FEMALES
20–29	175	165
30–39	195	180
40–49	210	200
50–59	215	225
60–69	215	230
70 +	205	230

*Adapted from "American Heart Association Special Report: Recommendation for the Treatment of Hyperlipidemia: A Joint Statement of the Nutrition Committee and the Council on Arteriosclerosis of the American Heart Association," *Circulation,* 69(1984):433a.

For adults, a cholesterol level over 200 milligrams is considered too high. If your cholesterol is above 200 milligrams your risk for heart disease and other problems is increased.

CHOLESTEROL VALUES THAT PLACE YOU AT RISK*

AGE	MODERATE RISK	HIGH RISK
20–29	200–220	Over 220
30–39	220–240	Over 240
40	240–260	Over 260

**"Lowering Blood Cholesterol to Prevent Heart Disease: Consensus Conference," *Journal of the American Medical Association,* 253(1985):2080.

If my cholesterol is higher than 200, what should I do?

In late 1987 the federal government, along with over twenty health organizations, issued guidelines to help identify and treat people whose blood cholesterol levels were too high. This will affect one in four Americans.

People with desirable cholesterol levels of under 200 milligrams were advised only to recheck the level every five years.

People with levels above 200 milligrams were advised to go on a cholesterol-lowering diet that is low in cholesterol, fats and saturated fats.

Many foods are high in all three—cholesterol, fats and saturated fats. By lowering your intake of high cholesterol foods, you reduce your intake of other fats as well and lower your risk for heart disease.

For each one percent decrease in blood cholesterol level, you reduce your risk of heart disease by two percent. Even the smallest change is to your benefit.

In the government guidelines for lowering cholesterol, the Step I diet for those whose cholesterol levels are 200 to 239 milligrams recommends eating less than 300 milligrams of cholesterol a day. Those people whose cholesterol levels are 240 milligrams and over are advised to restrict their cholesterol intake to less than 200 milligrams per day.

GUIDELINES FOR CHOLESTEROL INTAKE*

CHOLESTEROL LEVEL IN THE BLOOD	MG OF CHOLESTEROL YOU CAN EAT EACH DAY
200–239 mg	less than 300 mg a day
240 mg and over	less than 200 mg a day

*Adapted from material provided by National Cholesterol Education Program, National Heart, Lung and Blood Institute, National Institutes of Health, 1987

What about taking drugs to lower my cholesterol?

Some people who have a high cholesterol level may not be able to lower it enough by diet changes alone. They may need to use a drug in addition to making changes in the way they eat. Drugs used most often are cholestyramine, colestipol and niacin.

Cholestyramine (Questran) and colestipol (Colestid) are resins that increase the excretion of cholesterol from the body. Major side effects are constipation, bloating and gas. They are unpleasant to take.

Niacin (nicotinic acid, a B vitamin) causes intense flushing and itching of the skin right after you take it. Major side effects are rashes and upset stomach. It can worsen diabetes and gout.

Lovastatin (Mevacor), a new drug approved by the FDA in late 1987, is recommended to be used with caution because there has not yet been time to evaluate its long-term effects. It is recommended for use when other drugs do not work.

Probucol (Lorelco) and Gemfibrozil (Lopid) are reserved for use when diet and other medications are not effective.

COUNT UP
YOUR CHOLESTEROL

Most of us eat too much cholesterol each day.

We eat on the run and pick foods high in fat. By the end of the day we've eaten too much cholesterol.

You know that you shouldn't be eating a lot of cholesterol. You want to cut back. But it's not easy since you are not really sure which foods are high in cholesterol and which foods are not. With the *Cholesterol Counter* it's simple to find out which foods have cholesterol and to reduce the amount you are eating.

Let's look at a typical day. Are the food choices familiar? Let's see just how much cholesterol this sample day contains and how we can reduce the amount with better food choices.

CHOLESTEROL COUNTING:
A SAMPLE DAY OF POOR FOOD CHOICES

	CHOLESTEROL (MG)
Breakfast	
Orange juice (½ cup)	0
Scrambled eggs	427
Bacon (2 slices)	10
Toast (1 slice)	0
Butter (1 tsp)	10
Coffee & Cream (1 Tbsp)	6
Lunch	
Cheeseburger	
Hamburger (3 oz)	80
American cheese (1 slice)	25
Roll	0
Catsup	0
French fries	0
Vanilla shake	29
Snack	
Pound cake (1 slice)	46
Coffee &	0
Cream (1 Tbsp)	6
Dinner	
Batter-dipped fried chicken (½ breast)	119
Baked potato &	0
Sour cream (2 Tbsp)	14
Tossed salad &	0
Thousand Island dressing (¼ cup)	20
Apple pie (1 slice)	10
Tea &	0
Sugar	0
TV Snack	
Rich vanilla ice cream (1 cup)	88
Total Cholesterol:	**890**

This is too much cholesterol for one day—almost 3 times the recommended level of 300 milligrams a day. Now you can see how easy it is to take in more cholesterol than you need.

CHOLESTEROL COUNTING:
A SAMPLE DAY OF WISE FOOD CHOICES

	CHOLESTEROL (MG)
Breakfast	
Orange juice (4 oz)	0
Cheerios &	
Lowfat milk (½ cup)	5
Toast (1 slice) &	0
Jelly	0
Coffee &	0
Lowfat milk (2 Tbsp)	1
Lunch	
Hamburger (3 oz)	80
Roll	0
Catsup	0
French fries	0
Cola	0
Snack	
Pear	0
Dinner	
Roasted chicken breast, no skin (½ breast)	73
Baked potato &	0
Plain yogurt (2 Tbsp or 1 oz)	2
Tossed salad &	0
Oil & vinegar dressing (2 Tbsp)	0
Fruit cocktail (½ cup)	0
Tea &	0
Sugar	0
TV Snack	
Vanilla ice milk (1 cup)	18
Total Cholesterol:	**179**

Wise food choices! A much healthier intake of cholesterol for the day.

Now it's your turn to count your cholesterol. Note everything you eat today, then look up the cholesterol in each food you have eaten and see how much cholesterol you ate today. While you're at it, jot down the calories, too!

CHOLESTEROL COUNTING:
A SAMPLE WORKSHEET

FOOD	AMOUNT	CHOLESTEROL (MG)	CALORIES
Breakfast			
Snack			
Lunch			
Snack			
Dinner			
Snack			

TOTAL CHOLESTEROL: CALORIES:

Did your cholesterol total more than 300 milligrams for the day? If it did, you need to start counting cholesterol and making wiser food choices.

CHOLESTEROL COUNTING:
A SAMPLE WORKSHEET

FOOD	AMOUNT	CHOLESTEROL (MG)	CALORIES
Breakfast			
Snack			
Lunch			
Snack			
Dinner			
Snack			

TOTAL CHOLESTEROL: CALORIES:

Did your cholesterol total more than 300 milligrams for the day? If it did, you need to start counting cholesterol and making wiser food choices.

EIGHT STEPS
TO LOWER CHOLESTEROL

1. Use liquid vegetable oils. Choose olive, canola, corn, soybean, sunflower, safflower and cottonseed oils.

2. Limit amount of meat eaten. Do not use liver, brains or other organ meats. Poultry, shellfish and other fish also should be eaten in small portions.

3. Use lean cuts of meat; trim off all visible fat. Cook without added fat. Bake, broil or roast to further reduce fat. Remove skin from poultry and fish.

4. Use more beans, grains, pasta, rice and vegetables to make up for the smaller portions of meat, fish and poultry.

5. Avoid coffee whiteners (nondairy creamers) and whipped toppings.

6. Limit eggs to three a week, including those used in cooking and desserts. Two egg whites can be substituted for one egg.

7. Use skim milk, skim milk cheese, ice milk and lowfat yogurt. Avoid butter, cream, ice cream, sour cream and whole milk.

8. When using margarine, salad dressing or gravy, use a teaspoon or tablespoon to measure out a portion.

EIGHT STEPS
TO LOWER CHOLESTEROL

1. Use liquid vegetable oils. Choose olive, canola, corn, soybean, sunflower, safflower and cottonseed oils.

2. Limit amount of meat eaten. Do not use fatty brands of or often meats. Poultry, shellfish and other fish also should be eaten in small portions.

3. Use lean cuts of meat, trim off all visible fat. Cook without added fat. Bake, broil or roast to further reduce fat. Remove skin from poultry and fish.

4. Use more beans, grains, pasta, rice and vegetables to make up for the smaller portions of meat, fish, and poultry.

5. Avoid coffee whiteners (nondairy creamers) and whipped toppings.

6. Limit eggs to three a week, including those used in cooking and dessert. The egg white can be substituted for the egg.

7. Use skim milk, some milk cheese, ice milk and lowfat yogurt. Avoid butter, cream, ice cream, sour cream and whole milk.

8. When using margarine, salad dressing or gravy, use a teaspoon or tablespoon to measure out 1 portion.

are listed alphabetically beneath PRODUCT BRAND,

USING YOUR
CHOLESTEROL COUNTER

This book lists the cholesterol and calorie content of over 8000 foods. For the first time, information about cholesterol values is at your fingertips. Now you will find it easy to follow a low-cholesterol diet.

Before *Cholesterol Counter* it was impossible to tell how much cholesterol there was in prepared foods since most do not list cholesterol information on the label. Fresh foods like meat, chicken, fish and cheese do not even have a label. The same goes for take-out items like potato salad, coleslaw, quiche, or foods bought at the bakery. How can you tell how much cholesterol there is in a burger or taco that you enjoy at the local fast-food restaurant? *Cholesterol Counter* lists them all!

The second edition is divided into two main sections. Part I, Brand Name and Generic Foods, lists foods alphabetically. For each group, you will find brand-name foods listed first in alphabetical order, followed by an alphabetical listing of generic foods.

If you want to know how much cholesterol is in the hamburger you are having for lunch, look under BEEF, where you will find a beef patty or a microwave hamburger sandwich listed. If you are making a homemade hamburger, look under ROLL, where you will find the hamburger roll listed alphabetically. For foods like FRENCH TOAST, PASTA or TUNA, simply look for the specific food alphabetically in the complete listing. For example, FRENCH TOAST is found on page 178, listed alphabetically between FRENCH BEANS

and FROG LEG. Two slices have 224 milligrams of cho
lesterol.

Part II, Restaurant, Take-out and Fast-Food Chains, con
tains an alphabetical listing of 21 popular chains. Fast food
like BURGER KING, DOMINO'S PIZZA, TACO BELL an
WENDY'S are listed alphabetically under the chain's name
For example McDONALD'S is listed on page 483 unde
M.

If you are eating at home, simply look up the individua
foods you are eating and total the cholesterol for the meal
For example, your dinner may consist of:

	CHOLESTERO (MG)
2 rib lamb chops, broiled	132
Broccoli w/ Cheese Sauce (Birds Eye)	6
Long Grain & Wild Rice (Minute Rice)	10
Pecan Pie (Mrs. Smith's)	30
Glass of white wine	0
TOTAL CHOLESTEROL FOR THE MEAL	178

We have tried to include all foods for which cholestero
values are known. There will be some foods, however, tha
are not listed in *Cholesterol Counter* because the cholestero
values are not available for that particular food.

When you can't locate your favorite brand, look at othe
similar foods. You will probably find a brand food, a generi
product or a home recipe that is like your favorite food. Fo
example: You find that your favorite brand of vanilla yogurt is
not listed. Ask yourself, "Is my favorite brand made from
whole milk or is it lowfat?" If it is lowfat vanilla yogurt, or
pages 456–57 you will find a generic listing for lowfat vanilla

yogurt as well as an entry for Friendship Lowfat vanilla yogurt and Yoplait 150 vanilla yogurt. From these three entries you can quickly determine that lowfat vanilla yogurt has 14 milligrams or less cholesterol in a serving. You can then assume that your favorite brand has a comparable amount.

With your *Cholesterol Counter* as your guide, you will never again wonder how much cholesterol is in food. You will always be able to tell if a food is high in cholesterol, moderate in cholesterol or low in cholesterol. Your goal is to pick low-cholesterol foods each time you eat.

Finding Cholesterol in the Foods You Eat

When you know the ingredients in a food you can tell if that food contains cholesterol. Read the ingredients list on the label or, if you are using a home recipe, read through the recipe ingredients. To find cholesterol-containing ingredients you need only remember this simple rule:

If it grows in the ground, the food does not contain cholesterol.

If it has feet, fins, wings or claws and can walk, swim or fly, the food does contain cholesterol.

Try out the rule. Which of the following foods has cholesterol?

Is there cholesterol in:

	YES	NO
Hamburger	X	
Sardines	X	
Lobster	X	
Chicken leg	X	
Cheddar cheese	X	
Milk	X	
Egg	X	
Peanut butter		X
Apple		X
Olive oil		X

The first seven foods all contain cholesterol. Hamburger comes from a steer. Sardines and lobsters are seafood. Chicken leg comes from a chicken. All of these have either feet, fins, wings or claws. Therefore, they all contain cholesterol. Cheddar cheese, milk and egg have cholesterol because they all come from an animal that has feet.

Peanut butter, apples and olive oil are all from plants that grow in the ground. Therefore, they have no cholesterol.

Now you know why all of the ingredients on the following list have cholesterol. These are the ingredients to look for on a label or in a recipe.

INGREDIENTS THAT CONTAIN CHOLESTEROL
whole eggs
egg yolks
whole milk
lowfat milk
cream
ice cream
sour cream
yogurt (unless labeled nonfat)
cheese (unless labeled nonfat)
bacon or bacon fat
butter
lard
chicken fat
beef suet or tallow
liver
kidney
brains
meat (any variety)
fish (any variety)
poultry (any variety)

Here are some sample labels with the cholesterol containing ingredients in *italics*.

KEEBLER STONE CREEK HEARTY RYE CRACKERS
Enriched wheat flour containing niacin, reduced iron, thiamine mononitrate (vitamin B1) and riboflavin (vitamin B2), *animal* or vegetable shortening (*lard* or partially hydrogenated soybean oil), sugar, stone ground rye flour, stone ground corn flour, salt, molasses, dehydrated onion, leavening, spices, artificial color (caramel) and lecithin.

These crackers have only one ingredient that contains cholesterol, but it is the second ingredient listed after flour. This means that the crackers contain more lard or soybean oil than any other ingredient except flour. Note that lard or soybean oil may be used. You have no way of knowing which was used. It is safer to assume it is the lard and that the crackers contain cholesterol.

NOODLE RONI CHICKEN AND MUSHROOM FLAVOR
Egg noodles, food starch modified, natural flavors, *chicken fat,* hydrolyzed vegetable protein with dry yeast and soy flour, dried mushrooms, *dried chicken,* monosodium glutamate, dried onion, dried red pepper, onion tumeric, tricalcium phosphate, sugar, dried parsley, spice, dried garlic, disodium inosinate, disodium guanylate, freshness preserved with BHA, propylgallate, citric acid.

This side dish contains three sources of cholesterol: egg noodles, chicken fat and dried chicken.

FRENCH'S IDAHO MASHED POTATOES
Idaho potato granules (with sodium bisulfite, citric acid and BHA added to protect color and flavor), monoglycerides.

Although these instant mashed potatoes contain no cholesterol, the package directions tell you to add butter and milk. Both are sources of cholesterol. Even though you buy a cholesterol-free product, you may be adding cholesterol in the preparation.

To cut down on the cholesterol in the instant mashed potatoes, you could use margarine and skim milk in place of butter and whole milk.

DEFINITIONS

as prep (as prepared): refers to food that has been prepared according to package directions

cooked: refers to food cooked without the addition of fat (oil, butter, margarine, etc.); steaming, poaching, broiling and dry roasting are examples of this type of preparation

generic: describes a food without a brand name

home recipe: describes homemade dishes; those included can be used as a guide to the cholesterol and calorie values of similar products you may prepare or take-out food you buy ready-to-eat

lean and fat: describes meat with some fat on its edges that is not cut away before cooking or poultry prepared with skin and fat as purchased

lean only: lean portion, trimmed of all visible fat

tr (trace): value used when a food contains less than one calorie or less than one mg of cholesterol

ABBREVIATIONS

avg	=	average
diam	=	diameter
fl oz	=	fluid ounce
frzn	=	frozen
g	=	gram
lb	=	pound
lg	=	large
med	=	medium
mg	=	milligram
oz	=	ounce
pkg	=	package
prep	=	prepared
pt	=	pint
reg	=	regular
sm	=	small
sq	=	square
Tbsp	=	tablespoon
tr	=	trace
tsp	=	teaspoon
w/	=	with
w/o	=	without
"	=	inch
<	=	less than

EQUIVALENT MEASURES

1 tablespoon	=	3 teaspoons
4 tablespoons	=	¼ cup
8 tablespoons	=	½ cup
12 tablespoons	=	¾ cup
16 tablespoons	=	1 cup
1000 milligrams	=	1 gram
28 grams	=	1 ounce

LIQUID MEASUREMENTS

2 tablespoons	=	1 ounce
¼ cup	=	2 ounces
½ cup	=	4 ounces
¾ cup	=	6 ounces
1 cup	=	8 ounces
2 cups	=	1 pint
4 cups	=	1 quart

DRY MEASUREMENTS

16 ounces	=	1 pound
12 ounces	=	¾ pound
8 ounces	=	½ pound
4 ounces	=	¼ pound

THE
CHOLESTEROL
COUNTER

All cholesterol values of food are given in milligrams (mg).

PART I
Brand Name and Generic Foods

PART I

Brand-Name and Generic
Foods

FOOD	PORTION	CALORIES	CHOLESTEROL

ABALONE

FRESH

fried	3 oz	161	80
raw	3 oz	89	72

ACEROLA

FRESH

acerola	1 fruit	2	0

JUICE

acerola	1 oz	6	0

ADZUKI BEANS

CANNED

sweetened	½ cup	351	0

DRIED

cooked	1 cup	294	0
raw	1 cup	649	0

READY-TO-USE

yokan; sliced	¼" slice	36	0

ALE

(*see* BEER AND ALE)

ALFALFA

SPROUTS

alfalfa sprouts	1 cup	40	0
alfalfa sprouts	1 Tbsp	1	0

FOOD	PORTION	CALORIES	CHOLESTEROL
ALMONDS			
Almond Butter (Erewhon)	1 Tbsp	90	0
Blanched, Slivered, Whole or Sliced (Planters)	1 oz	170	0
Dry Roasted (Planters)	1 oz	170	0
Honey Roasted (Planters)	1 oz	170	0
Shelled Almonds (Dole)	1 oz	170	0
almond butter	1 Tbsp	101	0
almond butter, honey and cinnamon	1 Tbsp	96	0
almond meal, partially defatted	1 oz	116	0
almond paste	1 oz	127	0
dried, unblanched	1 oz	167	0
dried, unblanched	1 cup	837	0
dried, blanched	1 oz	166	0
dry roasted, unblanched	1 oz	167	0
oil roasted, blanched	1 oz	174	0
oil roasted, unblanched	1 oz	176	0
toasted, unblanched	1 oz	167	0
whole, dried, blanched	1 cup	850	0
AMARANTH			
Amaranth Flakes (Health Valley)	1 oz	110	0

FOOD	PORTION	CALORIES	CHOLESTEROL
Amaranth w/ Banana (Health Valley)	1 oz	100	0
Amaranth Crunch w/ Raisins (Health Valley)	1 oz	110	0
Amaranth Pilaf (Health Valley)	7.5 oz	178	0
amaranth; cooked	½ cup	59	0

APPLE

FOOD	PORTION	CALORIES	CHOLESTEROL
Spiced Apple Rings (White House)	3.5 oz	180	0
applesauce, sweetened	½ cup	97	0
applesauce, unsweetened	½ cup	53	0
sliced, sweetened	½ cup	68	0
DRIED			
Apples (Mariani)	¼ cup	150	0
cooked w/ sugar	½ cup	116	0
cooked w/o sugar	½ cup	172	0
rings	10	155	0
FRESH			
apple	1	81	0
w/o skin; cooked	1 cup	91	0
w/o skin; microwaved	1 cup	96	0
w/o skin; sliced	1 cup	62	0
FROZEN			
Apples, Glazed in Raspberry Sauce (Budget Gourmet)	5 oz	110	10
sliced	½ cup	41	0

FOOD	PORTION	CALORIES	CHOLESTER
JUICE			
Apple (Mott's)	6 oz	88	
Apple (Mott's)	8.5 oz	124	
Apple (Mott's)	9.5 oz	141	
Apple (Mott's)	10 oz	148	
Apple (Seneca)	6 oz	90	
Apple (Tree Top)	6 oz	90	
Apple frzn; as prep (Seneca)	6 oz	90	
Apple frzn; as prep (Tree Top)	6 oz	90	
Apple 100% Unsweetened (S&W)	6 oz	85	
Apple Cider (Tree Top)	6 oz	90	
Apple Cider frzn; as prep (Tree Top)	6 oz	90	
Apple Juice (Ocean Spray)	6 oz	90	
Apple Juice (White House)	6 oz	87	
Apple Juice 100% Pure (Kraft)	6 oz	80	0
Apple Natural Style (Mott's)	6 oz	88	0

FOOD	PORTION	CALORIES	CHOLESTEROL
Apple Unfiltered frzn; as prep (Tree Top)	6 oz	90	0
Natural Apple frzn; as prep (Seneca)	6 oz	90	0
apple	1 cup	116	0
frzn; as prep	1 cup	111	0
frzn; not prep	6 oz	349	0

APRICOTS

CANNED			
Apricot Halves Unpeeled in Heavy Syrup (S&W)	½ cup	110	0
Apricots Whole Peeled in Heavy Syrup (S&W)	½ cup	100	0
apricots, heavy syrup w/ skin	3 halves, 1¾ Tbsp liquid	70	0
apricots, juice pack w/ skin	3 halves, 1¾ Tbsp liquid	40	0
apricots, light syrup w/ skin	3 halves, 1¾ Tbsp liquid	54	0
apricots, water pack w/o skin	2 fruits, 2 Tbsp liquid	20	0
apricots, water pack w/ skin	3 halves	22	0
DRIED			
Apricots (Mariani)	¼ cup	140	0

FOOD	PORTION	CALORIES	CHOLESTEROL
halves	10	83	0
halves; cooked w/o sugar	½ cup	106	0
FRESH apricots	3	51	0
FROZEN apricots	½ cup	119	0
JUICE Nectar (S&W)	6 oz	100	0
nectar	1 cup	141	0

ARROWHEAD

FRESH boiled	1 med	9	0
raw	1 med	12	0

ARTICHOKE

CANNED Heart Marinated (S&W)	3.5 oz	225	0
FRESH artichoke; cooked	1 med	53	0
hearts; cooked	½ cup	37	0
jerusalem, raw; sliced	½ cup	57	0
raw	1 med	65	0
FROZEN Artichoke Hearts (Birds Eye)	½ cup	32	0

FOOD	PORTION	CALORIES	CHOLESTEROL
frzn; cooked	9 oz pkg	108	0
frzn; not prep	9 oz pkg	96	0

ASPARAGUS

CANNED			
Cut Spears (Owatonna)	½ cup	20	0
Spears Colossal Fancy (S&W)	½ cup	20	0
Spears Fancy (S&W)	½ cup	18	0
asparagus	½ cup spears	24	0
FRESH			
asparagus, raw	½ cup	15	0
asparagus; cooked	½ cup	22	0
asparagus; cooked	4 spears	15	0
FROZEN			
Cut (Birds Eye)	½ cup	23	0
Spears (Birds Eye)	½ cup	24	0
frzn; cooked	4 spears	17	0
frzn; not prep	10 oz	69	0

AVOCADO

FRESH			
Avocado (California Avocados)	½	153	0

FOOD	PORTION	CALORIES	CHOLESTEROL
Avocado; mashed (California Avocados)	1 cup	407	0
avocado	1	324	0

BACON
(*see also* BACON SUBSTITUTE)

FOOD	PORTION	CALORIES	CHOLESTEROL
Armour Lower Salt; cooked	1 strip	38	6
Armour Star; cooked	1 strip	38	6
Oscar Mayer Center Cut; cooked	1 strip (4.6 g)	24	5
Oscar Mayer Lower Salt; cooked	1 strip (6.1 g)	33	5
Oscar Mayer; cooked	1 strip (6 g)	35	5
bacon; cooked	3 strips (19 g)	109	16
breakfast strips, beef; cooked	3 strips (34 g)	153	40
breakfast strips, pork, raw	3 strips (3 oz)	264	47
breakfast strips; cooked	3 strips (34 g)	156	36
Canadian bacon; grilled	2 slices (1.7 oz)	86	27
Canadian bacon; unheated	1 pkg (6 oz)	268	85
pork	3 slices (2 oz)	378	46

BACON SUBSTITUTE

FOOD	PORTION	CALORIES	CHOLESTEROL
Bacon Bits (Oscar Mayer)	¼ oz	21	6

FOOD	PORTION	CALORIES	CHOLESTEROL
Breakfast Strips Lean 'N Tasty Beef; cooked (Oscar Mayer)	1 strip (12 g)	46	13
Breakfast Strips Lean 'N Tasty Pork; cooked (Oscar Mayer)	1 strip (12 g)	54	14
Strips, frzn (Morningstar Farms)	3.5 oz	333	1
bacon substitute	1 strip	25	0
breakfast strips, beef, raw	3 strips	276	56

BAGEL

Big 'N Crusty (Lenders)	1	230	0
Blueberry (Lenders)	1	190	0
Cinnamon & Raisin (Sara Lee)	1	240	0
Egg (Sara Lee)	1	250	20
Onion (Sara Lee)	1	230	0
Plain (Lenders)	1	150	0
Plain (Sara Lee)	1	230	0
Poppy Seed (Sara Lee)	1	230	0
Sesame Seed (Sara Lee)	1	260	0

BAKING POWDER

Calumet	1 tsp	3	0

FOOD	PORTION	CALORIES	CHOLESTEROL

BAKING SODA

FOOD	PORTION	CALORIES	CHOLESTEROL
Arm & Hammer (Church Dwight)	1 tsp	0	0

BAMBOO SHOOTS

FOOD	PORTION	CALORIES	CHOLESTEROL
CANNED			
bamboo shoots; sliced	1 cup	25	0
FRESH			
cooked	½ cup	15	0
raw	½ cup	21	0

BANANA

FOOD	PORTION	CALORIES	CHOLESTEROL
DRIED			
dehydrated powder	1 Tbsp	21	0
FRESH			
Chiquita	1 (3½ oz)	110	0
banana	1	105	0

BASS

FOOD	PORTION	CALORIES	CHOLESTEROL
FRESH			
freshwater	1 fillet (2.7 oz)	903	54
freshwater	3 oz	97	58
sea, raw	1 fillet (4.5 oz)	125	53
sea, raw	3 oz	82	35
sea; cooked	3 oz	105	45
sea; cooked	1 fillet (3.5 oz)	125	53

FOOD	PORTION	CALORIES	CHOLESTEROL
striped, raw	3 oz	82	68
striped, raw	1 fillet (5.6 oz)	154	127

BEANS
(see also individual names)

CANNED			
Boston Baked (Health Valley)	4 oz	110	0
Cut Green Beans (Hanover)	½ cup	20	0
Four Bean Salad (Hanover)	½ cup	80	0
Maple Sugar Beans (S&W)	½ cup	150	0
Mixed Bean Salad Marinated (S&W)	½ cup	90	0
Pork 'N Beans (S&W)	½ cup	130	0
Smokey Ranch Beans (S&W)	½ cup	130	0
Vegetarian (Libby)	½ cup	130	0
Vegetarian (Seneca)	½ cup	130	0
Vegetarian w/ Miso (Health Valley)	4 oz	90	0
baked beans, plain	½ cup	118	0
baked beans, vegetarian	½ cup	118	0
baked beans, w/ beef	½ cup	161	29
baked beans, w/ franks	½ cup	182	8

FOOD	PORTION	CALORIES	CHOLESTEROL
baked beans, w/ pork	½ cup	133	9
baked beans, w/ pork & sweet sauce	½ cup	140	9
baked beans, w/ pork & tomato sauce	½ cup	123	9
FROZEN Romano Bean Medley (Hanover)	½ cup	25	0
HOME RECIPE baked beans	½ cup	190	6
refried beans	½ cup	43	2
three bean salad	¾ cup	230	0
SPROUTS bean sprouts, canned	½ cup	8	0

BEECHNUTS

dried	1 oz	164	0

BEEF

(see also BEEF DISHES, VEAL)

Beef is graded according to its marbling, the little flecks of fat in the muscle. Beef graded "Prime" has the highest percentage of fat, followed by "Choice" with less fat and "Select" with the least fat.

CANNED			
corned beef	1 oz	71	24
corned beef	1 slice (21 g)	53	18
stew w/vegetables	1 cup	186	33

FOOD	PORTION	CALORIES	CHOLESTEROL

FRESH

Note that the values for cooked beef may differ slightly from values for raw beef. When meat is cooked some moisture and fat is lost, changing the nutrition value slightly. As a rule of thumb it can be assumed that a 4 oz raw portion will equal a 3 oz cooked portion of meat.

FOOD	PORTION	CALORIES	CHOLESTEROL
bottom round, lean & fat, Choice, raw	4 oz	256	72
bottom round, lean & fat, Choice; braised	3 oz	224	81
bottom round, lean & fat, Prime; braised	3 oz	253	81
bottom round, lean & fat, Prime, raw	4 oz	256	72
bottom round, lean & fat, Select, raw	4 oz	244	72
bottom round, lean & fat, Select; braised	3 oz	215	81
bottom round, lean only, Choice, raw	4 oz	172	68
bottom round, lean only, Choice; braised	3 oz	191	81
bottom round, lean only, Prime, raw	4 oz	180	68
bottom round, lean only, Prime; braised	3 oz	212	81
bottom round, lean only, Select, raw	4 oz	164	68
bottom round, lean only, Select; braised	3 oz	182	81
brisket, flat half, lean & fat; braised	3 oz	347	78

FOOD	PORTION	CALORIES	CHOLESTEROL
brisket, flat half, lean only; braised	3 oz	223	77
brisket, point half, lean & fat, raw	4 oz	336	80
brisket, point half, lean only, raw	4 oz	152	68
brisket, point half, lean only; braised	3 oz	181	81
brisket, point half; braised	3 oz	311	81
brisket, whole, lean & fat; braised	3 oz	332	79
brisket, whole, lean only; braised	3 oz	205	79
chuck arm pot roast, lean only, Choice; braised	3 oz	199	85
chuck arm pot roast, lean only, Prime; braised	3 oz	222	85
chuck arm pot roast, lean only, Select; braised	3 oz	189	85
chuck arm pot roast, lean & fat, Choice; braised	3 oz	301	84
chuck arm pot roast, lean & fat, Choice, raw	4 oz	296	80
chuck arm pot roast, lean & fat, Prime, raw	4 oz	332	80
chuck arm pot roast, lean & fat, Prime; braised	3 oz	332	84
chuck arm pot roast, lean & fat, Select, raw	4 oz	268	76
chuck arm pot roast, lean & fat, Select; braised	3 oz	287	84
chuck arm pot roast, lean only, Choice, raw	4 oz	156	68

FOOD	PORTION	CALORIES	CHOLESTEROL
chuck arm pot roast, lean only, Prime, raw	4 oz	176	68
chuck arm pot roast, lean only, Select, raw	4 oz	148	68
chuck blade roast, Select, raw	4 oz	296	80
chuck blade roast, lean only, Choice; braised	3 oz	234	90
chuck blade roast, lean only, Prime; braised	3 oz	270	90
chuck blade roast, lean only, Select; braised	3 oz	218	90
chuck blade roast, lean & fat, Choice, raw	4 oz	328	84
chuck blade roast, lean & fat, Choice; braised	3 oz	330	87
chuck blade roast, lean & fat, Prime, raw	4 oz	372	84
chuck blade roast, lean & fat, Prime; braised	3 oz	354	87
chuck blade roast, lean & fat, Select; braised	3 oz	311	88
chuck blade roast, lean only, Choice, raw	4 oz	192	72
chuck blade roast, lean only, Prime, raw	4 oz	232	72
chuck blade roast, lean only, Select, raw	4 oz	172	72
corned beef brisket, raw	4 oz	224	60
corned beef brisket; cooked	3 oz	213	83
eye of round, lean & fat, Choice, raw	4 oz	228	68

FOOD	PORTION	CALORIES	CHOLESTEROL
eye of round, lean & fat, Choice; roasted	3 oz	207	62
eye of round, lean & fat, Prime, raw	4 oz	252	68
eye of round, lean & fat, Select, raw	4 oz	212	68
eye of round, lean & fat, Select; roasted	3 oz	201	62
eye of round, lean and fat, Prime; roasted	3 oz	213	61
eye of round, lean only, Choice, raw	4 oz	152	60
eye of round, lean only, Choice; roasted	3 oz	156	59
eye of round, lean only, Prime; roasted	3 oz	168	59
eye of round, lean only, Select, raw	4 oz	144	60
eye of round, lean only, Select; roasted	3 oz	151	59
eye of round, lean only, Prime, raw	4 oz	168	60
flank, lean only, Choice; broiled	3 oz	207	60
flank, lean only, Choice, raw	3 oz	192	56
flank, lean only, Choice; braised	3 oz	208	60
flank, lean & fat, Choice, raw	4 oz	220	60
flank, lean & fat, Choice; braised	3 oz	218	61
flank, lean & fat, Choice; broiled	3 oz	216	60

FOOD	PORTION	CALORIES	CHOLESTEROL
ground, extra lean, raw	4 oz	265	78
ground, extra lean; cooked medium	3 oz	213	70
ground, extra lean; cooked well-done	3 oz	232	91
ground, lean, raw	4 oz	298	85
ground, lean; cooked medium	3 oz	227	66
ground, lean; cooked well-done	3 oz	248	84
ground, regular, raw	4 oz	351	96
ground, regular; cooked medium	3 oz	244	74
ground, regular; cooked well-done	3 oz	269	92
lungs, raw	4 oz	104	274
lungs; braised	3 oz	102	236
porterhouse steak, lean only, Choice, raw	4 oz	180	68
porterhouse steak, lean only, Choice; broiled	3 oz	185	68
porterhouse steak, lean & fat, Choice, raw	4 oz	324	80
porterhouse steak, lean & fat, Choice; broiled	3 oz	254	70
rib eye small end, lean only, Choice, raw	4 oz	184	68
rib eye small end, lean & fat, Choice, raw	4 oz	284	76
rib eye small end, lean & fat, Choice; broiled	3 oz	250	70
rib large end, lean & fat, Choice, raw	4 oz	404	84

FOOD	PORTION	CALORIES	CHOLESTEROL
rib large end, lean & fat, Choice; broiled	3 oz	327	74
rib large end, lean & fat, Choice; roasted	3 oz	316	72
rib large end, lean & fat, Prime; broiled	3 oz	361	74
rib large end, lean & fat, Prime, raw	4 oz	436	84
rib large end, lean & fat, Prime; roasted	3 oz	346	72
rib large end, lean & fat, Select, raw	4 oz	372	80
rib large end, lean & fat, Select; broiled	3 oz	301	73
rib large end, lean & fat, Select; roasted	3 oz	304	72
rib large end, lean only, Choice, raw	4 oz	196	68
rib large end, lean only, Choice; broiled	3 oz	203	70
rib large end, lean only, Choice; roasted	3 oz	210	68
rib large end, lean only, Prime; broiled	3 oz	250	70
rib large end, lean only, Prime; roasted	3 oz	241	68
rib large end, lean only, Select, raw	4 oz	180	68
rib large end, lean only, Select; broiled	3 oz	183	70
rib large end, lean only, Select; roasted	3 oz	197	68

FOOD	PORTION	CALORIES	CHOLESTEROL
rib large end, lean only, Prime, raw	4 oz	240	68
rib small end, lean & fat, Choice, raw	4 oz	356	80
rib small end, lean & fat, Choice; broiled	3 oz	282	71
rib small end, lean & fat, Choice; roasted	3 oz	312	72
rib small end, lean & fat, Prime, raw	4 oz	396	80
rib small end, lean & fat, Prime; broiled	3 oz	309	71
rib small end, lean & fat, Prime; roasted	3 oz	357	72
rib small end, lean & fat, Select, raw	4 oz	324	80
rib small end, lean & fat, Select; broiled	3 oz	263	71
rib small end, lean & fat, Select; roasted	3 oz	283	72
rib small end, lean only, Choice, raw	4 oz	184	68
rib small end, lean only, Choice; broiled	3 oz	191	68
rib small end, lean only, Choice; broiled	3 oz	191	68
rib small end, lean only, Choice; roasted	3 oz	206	68
rib small end, lean only, Prime; broiled	3 oz	221	68
rib small end, lean only, Prime; roasted	3 oz	259	68

FOOD	PORTION	CALORIES	CHOLESTEROL
rib small end, lean only, Select, raw	4 oz	168	68
rib small end, lean only, Select; broiled	3 oz	178	68
rib small end, lean only, Select; roasted	3 oz	183	68
rib small end, lean only, Prime, raw	4 oz	228	68
rib whole, lean & fat, Choice, raw	4 oz	384	80
rib whole, lean & fat, Choice; broiled	3 oz	313	73
rib whole, lean & fat, Choice; roasted	3 oz	328	72
rib whole, lean & fat, Prime, raw	4 oz	420	84
rib whole, lean & fat, Prime; broiled	3 oz	347	73
rib whole, lean & fat, Prime; roasted	3 oz	361	73
rib whole, lean & fat, Select, raw	4 oz	352	80
rib whole, lean & fat, Select; broiled	3 oz	289	72
rib whole, lean & fat, Select; roasted	3 oz	306	72
rib whole, lean only, Choice, raw	4 oz	192	68
rib whole, lean only, Choice; broiled	3 oz	198	69
rib whole, lean only, Choice; roasted	3 oz	209	68

FOOD	PORTION	CALORIES	CHOLESTEROL
rib whole, lean only, Prime, raw	4 oz	232	68
rib whole, lean only, Prime; broiled	3 oz	238	69
rib whole, lean only, Prime; roasted	3 oz	248	68
rib whole, lean only, Select, raw	4 oz	172	68
rib whole, lean only, Select; broiled	3 oz	181	69
rib whole, lean only, Select; roasted	3 oz	191	68
round, lean only, Choice, raw	4 oz	156	64
round, lean only, Choice; broiled	3 oz	165	70
round, lean only, Select, raw	4 oz	152	64
round, lean only, Select; broiled	3 oz	157	70
round, lean & fat, Choice, raw	4 oz	272	76
round, lean & fat, Choice; broiled	3 oz	233	71
round, lean & fat, Select, raw	4 oz	260	76
round, lean & fat, Select; broiled	3 oz	222	71
shank crosscut, lean & fat, Choice, raw	4 oz	180	48
shank crosscut, lean only, Choice, raw	4 oz	144	44
shank, crosscut, lean & fat, Choice; simmered	3 oz	208	67

FOOD	PORTION	CALORIES	CHOLESTEROL
shank, crosscut, lean only, Choice; simmered	3 oz	171	66
short loin tenderloin, lean & fat, Choice, raw	1 steak (6.6 oz)	391	110
short loin tenderloin, lean & fat, Prime, raw	1 steak (5.5 oz)	450	111
short loin tenderloin, lean & fat, Prime; broiled	1 steak (4 oz)	362	99
short loin tenderloin, lean & fat, Select, raw	1 steak (5.5 oz)	364	108
short loin tenderloin, lean & fat, Select; broiled	1 steak (4 oz)	286	97
short loin tenderloin, lean only, Choice, raw	4 oz	168	72
short loin tenderloin, lean only, Prime, raw	4 oz	192	72
short loin tenderloin, lean only, Select, raw	4 oz	160	72
short loin top loin, lean & fat, Choice, raw	1 steak (10.7 oz)	886	212
short loin top loin, lean & fat, Choice; broiled	1 steak (8.2 oz)	672	187
short loin top loin, lean & fat, Prime, raw	1 steak (10.7 oz)	980	212
short loin top loin, lean & fat, Prime; broiled	1 steak (8 oz)	774	183
short loin top loin, lean & fat, Select, raw	1 steak (10.7 oz)	804	208
short loin top loin, lean & fat, Select; broiled	1 steak (8.1 oz)	603	182
short loin top loin, lean only, Choice, raw	4 oz	176	68

FOOD	PORTION	CALORIES	CHOLESTEROL
short loin top loin, lean only, Prime, raw	4 oz	212	68
short loin top loin, lean only, Select, raw	4 oz	156	68
short loin, tenderloin, lean & fat, Choice; broiled	3 oz	230	73
short loin, tenderloin, lean & fat, Choice; roasted	3 oz	262	74
short loin, tenderloin, lean & fat, Choice; broiled	1 steak (4.1 oz)	314	100
short loin, tenderloin, lean & fat, Prime; broiled	3 oz	270	73
short loin, tenderloin, lean & fat, Prime; roasted	3 oz	305	75
short loin, tenderloin, lean & fat, Select; broiled	3 oz	216	73
short loin, tenderloin, lean & fat, Select; roasted	3 oz	245	74
short loin, tenderloin, lean only, Choice; broiled	3 oz	176	72
short loin, tenderloin, lean only, Choice; roasted	3 oz	189	73
short loin, tenderloin, lean only, Prime; broiled	3 oz	197	72
short loin, tenderloin, lean only, Prime; roasted	3 oz	217	73
short loin, tenderloin, lean only, Select; broiled	3 oz	167	72
short loin, tenderloin, lean only, Select; roasted	3 oz	177	73
short loin, top loin, lean & fat, Choice; roasted	3 oz	243	68

FOOD	PORTION	CALORIES	CHOLESTEROL
short loin, top loin, lean & fat, Prime; broiled	3 oz	288	68
short loin, top loin, lean & fat, Select; broiled	3 oz	223	67
short loin, top loin, lean only, Choice; broiled	3 oz	176	65
short loin, top loin, lean only, Prime; broiled	3 oz	208	65
short loin, top loin, lean only, Select; broiled	3 oz	162	65
shortribs, lean & fat, Choice, raw	4 oz	440	88
shortribs, lean & fat, Choice; braised	3 oz	400	80
shortribs, lean only, Choice, raw	4 oz	196	68
shortribs, lean only, Choice; braised	3 oz	251	79
sirloin, wedge-bone, lean & fat, Choice; broiled	3 oz	240	77
sirloin, wedge-bone, lean & fat, Choice; pan-fried	3 oz	288	84
sirloin, wedge-bone, lean & fat, Prime; broiled	3 oz	271	77
sirloin, wedge-bone, lean & fat, Select; broiled	3 oz	232	77
sirloin, wedge-bone, lean only, Choice; broiled	3 oz	180	76
sirloin, wedge-bone, lean only, Choice; pan-fried	3 oz	202	85
sirloin, wedge-bone, lean only, Prime; broiled	3 oz	201	76

OOD	PORTION	CALORIES	CHOLESTEROL
sirloin, wedge-bone, lean only, Select; broiled	3 oz	170	76
spleen, raw	4 oz	119	298
spleen; braised	3 oz	123	295
T-bone steak, lean & fat, Choice, raw	4 oz	348	80
T-bone steak, lean only, Choice, raw	4 oz	180	68
T-bone steak, lean & fat, Choice; broiled	3 oz	276	71
T-bone steak, lean only, Choice; broiled	3 oz	182	68
thymus, raw	4 oz	266	252
thymus; braised	3 oz	271	250
tip round, lean & fat, Choice, raw	4 oz	240	72
tip round, lean & fat, Choice; roasted	3 oz	216	70
tip round, lean & fat, Prime, raw	4 oz	256	76
tip round, lean & fat, Prime; roasted	3 oz	242	71
tip round, lean & fat, Select, raw	4 oz	220	72
tip round, lean & fat, Select; roasted	3 oz	205	70
tip round, lean only, Choice, raw	4 oz	152	68
tip round, lean only, Choice; roasted	3 oz	164	69
tip round, lean only, Prime, raw	4 oz	164	68

FOOD	PORTION	CALORIES	CHOLESTEROL
tip round, lean only, Prime; roasted	3 oz	181	69
tip round, lean only, Select, raw	4 oz	144	68
tip round, lean only, Select; roasted	3 oz	156	69
top round, lean & fat, Choice, raw	4 oz	196	68
top round, lean & fat, Choice; pan-fried	3 oz	246	82
top round, lean & fat, Choice; roasted	3 oz	181	72
top round, lean & fat, Prime, raw	4 oz	212	68
top round, lean & fat, Prime; broiled	3 oz	201	72
top round, lean & fat, Select, raw	4 oz	188	68
top round, lean & fat, Select; broiled	3 oz	176	72
top round, lean only, Choice, raw	4 oz	152	64
top round, lean only, Choice; broiled	3 oz	165	72
top round, lean only, Choice; pan-fried	3 oz	193	83
top round, lean only, Prime, raw	4 oz	176	64
top round, lean only, Prime; broiled	3 oz	183	72
top round, lean only, Select, raw	4 oz	144	64

OOD	PORTION	CALORIES	CHOLESTEROL
op round, lean only, Select; roiled	3 oz	156	72
ripe, raw	4 oz	111	107
wedge-bone sirloin, lean only, Choice, raw	4 oz	156	68
wedge-bone sirloin, lean only, Prime, raw	4 oz	176	68
wedge-bone sirloin, lean only, Select, raw	4 oz	148	68
wedge-bone sirloin, lean & fat, Choice, raw	4 oz	300	80
wedge-bone sirloin, lean & fat, Prime, raw	4 oz	328	80
wedge-bone sirloin, lean & fat, Select, raw	4 oz	280	80

BEEF DISHES

FROZEN			
Beef w/ Barbeque Sauce Sandwich (Microwave Chefwich)	1 (5 oz)	360	23
Cheeseburger (Micro Magic)	1 (4.75 oz)	450	80
Hamburger (Micro Magic)	1 (4.75 oz)	350	55
ground patties, frzn, raw	4 oz	319	89
patties; cooked medium	3 oz	240	80
Hamburger Helper Beef Noodle; as prep (General Mills)	6 oz	326	61

FOOD	PORTION	CALORIES	CHOLESTEROL
Hamburger Helper Cheeseburger Macaroni; as prep (General Mills)	6 oz	366	61
Hamburger Helper Chili Tomato; as prep (General Mills)	6 oz	336	61
Hamburger Helper Lasagne; as prep (General Mills)	6 oz	336	61
HOME RECIPE			
sauerbraten	3.5 oz	190	75
stew w/ vegetables	1 cup	209	61
stroganoff	¾ cup	260	69
swiss steak	4.6 oz	214	61

BEER AND ALE

FOOD	PORTION	CALORIES	CHOLESTEROL
Amstel Light	12 oz	95	0
Anheuser Busch Natural Light	12 oz	110	0
Bud Light	12 oz	108	0
Coors Light	12 oz	105	0
Guiness Kaliber (nonalcoholic)	12 oz	43	0
Michelob Light	12 oz	134	0
Miller Lite	12 oz	96	0
Molson Light	12 oz	109	0
Piels Light	12 oz	136	0
Schlitz Light	12 oz	96	0
Schaefer Light	12 oz	112	0
Schmidts Light	12 oz	96	0

FOOD	PORTION	CALORIES	CHOLESTEROL
ale	12 oz	155	0
beer, light	12 oz can	100	0
beer, regular	12 oz can	146	0
light	12 oz	95	0
malt beverage	12 oz	32	0
regular	12 oz	150	0

BEETS

FOOD	PORTION	CALORIES	CHOLESTEROL
Cuts (Libby)	½ cup	35	0
Cuts (Seneca)	½ cup	35	0
Diced (Libby)	½ cup	35	0
Diced (Seneca)	½ cup	35	0
Diced Tender (S&W)	½ cup	40	0
Harvard (Libby)	½ cup	80	0
Harvard (Seneca)	½ cup	80	0
Julienne French Style (S&W)	½ cup	40	0
Pickled (Libby)	½ cup	35	0
Pickled (Seneca)	½ cup	35	0
Sliced (Libby)	½ cup	35	0

FOOD	PORTION	CALORIES	CHOLESTEROL
Sliced (Seneca)	½ cup	35	0
Sliced Pickled w/ Red Wine Vinegar (S&W)	½ cup	70	0
CANNED			
Sliced Small Premium (S&W)	½ cup	40	0
Whole (Libby)	½ cup	35	0
Whole (Seneca)	½ cup	35	0
Whole Extra Small Pickled (S&W)	½ cup	70	0
Whole Small (S&W)	½ cup	40	0
beets, harvard	½ cup	89	0
beets, pickled	½ cup	75	0
beets, sliced	½ cup	27	0
FRESH			
beet greens, raw; chopped	½ cup	4	0
beet greens; cooked	½ cup	20	0
cooked	½ cup	26	0
raw	2 (5.7 oz)	30	0

BEVERAGES

(*see* BEER AND ALE, COFFEE, DRINK MIXER, FRUIT DRINKS, LIQUOR/ LIQUEUR, MINERAL WATER/BOTTLED WATER, SODA, TEA/HERBAL TEA, WINE, WINE COOLERS)

FOOD	PORTION	CALORIES	CHOLESTEROL

BISCUIT

| Buttermilk Biscuit Mix; not prep (Health Valley) | 1 oz | 100 | 0 |
| biscuit (home recipe) | 1.5 oz | 155 | 3 |

BLACK BEANS

| cooked | 1 cup | 227 | 0 |
| raw | 1 cup | 661† | 0 |

BLACKBERRIES

CANNED in heavy syrup	½ cup	118	0
FRESH blackberries	½ cup	37	0
FROZEN blackberries	1 cup	97	0

BLACKEYE PEAS

| DRIED Blackeye Peas (Hurst Brand) | 1 cup | 233 | 0 |

BLINTZE

| cheese (home recipe) | 2 | 186 | 149 |

BLUEBERRIES

| CANNED Blueberries in Heavy Syrup (S&W) | ½ cup | 111 | 0 |

FOOD	PORTION	CALORIES	CHOLESTEROL
blueberries in heavy syrup	½ cup	112	0
FRESH blueberries	1 cup	82	0
FROZEN blueberries, unsweetened	1 cup	78	0
sweetened	1 cup	187	0

BLUEFISH

FRESH raw	3 oz	105	50
raw	1 fillet (5.3 oz)	186	88

BORAGE

FRESH cooked; chopped	3½ oz	25	0
raw; chopped	½ cup	9	0

BOYSENBERRIES

CANNED in heavy syrup	½ cup	113	0
FROZEN unsweetened	1 cup	66	0
JUICE Boysenberry (Smucker's)	8 oz	120	0

BRAINS

FRESH beef, raw	4 oz	142	1890

FOOD	PORTION	CALORIES	CHOLESTEROL
beef; pan-fried	3 oz	167	1696
beef; simmered	3 oz	136	1746
pork, raw	3 oz	108	1866
pork; braised	3 oz	117	2169

BRAN
(see CEREAL)

BRAZIL NUTS

dried, unblanched	1 oz	186	0

BREAD
(see also BAGEL, BISCUIT, BREADSTICK, CROISSANT, ENGLISH MUFFIN, MUFFIN, ROLL, SCONE)

CANNED

Brown Bread New England Recipe (S&W)	2 slices	76	0

FROZEN

OH Boy! Garlic Bread	2 oz	202	0

HOME RECIPE

banana	½" slice	116	25
cornbread	2"x2" piece (1.4 oz)	107	28
cornstick	1 (1.3 oz)	101	30
date-nut	½" slice	92	15
hush puppies	1 (2 oz)	147	45
nut	1 slice (1½ oz)	127	13
pita, whole wheat	1 (6" diam)	247	0

FOOD	PORTION	CALORIES	CHOLESTEROL
pumpkin	1 slice (1½ oz)	127	28
raisin	1 slice (1½ oz)	140	6
whole wheat	1 slice	71	0
READY-TO-EAT Bran'nola Country Oat	1 slice	90	tr
Bran'nola Dark Wheat (Arnold)	1 slice	80	tr
Bran'nola Hearty Wheat (Arnold)	1 slice	90	tr
Bran'nola Nutty Grains (Arnold)	1 slice	90	tr
Bran'nola Original (Arnold)	1 slice	70	tr
Butter Crust (Freihofer's)	1 slice	70	0
Canadian Oat (Freihofer's)	1 slice	80	0
Cinnamon Oatmeal (Oatmeal Goodness)	1 slice	90	0
Club Pullman (Freihofer's)	1 slice	70	0
Cracked Wheat (Roman Meal)	1 slice	66	0
Garlic Bread (Arnold)	1 slice	80	0
Harvest Recipe 100% Whole Wheat (Roman Meal)	1 slice	66	0
Hi-Fibre (Monks' Bread)	1 slice	50	0

FOOD	PORTION	CALORIES	CHOLESTEROL
Honey Wheat Berry (Roman Meal)	1 slice	66	0
Honey Wheat Berry Light (Roman Meal)	1 slice	40	0
Honeybran Light (Roman Meal)	1 slice	40	0
Italian, Francisco (Arnold)	1 slice	70	0
Italian, Francisco, Thick Sliced (Arnold)	1 slice	70	0
Italian, Light (Arnold)	1 slice	40	tr
Italian, No Seeds (Freihofer's)	1 slice	70	0
Italian, Seeded (Freihofer's)	1 slice	70	0
Italian, Stick, unsliced (Arnold)	1 oz	90	0
Lite Diet (Freihofer's)	1 slice	40	0
Oat (Roman Meal)	1 slice	71	0
Oat, Milk & Honey (Arnold)	1 slice	60	tr
Oatmeal & Sunflower Seeds (Oatmeal Goodness)	1 slice	90	0
Oatmeal & Bran (Oatmeal Goodness)	1 slice	90	0
Oatmeal, Light (Arnold)	1 slice	40	tr
Old Fashion (Freihofer's)	1 slice	70	0

FOOD	PORTION	CALORIES	CHOLESTEROL
Pita, White, Regular Size (Sahara Bread)	1 pocket (2 oz)	160	0
Pita, White, Mini Loaf (Sahara Bread)	1 pocket (1 oz)	80	0
Pita, White, Large Size (Sahara Bread)	1 pocket (3 oz)	240	0
Pita, Whole Wheat, Mini Loaf (Sahara Bread)	1 pocket (1 oz)	80	0
Pita, Whole Wheat, Regular Size (Sahara Bread)	1 pocket (2 oz)	150	0
Pumpernickel (Arnold)	1 slice	80	0
Pumpernickel, Levy's (Arnold)	1 slice	80	0
Raisin (Monks' Bread)	1 slice	70	0
Raisin Tea Loaf (Arnold)	1 slice	70	2
Raisin Orange (Arnold)	1 slice	70	tr
Raisin, Sun Maid (Arnold)	1 slice	70	2
Rite Diet (Freihofer's)	2 slices	90	0
Rite Diet Wheat (Freihofer's)	2 slices	90	0
Round Top (Roman Meal)	1 slice	67	0
Rye, Dill, Seeded (Arnold)	1 slice	80	0
Rye, Jewish, Seeded (Arnold)	1 slice	80	0

FOOD	PORTION	CALORIES	CHOLESTEROL
Rye, Jewish, Unseeded (Arnold)	1 slice	80	0
Rye, Levy's Real Jewish, Seeded (Arnold)	1 slice	80	0
Rye, Levy's Real Jewish, Unseeded (Arnold)	1 slice	80	0
Rye, Melba Thin (Arnold)	1 slice	40	0
Rye, Stub Pullman (Freihofer's)	1 slice	70	0
Sandwich Bread (Roman Meal)	1 slice	55	0
Seven Grain (Roman Meal)	1 slice	68	0
Seven Grain Light (Roman Meal)	1 slice	40	0
Soft Rye Pumpernickel (Freihofer's)	1 slice	70	0
Soft Rye, No Seeds (Freihofer's)	1 slice	70	0
Soft Rye, Seeded (Freihofer's)	1 slice	70	0
Soft Rye, Dill & Onion (Freihofer's)	1 slice	70	0
Split Top Wheat (Freihofer's)	1 slice	70	0
Split Top White (Freihofer's)	1 slice	70	0
Sun Grain (Roman Meal)	1 slice	68	0

FOOD	PORTION	CALORIES	CHOLESTEROL
Sunbeam King (Freihofer's)	1 slice	70	0
Sunflower & Bran (Monks' Bread)	1 slice	70	0
The Original (Freihofer's)	1 slice	70	0
Wheat (Freihofer's)	1½ slices	70	0
Wheat (Fresh Horizons)	1 slice	49	0
Wheat Berry, Honey (Arnold)	1 slice	80	tr
Wheat Cottage (America's Own)	1 slice	70	0
Wheat Light (Roman Meal)	1 slice	40	0
Wheat Oatmeal (Oatmeal Goodness)	1 slice	90	0
Wheat, Brick Oven (Arnold)	1 slice of 8 oz loaf	60	tr
Wheat, Brick Oven (Arnold)	1 slice of 16 oz loaf	60	tr
Wheat, Brick Oven (Arnold)	1 slice of 32 oz loaf	90	tr
Wheat, Golden Light (Arnold)	1 slice	40	tr
Wheat, Less (Arnold)	1 slice	40	0
Wheat, Small (Freihofer's)	1½ slices	70	0
Wheat, Stone Ground 100% Whole (Arnold)	1 slice	50	tr

FOOD	PORTION	CALORIES	CHOLESTEROL
Wheat, Stub Pullman (Freihofer's)	1 slice	70	0
Wheat, Very Thin (Arnold)	1 slice	40	tr
White (Freihofer's)	1 slice	70	0
White (Fresh Horizons)	1 slice	50	0
White (Monks' Bread)	1 slice	60	0
White (Roman Meal)	1 slice	71	0
White Cottage (America's Own)	1 slice	70	0
White Light (Roman Meal)	1 slice	40	0
White ½" Stub Pullman (Freihofer's)	1 slice	70	0
White, 7/16" Stub Pullman (Freihofer's)	1½ slices	70	0
White, Brick Oven (Arnold)	1 slice of 8 oz loaf	60	tr
White, Brick Oven (Arnold)	1 slice of 16 oz loaf	60	tr
White, Brick Oven (Arnold)	1 slice of 32 oz loaf	90	tr
White, Country (Arnold)	1 slice	100	tr
White, Less (Arnold)	1 slice	40	0
White, Milk & Honey (Arnold)	1 slice	60	tr

FOOD	PORTION	CALORIES	CHOLESTEROL
White, Very Thin (Arnold)	1 slice	40	tr
Whole Wheat 100% (Freihofer's)	1 slice	75	0
Whole Wheat 100% Stone Ground (Monks' Bread)	1 slice	70	0
whole wheat	1 slice	56	1

BREAD COATING

FOOD	PORTION	CALORIES	CHOLESTEROL
Oven Fry Extra Crispy Recipe for Chicken (General Foods)	¼ pkg (1 oz)	111	0
Oven Fry Extra Crispy Recipe for Pork (General Foods)	¼ pkg (1 oz)	115	0
Oven Fry Light Crispy Homestyle Recipe (General Foods)	¼ pkg (1 oz)	107	0
Shake 'N Bake Country Mild Recipe	¼ pkg (½ oz)	65	0
Shake 'N Bake Italian Herb Recipe	¼ pkg (½ oz)	75	tr
Shake 'N Bake Original Barbecue Recipe for Chicken	¼ pkg (½ oz)	90	0
Shake 'N Bake Original Barbecue Recipe for Pork	¼ pkg (½ oz)	75	0
Shake 'N Bake Original Recipe for Chicken	¼ pkg (½ oz)	75	0
Shake 'N Bake Original Recipe for Fish	¼ pkg (½ oz)	74	0
Shake 'N Bake Original Recipe for Pork	¼ pkg (½ oz)	80	0

FOOD	PORTION	CALORIES	CHOLESTEROL

BREAD CRUMBS

FOOD	PORTION	CALORIES	CHOLESTEROL
Contadina Seasoned	1 rounded Tbsp	35	tr
Contadina Seasoned	1 cup	426	tr

BREADFRUIT

FOOD	PORTION	CALORIES	CHOLESTEROL
breadfruit	¼ small	99	0
breadfruit	3.5 oz	109	0
seeds; roasted	1 oz	59	0

BREADSTICK

FOOD	PORTION	CALORIES	CHOLESTEROL
Cheese Breadsticks (Lance)	2	20	0
Dunking Sticks (Lance)	1⅜ oz	190	0
Garlic Breadsticks (Lance)	2	30	0
Plain Breadsticks (Lance)	2	30	0
Sesame Breadsticks (Lance)	2	30	0
breadstick	1 med	19	0
onion poppyseed (home recipe)	1	64	10

BREAKFAST BAR
(see also BREAKFAST DRINKS, NUTRITIONAL SUPPLEMENTS)

FOOD	PORTION	CALORIES	CHOLESTEROL
Chocolate Chip (Carnation)	1 bar (1.44 oz)	200	tr
Chocolate Crunch (Carnation)	1 bar (1.34 oz)	190	tr

FOOD	PORTION	CALORIES	CHOLESTEROL
Oat Bran Fruit Bar (Health Valley)	1.5 oz	140	0
Peanut Butter Crunch (Carnation)	1 bar (1.35 oz)	190	tr
Peanut Butter w/ Chocolate Chips (Carnation)	1 bar (1.39 oz)	200	tr

BREAKFAST DRINKS

(see also BREAKFAST BAR, NUTRITIONAL SUPPLEMENTS)

FOOD	PORTION	CALORIES	CHOLESTEROL
Chocolate Instant Breakfast (Carnation)	1 pkg (1.25 oz)	130	3
Chocolate Instant Breakfast; as prep w/ whole milk (Carnation)	1 pkg + 8 oz milk	280	36
Chocolate Instant Breakfast; as prep w/ skim milk (Carnation)	1 pkg + 8 oz milk	220	8
Chocolate Instant Breakfast No Sugar Added (Carnation)	1 pkg (.69 oz)	70	2
Chocolate Instant Breakfast No Sugar Added; as prep w/ skim milk (Carnation)	1 pkg + 8 oz milk	160	7
Chocolate Malt Instant Breakfast (Carnation)	1 pkg (1.24 oz)	130	3
Chocolate Malt Instant Breakfast; as prep w/ whole milk (Carnation)	1 pkg + 8 oz milk	280	36

FOOD	PORTION	CALORIES	CHOLESTEROL
Chocolate Malt Instant Breakfast; as prep w/ skim milk (Carnation)	1 pkg + 8 oz milk	220	8
Chocolate Malt Instant Breakfast No Sugar Added (Carnation)	1 pkg (.71 oz)	70	1
Chocolate Malt Instant Breakfast No Sugar Added; as prep w/ skim milk (Carnation)	1 pkg + 8 oz milk	160	6
Coffee Instant Breakfast (Carnation)	1 pkg (1.26 oz)	130	4
Coffee Instant Breakfast; as prep w/ skim milk (Carnation)	1 pkg + 8 oz milk	220	9
Coffee Instant Breakfast; as prep w/ whole milk (Carnation)	1 pkg + 8 oz milk	280	37
Eggnog Instant Breakfast (Carnation)	1 pkg (1.2 oz)	130	15
Eggnog Instant Breakfast; as prep w/ skim milk (Carnation)	1 pkg + 8 oz milk	220	20
Eggnog Instant Breakfast; as prep w/ whole milk (Carnation)	1 pkg + 8 oz milk	280	48
Strawberry Instant Breakfast (Carnation)	1 pkg (1.25 oz)	130	4
Strawberry Instant Breakfast No Sugar Added (Carnation)	1 pkg (.68 oz)	70	3
Strawberry Instant Breakfast; as prep w/ skim milk (Carnation)	1 pkg + 8 oz milk	220	9

FOOD	PORTION	CALORIES	CHOLESTEROL
Strawberry Instant Breakfast; as prep w/ whole milk (Carnation)	1 pkg + 8 oz milk	280	37
Strawberry Instant Breakfast No Sugar Added; as prep w/ skim milk (Carnation)	1 pkg + 8 oz milk	160	8
Vanilla Instant Breakfast No Sugar Added (Carnation)	1 pkg (.67 oz)	70	3
Vanilla Instant Breakfast No Sugar Added; as prep w/ skim milk (Carnation)	1 pkg + 8 oz milk	160	8
Vanilla, Instant Breakfast (Carnation)	1 pkg (1.23 oz)	130	4
Vanilla, Instant Breakfast: as prep w/ skim milk (Carnation)	1 pkg + 8 oz skim milk	220	9
Vanilla, Instant Breakfast; as prep w/ whole milk (Carnation)	1 pkg + 8 oz milk	280	37
orange drink powder; as prep w/ water	6 oz	86	0
orange drink, powder	3 rounded tsp	93	0

BROAD BEANS

CANNED broad beans	1 cup	183	0
DRIED cooked	1 cup	186	0
raw	1 cup	511	0

OD	PORTION	CALORIES	CHOLESTEROL
RESH			
ooked	3½ oz	56	0
w	1 cup	79	0
ROCCOLI			
RESH			
w; chopped	½ cup	12	0
hole; cooked	½ cup	23	0
ROZEN			
aby Spears (Birds Eye)	⅔ cup	29	0
roccoli (Health Valley)	3 oz	24	0
roccoli Vegetable Crisp (Ore Ida)	3 oz	190	5
roccoli w/ Cheese Sauce (Birds Eye)	½ cup	115	6
roccoli w/ Creamy Italian heese Sauce (Birds Eye)	½ cup	90	14
hopped (Birds Eye)	⅔ cup	26	0
ut (Hanover)	½ cup	25	0
uts (Birds Eye)	⅔ cup	25	0
lorets (Birds Eye)	⅔ cup	26	0
lorets (Hanover)	½ cup	30	0
Spears (Birds Eye)	⅔ cup	26	0

FOOD	PORTION	CALORIES	CHOLESTERO
frzn; cooked	½ cup	25	
frzn; not prep	10 oz pkg	75	
spears; cooked	½ cup	69	
spears; not prep	10 oz pkg	84	

BROWNIE

FOOD	PORTION	CALORIES	CHOLESTERO
Estee Brownie Mix; as prep	1 (2"x2")	45	30
Lance Brownie	1 pkg (1¾ oz)	200	5
Little Debbie Fudge Brownies	1 pkg (2 oz)	240	t
Little Debbie Fudge Brownies	1 pkg (2.9 oz)	350	t
brownie w/ nuts (home recipe)	1 (.8 oz)	97	15

BRUSSELS SPROUTS

FOOD	PORTION	CALORIES	CHOLESTERO
FRESH			
cooked	½ cup	30	0
raw	½ cup	19	0
FROZEN			
Baby Brussels Sprouts w/ Cheese Sauce (Birds Eye)	½ cup	113	5
Brussels Sprouts (Birds Eye)	½ cup	37	0
Brussels Sprouts (Hanover)	½ cup	40	0
frzn; cooked	½ cup	33	0
frzn; not prep	10 oz	116	0

FOOD	PORTION	CALORIES	CHOLESTEROL

BULGUR

bulgur; not prep	1 cup	605	0

BURBOT (FISH)

FRESH

raw	1 fillet (4.1 oz)	104	69
raw	3 oz	76	51

BURDOCK ROOT

cooked	1 cup	110	0
raw	1 cup	85	0

BUTTER

(see also BUTTER BLENDS, BUTTER SUBSTITUTE, MARGARINE)

REGULAR

Land O'Lakes, Lightly Salted	1 Tbsp	100	30
Land O'Lakes, Unsalted	1 Tbsp	100	30
butter	4 oz	813	248
butter	1 pat	36	11
butter	1 stick	813	248
butter	1 tsp	36	11
butter oil	1 cup	1795	524
butter oil	1 Tbsp	112	33
clarified butter	3½ oz	876	256

WHIPPED

Land O'Lakes, Lightly Salted	1 Tbsp	60	20
Land O'Lakes, Unsalted	1 Tbsp	60	20
butter	1 tsp	27	8
butter	4 oz	542	165

FOOD	PORTION	CALORIES	CHOLESTEROL

BUTTER BEANS

CANNED
Butter Beans (Hanover)	½ cup	80	0
Butter Beans in Sauce (Hanover)	½ cup	100	0
Butter Beans Tender Cooked (S&W)	½ cup	100	0

BUTTER BLENDS
(*see also* BUTTER, BUTTER SUBSTITUTE, MARGARINE)

REGULAR
Blue Bonnet	1 Tbsp	90	5
Blue Bonnet, Unsalted	1 Tbsp	90	5
Country Morning Blend, Lightly Salted	1 Tbsp	100	10
Country Morning Blend, Unsalted	1 Tbsp	100	10

SOFT
Blue Bonnet	1 Tbsp	90	5
Country Morning Blend, Lightly Salted	1 Tbsp	90	10
Country Morning Blend, Unsalted	1 Tbsp	90	10

BUTTER SUBSTITUTE
(*see also* BUTTER, BUTTER BLENDS, MARGARINE)

Butter Buds	⅛ oz	12	0
Butter Buds Sprinkles	½ tsp	4	0
Molly McButter All Natural Butter Flavor Sprinkles	½ tsp	4	0

FOOD	PORTION	CALORIES	CHOLESTEROL
Molly McButter Natural Sour Cream & Butter Flavor Sprinkles	½ tsp	4	0

BUTTERFISH

raw	3 oz	124	55
raw	1 fillet (1.1 oz)	47	21

BUTTERNUTS

dried	1 oz	174	0

CABBAGE

FRESH

chinese cabbage (pak-choi), raw; shredded	1 cup	9	0
chinese cabbage (pe-tsai), raw; shredded	1 cup	12	0
chinese cabbage (pe-tsai); shredded, cooked	1 cup	16	0
chinese cabbage; shredded, cooked	½ cup	10	0
coleslaw	½ cup	42	0
green, raw; shredded	½ cup	8	0
green; shredded, cooked	½ cup	16	0
red, raw; shredded	½ cup	10	0
red; shredded, cooked	½ cup	16	0
savoy, raw; shredded	½ cup	10	0
savoy; shredded, cooked	½ cup	18	0

HOME RECIPE

stuffed cabbage	1 (6 oz)	373	95

FOOD	PORTION	CALORIES	CHOLESTEROL

CAKE
(*see also* BROWNIE, COOKIE, DANISH PASTRY, DOUGHNUT, PIE)

FOOD	PORTION	CALORIES	CHOLESTEROL
FROSTING/ICING			
Frosting Mix; as prep (Estee)	1½ Tbsp	50–60	0
caramel (home recipe)	1 cup	895	0
chocolate (home recipe)	1 cup	1123	75
coconut fluff (home recipe)	1 cup	533	77
white boiled (home recipe)	1 cup	247	0
white uncooked (home recipe)	1 cup	813	60
FROZEN			
Cheese Cherry French Cream (Sara Lee)	1 piece (3 oz)	254	68
Pound Cake Cholesterol Free (Pepperidge Farm)	1 slice (1 oz)	110	0
eclair w/ chocolate icing & custard filling, frzn	1	205	35
HOME RECIPE			
apple cake	1.5 oz piece	145	21
baklava	1 oz	126	23
Boston cream	⅛ of 9" cake	433	158
carrot w/ cream cheese icing	1 cake, 10" diam tube	6175	1183
carrot w/ cream cheese icing	1/16 of cake	385	74
chocolate cupcake	1 (1.1 oz)	103	21

FOOD	PORTION	CALORIES	CHOLESTEROL
chocolate cupcake w/ chocolate icing	1 (1.6 oz)	175	32
cobbler, peach	½ cup	201	35
cream puff, shell only	1 (2.3 oz)	156	100
hot cross bun	1 (1.8 oz)	172	39
kuchen	2¼"x2¼" (3.3 oz)	315	84
peanut butter	1 piece (1.8 oz)	211	22
spice w/ caramel icing	1/10 of 9" cake	411	61
sponge	1/12 of 8½" cake	135	48
strudel	1 piece (4.1 oz)	272	39
torte, chocolate	1/16 of 8½" diam (3.2 oz)	317	61
white cupcake	1 (1.1 oz)	114	1
white cupcake w/ white icing	1 (1.6 oz)	164	6
yellow cupcake	1 (1.1 oz)	127	17
yellow cupcake w/ chocolate icing	1 (1.6 oz)	186	28
MIX			
Angel Food; as prep (Duncan Hines)	1/12 cake	140	0
Angel Food Chocolate (General Mills)	1/12 cake	150	0
Angel Food Confetti (General Mills)	1/12 cake	160	0
Angel Food Lemon Custard (General Mills)	1/12 cake	150	0

FOOD	PORTION	CALORIES	CHOLESTEROL
Angel Food Strawberry (General Mills)	1/12 cake	150	0
Angel Food Traditional (General Mills)	1/12 cake	130	0
Angel Food White (General Mills)	1/12 cake	150	0
Bisquick (General Mills)	2 oz	230	0
Cheesecake No Bake Dessert; as prep (Jell-O)	1/8 cake	281	28
Chocolate Lite Cake & Frosting Mix (Batter Lite)	1/9 of cake	110	0
Chocolate; as prep (Estee)	1/10 cake	100	0
Coffee Cake Easy Mix; as prep (Aunt Jemima)	1/8 cake	170	12
White Lite Cake & Frosting Mix (Batter Lite)	1/9 of cake	110	0
Yellow Cake Mix Microwave; as prep (Pillsbury)	1/8 cake	220	10
yellow w/ chocolate frosting; as prep	1 cake, 9" diam	3735	576
yellow w/ chocolate frosting; as prep	1/16 of cake	235	36
READY-TO-USE Cheesecake La Creame Amaretto Almond (Formagg)	2 oz	115	0

FOOD	PORTION	CALORIES	CHOLESTEROL
Cheesecake La Creame Pineapple (Formagg)	2 oz	115	0
Cheesecake La Creame Plain (Formagg)	2 oz	115	0
Cheesecake La Creame Strawberry (Formagg)	2 oz	115	0
angel food	1 cake, 9¾" diam	1510	0
angel food	¹⁄₁₂ of cake	125	0
cheesecake	1 cake, 9" diam	3350	2053
cheesecake	¹⁄₁₂ of cake	280	170
cream puff w/ custard filling	1 (4.6 oz)	303	187
crumb coffeecake	1 cake, 7¾" × 5⅝"	1385	279
crumb coffeecake	⅙ of cake	230	47
devil's food w/ chocolate frosting	1 cake, 2" layers	3755	598
devil's food cupcake w/ chocolate frosting	1	120	19
devil's food w/ chocolate frosting	¹⁄₁₆ of cake	235	37
fruitcake, dark	1 cake, 7½"x2¼" tube	5185	640
fruitcake, dark	⅔ slice	165	20
gingerbread	1 cake, 8" sq	1575	6

FOOD	PORTION	CALORIES	CHOLESTEROL
gingerbread	⅑ cake	175	1
pound	1 loaf, 8½"x3½"	1935	1100
sheet cake w/ white frosting	⅑ of cake	445	70
sheet cake w/ white frosting	1 cake, 9" sq	4020	636
sheet cake w/o frosting	1 cake, 9" sq	2830	552
sheet cake w/o frosting	⅑ of cake	315	61

SNACK

FOOD	PORTION	CALORIES	CHOLESTEROL
Apple Delights (Little Debbie)	1 pkg (1.25 oz)	140	tr
Banana Slices (Little Debbie)	1 pkg (3 oz)	340	tr
Banana Twins (Little Debbie)	1 pkg (2.2 oz)	250	tr
Be My Valentine (Little Debbie)	1 pkg (2.5 oz)	330	tr
Big Wheels (Hostess)	2	345	14
Caravella (Little Debbie)	1 pkg (1.2 oz)	170	tr
Choc-O-Jel (Little Debbie)	1 pkg (1.16 oz)	150	tr
Chocolate Cakes (Little Debbie)	1 pkg (2.4 oz)	320	tr
Chocolate Twins (Little Debbie)	1 pkg (2.2 oz)	240	tr
Christmas Tree Cakes (Little Debbie)	1 pkg (1.6 oz)	220	tr

FOOD	PORTION	CALORIES	CHOLESTEROL
Coconut Crunch (Little Debbie)	1 pkg (2 oz)	320	1
Coconut Rounds (Little Debbie)	1 pkg (1.13 oz)	150	1
Crumb Cake (Hostess)	2 cakes	259	21
Cupcake Chocolate (Hostess)	2 cupcakes	314	10
Cupcake Orange (Hostess)	2 cupcakes	294	25
Debbie Doodle Dandies (Little Debbie)	1 pkg (2.5 oz)	320	tr
Dessert Cups (Little Debbie)	1 pkg (.79 oz)	80	tr
Devil Cremes (Little Debbie)	1 pkg (1.3 oz)	160	tr
Devil Slices (Little Debbie)	1 pkg (3 oz)	320	tr
Devil Squares (Little Debbie)	1 pkg (2.2 oz)	270	tr
Devil's Food Cupcake (Hostess)	1 (1.5 oz)	136	4
Ding Dongs (Hostess)	2	345	14
Dutch Apple (Little Debbie)	1 pkg (2.17 oz)	230	tr
Dutch Apple (Little Debbie)	1 pkg (2.5 oz)	270	tr
Easter Bunny Cakes (Little Debbie)	1 pkg (2.5 oz)	320	tr
Fancy Cakes (Little Debbie)	1 pkg (2.6 oz)	340	tr

FOOD	PORTION	CALORIES	CHOLESTEROL
Fig Cake (Lance)	2⅛ oz	210	0
Figaroos (Little Debbie)	1 pkg (1.5 oz)	160	tr
Fudge Crispy (Little Debbie)	1 pkg (2.08 oz)	260	tr
Fudge Rounds (Little Debbie)	1 pkg (1.19 oz)	150	tr
Fudge Rounds (Little Debbie)	1 pkg (2.75 oz)	330	tr
Golden Cremes (Little Debbie)	1 pkg (1.4 oz)	150	tr
Golden Cremes (Little Debbie)	1 pkg (2.5 oz)	270	tr
Hoho (Hostess)	1 (1 oz)	119	13
Holiday Cakes Chocolate (Little Debbie)	1 pkg (2.5 oz)	320	tr
Holiday Cakes Vanilla (Little Debbie)	1 pkg (2.5 oz)	320	tr
Ice Cream Cups (Little Debbie)	1 pkg (.15 oz)	15	tr
Jelly Rolls (Little Debbie)	1 pkg (2.2 oz)	250	tr
Lemon Stix (Little Debbie)	1 pkg (1.5 oz)	220	tr
Marshmallow Supremes (Little Debbie)	1 pkg (1.1 oz)	130	tr
Mint Sprints (Little Debbie)	1 pkg (1.33 oz)	200	tr
Nutty Bar (Little Debbie)	1 pkg (2 oz)	310	tr

FOOD	PORTION	CALORIES	CHOLESTEROL
Nutty Bar (Little Debbie)	1 pkg (2.5 oz)	390	tr
Nutty Wafers (Little Debbie)	1 pkg (2 oz)	310	tr
Peanut Butter Bars (Little Debbie)	1 pkg (1.83 oz)	260	tr
Peanut Butter Bars (Little Debbie)	1 pkg (2.5 oz)	370	tr
Peanut Clusters (Little Debbie)	1 pkg (1.5 oz)	220	tr
Pecan Twins (Little Debbie)	1 pkg (2 oz)	220	tr
Pumpkin Delights (Little Debbie)	1 pkg (1.1 oz)	140	tr
Snack Cakes Chocolate (Little Debbie)	1 pkg (2.5 oz)	320	tr
Snack Cakes Chocolate (Little Debbie)	1 pkg (3 oz)	390	tr
Snack Cakes Vanilla (Little Debbie)	1 pkg (2.6 oz)	330	tr
Snack Cakes Vanilla (Little Debbie)	1 pkg (3 oz)	390	tr
Snoball (Hostess)	1 (1.5 oz)	136	2
Spice Cakes (Little Debbie)	1 pkg (2.2 oz)	270	tr
Star Crunch (Little Debbie)	1 pkg (1.08 oz)	150	tr
Swiss Cake Roll (Little Debbie)	1 pkg (2.17 oz)	270	tr
Swiss Rolls (Little Debbie)	1 pkg (2.25 oz)	280	tr

FOOD	PORTION	CALORIES	CHOLESTEROL
Turnover Apple, frzn (Lamb-Weston)	3 oz	230	10
Turnover Blueberry, frzn (Lamb-Weston)	3 oz	260	10
Turnover Cherry, frzn (Lamb-Weston)	3 oz	260	10
Twinkie (Hostess)	1 (1.5 oz)	144	21
toaster pastries	1 (1.9 oz)	210	0

CANADIAN BACON

Oscar Mayer	1 slice (28 g)	35	12
Canadian bacon; grilled	2 slices (1.7 oz)	86	27
Canadian bacon; unheated	2 slices (1.9 oz)	89	28

CANDY

3 Musketeers Bar	2.1	260	5
Baby Ruth (Nabisco)	1 oz	130	0
Bar None Candy Bar (Hershey)	1.5 oz	240	5
Barat Bar	1 (2 oz)	340	0
Bridge Mix (Nabisco)	1 oz	126	tr
Butter Mints (Kraft)	1	8	0
Butterfinger	1 oz	130	0

FOOD	PORTION	CALORIES	CHOLESTEROL
Caramels (Kraft)	1	35	0
Chocolate Fudgies (Kraft)	1	35	0
Chocolate Bar (Estee)	2 squares	60	2
Chocolate Coated Raisins (Estee)	6 pieces	30	tr
Chocolaty Peanut Bar (Lance)	2 oz	320	0
Crunch 'N Munch Candied (Franklin)	1.25 oz	170	0
Crunch 'N Munch Caramel (Franklin)	1.25 oz	160	13
Crunch 'N Munch Maple Walnut (Franklin)	1.25 oz	160	6
Crunch 'N Munch Toffee (Franklin)	1.25 oz	160	6
Crunch Chocolate Bar (Estee)	2 squares	45	2
Estee-ets (Estee)	5 pieces	35	tr
Fruit and Nut Mix (Estee)	4 pieces	35	tr
Gum Drops (Estee)	4 pieces	25	0
Gummy Bears (Estee)	4 pieces	20	0
Hard Candy (Estee)	2	25	0
Hard Candy Sugar Free (Louis Sherry)	2 pieces	25	0

FOOD	PORTION	CALORIES	CHOLESTEROL
Hershey's Kisses	9 pieces	220	10
Kit Kat Wafer (Hershey)	1.625 oz	250	10
Krackel Chocolate Bar (Hershey)	1.65 oz	250	10
Life Saver	1 piece	8	0
Lollipops (Estee)	2	12	0
Lollipops Sugar Free (Louis Sherry)	1	18	0
M&M's, Peanut	1.7 oz	250	5
M&M's, Plain	1.7 oz	240	8
Mars Bar	1.8 oz	240	6
Milk Chocolate Bar (Hershey)	1.65 oz	250	15
Milk Way Bar	2.2 oz	290	9
Mints (Estee)	1	4	0
Mr. GoodBar Chocolate Bar (Hershey)	1.85 oz	300	15
Munch Bar	1.4 oz	220	6
NECCO Mint Lozenges	1 piece	12	0
Party Mints (Kraft)	1	8	0
Peanut Bar (Lance)	1¾ oz	260	0
Peanut Brittle (Kraft)	1 oz	140	0
Peanut Butter Cups (Estee)	1	45	tr

FOOD	PORTION	CALORIES	CHOLESTEROL
Peppermint Pattie Chocolate Covered (Nabisco)	1 (½ oz)	64	tr
Reese's Pieces Candy (Hershey)	1.95 oz	270	5
Rolo Caramels in Milk Chocolate (Hershey)	9 pieces	270	15
Skittles	2 oz	320	0
Skor Toffee Bar (Hershey)	1.4 oz	220	25
Snickers Bar	2.2 oz	290	9
Special Dark Sweet Chocolate Bar (Hershey)	1.45	220	5
Starburst Fruit Chews	2 oz	240	0
Starburst Fruit Fruit Chews Strawberry	2.07 oz	240	0
Thin Mint (Nabisco)	1 (10 g)	42	0
Toffee (Kraft)	1	30	0
Tootsie Roll Miniature	1 (6 g)	24	0
Twix Cookie Bar, Caramel	2 bars (2 oz)	140	3
Twix Cookie Bar, Peanut Butter	2 bars (1.8 oz)	130	tr
Velamints	1 mint	9	0
Velamints Cocoamint	1 mint	8	0
candy corn	¼ cup	182	0
chocolate covered raisins	1 oz	121	2

FOOD	PORTION	CALORIES	CHOLESTER
gum drop	1	7	
hard candy ball	1	19	
jelly beans	¼ cup	202	
licorice	1 stick (10 g)	35	
lollipop	1 (1 oz)	110	
malted milk balls, chocolate coated	1	25	
mint fondant pattie	1 (9 g)	32	
peanut brittle	1 oz	120	

CANTALOUPE

FRESH

Chiquita	1 cup	70	
cantaloupe	½	94	
cubed	1 cup	57	

CARAMBOLA

FRESH

carambola	1	42	0

CARDOON

FRESH

cooked	3½ oz	22	0
raw; shredded	1 cup	36	0

CAROB

carob flavor mix; as prep w/ whole milk	8 oz	195	33

FOOD	PORTION	CALORIES	CHOLESTEROL
carob mix	3 tsp	45	0
flour	1 cup	185	0
flour	1 Tbsp	14	0

CARP

FRESH

cooked	3 oz	138	72
cooked	1 fillet (6 oz)	276	143
raw	1 fillet (7.6 oz)	276	143
raw	3 oz	108	56
roe, raw	3½ oz	130	360

CARROT

CANNED

Diced (Libby)	½ cup	20	0
Diced (Seneca)	½ cup	20	0
Diced Fancy (S&W)	½ cup	30	0
Julienne French Style Fancy (S&W)	½ cup	30	0
Sliced (Libby)	½ cup	20	0
Sliced (Seneca)	½ cup	20	0
Whole Tiny Fancy (S&W)	½ cup	30	0
carrots	½ cup	17	0

FOOD	PORTION	CALORIES	CHOLESTEROL
FRESH			
cooked	½ cup	35	0
raw	1	31	0
FROZEN			
Crinkle Sliced (Hanover)	½ cup	35	0
Whole Baby (Birds Eye)	½ cup	40	0
carrots; cooked	½ cup	26	0
sliced; not prep	½ cup	25	0
JUICE			
carrot juice	6 fl oz	73	0

CASABA

FRESH			
cubed	1 cup	45	0

CASHEWS

Cashews (Beer Nuts)	1 oz	170	0
Cashews (Lance)	1⅛ oz	190	0
Cashews, Long Tube (Lance)	1¼ oz	200	0
Dry Roasted (Planters)	1 oz	160	0
Dry Roasted, Unsalted (Planters)	1 oz	160	0
Fancy Oil Roasted (Planters)	1 oz	170	0

FOOD	PORTION	CALORIES	CHOLESTEROL
Halves Oil Roasted, Unsalted (Planters)	1 oz	170	0
Halves Oil Roasted (Planters)	1 oz	170	0
Honey Roasted (Planters)	1 oz	170	0
Honey Toasted (Lance)	1⅛ oz	200	0
Honey Toasted Tube (Lance)	1¹⁄₁₆ oz	200	0
Whole, Salted (Guy's)	1 oz	170	0
cashew butter	1 oz	167	0
cashew butter	1 Tbsp	94	0
dry roasted	1 oz	163	0
oil roasted	1 oz	163	0

CASSAVA

FRESH			
raw	3½ oz	120	0

CATFISH

FRESH			
channel, raw	1 fillet (2.8 oz)	92	46
channel, raw	3 oz	99	49
HOME RECIPE			
channel; breaded & fried	3 oz	194	69
channel; breaded & fried	1 fillet (3.1 oz)	199	70

FOOD	PORTION	CALORIES	CHOLESTEROL

CATSUP

FOOD	PORTION	CALORIES	CHOLESTEROL
Estee	1 Tbsp	6	0
Health Valley	1 Tbsp	16	0
Health Valley No Salt Added	1 Tbsp	16	0
Smucker's	1 tsp	8	0
Tillie Lewis Low Sodium, Low Calorie	1 Tbsp	8	0

CAULIFLOWER

FOOD	PORTION	CALORIES	CHOLESTEROL
FRESH			
cooked	½ cup	15	0
raw	½ cup	12	0
FROZEN			
Cauliflower (Birds Eye)	⅔ cup	23	0
Cauliflower (Hanover)	½ cup	20	0
Cauliflower Vegetable Crisp (Ore Ida)	3 oz	150	5
Cauliflower in Cheddar Cheese Sauce (Budget Gourmet)	5 oz	110	25
Cauliflower w/ Cheese Sauce (Birds Eye)	½ cup	113	6
Florets (Hanover)	½ cup	20	0
frzn; cooked	½ cup	17	0
frzn; not prep	½ cup	16	0

FOOD	PORTION	CALORIES	CHOLESTEROL

CAVIAR

red granular	1 Tbsp	40	94
red granular	1 oz	71	165
sturgeon, granular	1 Tbsp	42	48

CELERIC

FRESH

cooked	3½ oz	25	0
raw	½ cup	31	0

CELERY

FRESH

diced, cooked	½ cup	11	0
raw	1 stalk	6	0

CELTUCE

FRESH

raw	3½ oz	22	0

CEREAL
(*see also* GRANOLA)

Cup measurements represent approximately a 1 oz serving.

COOKED

Barley Plus (Erewhon)	1 oz	110	0
Brown Rice Cream (Erewhon)	1 oz	110	0
Cream of Wheat Instant (Nabisco)	¾ cup	110	0

FOOD	PORTION	CALORIES	CHOLESTEROL
Cream of Wheat Mix 'n Eat, flavored; not prep (Nabisco)	1 pkg (1¼ oz)	132	0
Cream of Wheat Mix 'n Eat, plain; not prep (Nabisco)	1 pkg (1 oz)	103	0
Cream of Wheat Quick (Nabisco)	¾ cup	110	0
Cream of Wheat Regular (Nabisco)	¾ cup	114	0
Farina Hot 'n Creamy; not prep (Quaker)	1 oz	101	0
Hominy Quick Grits; uncooked (Albers)	¼ cup	150	0
Maltex (Standard Milling)	½ cup	86	0
Maypo 30 Second (Standard Milling)	½ cup	110	0
Maypo Vermont Style (Standard Milling)	½ cup	90	0
Oat Bran Hot Cereal (Health Valley)	1 oz	100	0
Oat Bran w/ Toasted Wheat Germ (Erewhon)	1 oz	115	0
Oat Bran; not prep (Quaker)	⅓ cup	90	0
Oatmeal Instant Apple Cinnamon (Erewhon)	1 oz	145	0
Oatmeal Instant Apple Raisin (Erewhon)	1 oz	150	0

FOOD	PORTION	CALORIES	CHOLESTEROL
Oatmeal Instant Maple Spice (Erewhon)	1 oz	140	0
Oatmeal Instant w/ Apples & Cinnamon; not prep (Quaker)	1 pkg (1¼ oz)	133	0
Oatmeal Instant w/ Cinnamon & Spices; not prep (Quaker)	1 pkg (1⅝ oz)	176	0
Oatmeal Instant w/ Cinnamon Spice; not prep (Ralston)	1 pkg (1⅝ oz)	176	0
Oatmeal Instant w/ Maple & Brown Sugar; not prep (Quaker)	1 pkg (1½ oz)	161	0
Oatmeal Instant w/ Maple & Brown Sugar; not prep (Ralston)	1 pkg (1⅝ oz)	175	0
Oatmeal Instant; not prep (Quaker)	1 pkg (½ oz)	105	0
Oatmeal Instant; not prep (Ralston)	1 pkg (1 oz)	110	0
Oatmeal Quick or Old Fashioned; not prep (Quaker)	1 cup	307	0
Oatmeal Quick or Regular; not prep (Quaker)	1 cup	442	0
Oats, Old Fashioned; not prep (Roman Meal)	⅓ cup (1 oz)	100	0
Oats, Quick; not prep (Roman Meal)	⅓ cup (1 oz)	100	0
Oats, Quick & Regular (Ralston)	⅔ cup	110	0

FOOD	PORTION	CALORIES	CHOLESTEROL
Oats, Wheat, Dates, Raisins, Almonds Cereal; not prep (Roman Meal)	⅓ cup (1.3 oz)	140	0
Oats, Wheat, Honey, Coconut, Almonds Cereal; not prep (Roman Meal)	⅓ cup (1.3 oz)	150	0
Oats, Wheat, Rye Flax Cereal; not prep (Roman Meal)	⅓ cup (1 oz)	90	0
Original Cereal w/ Wheat, Rye, Bran, Flax; not prep (Roman Meal)	⅓ cup (1 oz)	80	0
Pettijohns (Quaker)	½ cup	93	0
Ralston Instant & Regular (Ralston)	¾ cup	110	0
Total Oatmeal Apple Cinnamon Almond Instant (General Mills)	1.5 oz pkg	150	0
Total Oatmeal Apple Cinnamon Instant (General Mills)	1.25 oz pkg	130	0
Total Oatmeal Mixed Nut Instant (General Mills)	1.3 oz pkg	140	0
Total Oatmeal Quick (General Mills)	1 oz pkg	90	0
Total Oatmeal Regular Flavor Instant (General Mills)	1 oz pkg	90	0
Wheat Hearts; as prep (General Mills)	¾ cup	110	0

FOOD	PORTION	CALORIES	CHOLESTEROL
Wheatena (Standard Milling)	½ cup	79	0
barley pearled light; not prep	2 tsp (1 oz)	99	0
bulgur	¼ cup	63	0
corn grits	½ cup	54	0
corn grits, instant; as prep	1 pkg (.8 oz)	82	0
corn grits, instant; not prep	1 pkg (.8 oz)	82	0
corn grits, regular & quick; cooked	1 cup	146	0
corn grits, regular & quick; not prep	1 tbsp	36	0
corn grits, regular & quick; not prep	1 cup	579	0
cornmeal, white or yellow	½ cup	60	0
READY-TO-EAT			
7-Grain Crunchy (Loma Linda)	½ cup	110	0
7-Grain No Sugar Added (Loma Linda)	1 cup	110	0
All-Bran (Kellogg's)	⅓ cup	70	0
All-Bran Fruit & Almonds (Kellogg's)	⅔ cup	100	0
All-Bran with Extra Fiber (Kellogg's)	½ cup	60	0
Alpha-Bits (Post)	1 cup	112	0
Apple Cinnamon Squares (Kellogg's)	½ cup	90	0

FOOD	PORTION	CALORIES	CHOLESTEROL
Apple Jacks (Kellogg's)	1 cup	110	0
Apple Raisin Crisp (Kellogg's)	⅔ cup	130	0
Aztec Corn and Amaranth (Erewhon)	1 oz	100	0
BooBerry (General Mills)	1 cup	110	0
Bran (Loma Linda)	⅓ cup	90	0
Bran Buds (Kellogg's)	⅓ cup	70	0
Bran Cereal w/ Raisins (Health Valley)	1 oz	70	0
Bran Flakes (Kellogg's)	⅔ cup	90	0
Brown Sugar & Honey Body Buddies (General Mills)	1 cup	110	0
Cap'n Crunch (Quaker)	¾ cup	120	0
Cap'n Crunch's Crunchberries (Quaker)	¾ cup	127	0
Cheerios (General Mills)	1¼ cup	110	0
Chex (Ralston)	⅔ cup	90	0
Cinnamon Toast Crunch (General Mills)	1 cup	120	0
Circus Fun (General Mills)	1 cup	110	0

FOOD	PORTION	CALORIES	CHOLESTEROL
Clusters (General Mills)	½ cup	100	0
Cocoa Krispies (Kellogg's)	¾ cup	110	0
Cocoa Pebbles (Post)	⅞ cup	112	0
Cocoa Puffs (General Mills)	1 cup	110	0
Corn Flakes (Kellogg's)	1 cup	100	0
Corn Flakes Blue (Health Valley)	1 oz	90	0
Corn Pops (Kellogg's)	1 cup	110	0
Country Corn Flakes (General Mills)	1 cup	110	0
Cracklin' Oat Bran (Kellogg's)	½ cup	110	0
Crispix (Kellogg's)	1 cup	110	0
Crispy Brown Rice (Erewhon)	1 oz	110	0
Crispy Brown Rice Cereal, Low Sodium (Erewhon)	1 oz	110	0
Crispy Critters (Post)	1 cup	112	0
Crispy Wheats 'n Raisins (General Mills)	¾ cup	110	0
Fiber 7 Flakes (Health Valley)	1 oz	100	0

FOOD	PORTION	CALORIES	CHOLESTEROL
Fortified Oat Flakes (Post)	⅔ cup	105	0
Frankenberry (General Mills)	1 cup	110	0
Froot Loops (Kellogg's)	1 cup	110	0
Frosted Flakes (Kellogg's)	¾ cup	110	0
Frosted Krispies (Kellogg's)	¾ cup	110	0
Frosted Mini-Wheats (Kellogg's)	4 biscuits	100	0
Fruit & Fiber Dates Raisins & Walnuts (Post)	½ cup	89	0
Fruit & Fiber Harvest Medley (Post)	½ cup	88	0
Fruit & Fiber Mountain Trail (Post)	½ cup	87	tr
Fruit & Fiber Peach Raisin Almond (Post)	½ cup	85	0
Fruit & Fiber Tropical Fruit (Post)	½ cup	90	0
Fruit 'n Wheat (Erewhon)	1 oz	100	0
Fruitful Bran (Kellogg's)	⅔ cup	110	0
Fruity Marshmallow Krispies (Kellogg's)	1¼ cups	140	0
Fruity Pebbles (Post)	⅞ cup	112	0

FOOD	PORTION	CALORIES	CHOLESTEROL
Golden Grahams (General Mills)	¾ cup	110	0
Grape-Nuts (Post)	¼ cup	104	0
Grape-Nuts Flakes (Post)	⅞ cup	104	0
Healthy Crunch w/ Almonds & Dates (Health Valley)	1 oz	110	0
Healthy Crunch w/ Apples & Cinnamon (Health Valley)	1 oz	110	0
Heartland Natural (Pet)	¼ cup	112	0
Honey Buc Wheat Crisp (General Mills)	¾ cup	110	0
Honey Nut Cheerios (General Mills)	1 cup	110	0
Honey Smacks (Kellogg's)	¾ cup	110	0
Honeycomb (Post)	1⅓ cups	110	0
Ice Cream Cones Chocolate Chip (General Mills)	¾ cup	110	0
Ice Cream Cones Vanilla (General Mills)	¾ cup	110	0
Just Right Nugget & Flake (Kellogg's)	⅔ cup	100	0
Just Right Fruit Nut & Flake (Kellogg's)	¾ cup	140	0
Kaboom (General Mills)	1 cup	110	0

FOOD	PORTION	CALORIES	CHOLESTEROL
Lucky Charms (General Mills)	1 cup	110	0
Muesli (Ralston)	½ cup	160	0
Muesli Unsweetened (Kentaur)	1.2 oz	120	0
Muesli Sweetened (Kentaur)	1.2 oz	120	0
Mueslix Bran (Kellogg's)	½ cup	130	0
Mueslix Five Grain (Kellogg's)	½ cup	150	0
Natural Bran Flakes (Post)	⅔ cup	87	0
Natural Raisin Bran (Post)	½ cup	83	0
Natural Sugar & Honey Body Buddies (General Mills)	1 cup	110	0
Nut & Honey Crunch (Kellogg's)	⅔ cup	110	0
Nutri-Grain Almond Raisin (Kellogg's)	⅔ cup	140	0
Nutri-Grain Corn (Kellogg's)	½ cup	100	0
Nutri-Grain Nuggets (Kellogg's)	¼ cup	90	0
Nutri-Grain Wheat (Kellogg's)	⅔ cup	100	0
Nutri-Grain Wheat & Raisins (Kellogg's)	⅔ cup	130	0
Nutrific (Kellogg's)	1 cup	120	0

FOOD	PORTION	CALORIES	CHOLESTEROL
Oat Bran Flakes (Health Valley)	1 oz	110	0
Oat Bran Flakes w/ Almonds & Dates (Health Valley)	1 oz	100	0
Oat Bran Flakes w/ Raisins (Health Valley)	1 oz	100	0
Oat Bran O'S (Health Valley)	1 oz	90	0
Oat Bran O'S Fruit & Nuts (Health Valley)	1 oz	90	0
Pac-Man (General Mills)	1 cup	110	0
Post Toasties (Post)	1¼ cup	108	0
Pro Grain (Kellogg's)	¾ cup	100	0
Product 19 (Kellogg's)	1 cup	100	0
Puffed Corn (Health Valley)	½ oz	50	0
Puffed Rice (Health Valley)	½ oz	50	0
Puffed Rice (Quaker)	1 cup	40	0
Puffed Wheat (Health Valley)	½ oz	50	0
Puffed Wheat (Quaker)	1 cup	35	0
Quisp (Quaker)	1⅛ cup	121	0
Raisin Grape-Nuts (Post)	¼ cup	101	0

FOOD	PORTION	CALORIES	CHOLESTEROL
Raisin Bran (Erewhon)	1 oz	100	0
Raisin Bran (Kellogg's)	¾ cup	120	0
Raisin Bran (Quaker)	½ cup	90	0
Raisin Bran (Skinner's)	1 oz	100	0
Raisin Bran Flakes (Health Valley)	1 oz	100	0
Raisin Bran, No Salt Added (Skinner's)	1 oz	100	0
Raisin Squares (Kellogg's)	½ cup	90	0
Rice Crispy (Ralston)	1 cup	110	0
Rice Krispies (Kellogg's)	1 cup	110	0
Rice Toasties (Post)	¾ oz	81	2
Ruskets Biscuits (Loma Linda)	2 biscuits	110	0
Shredded Wheat (Nabisco)	1 biscuit	84	0
Shredded Wheat (Sunshine)	1 biscuit	90	0
Shredded Wheat Bite Size (Sunshine)	⅔ cup	110	0
Shredded Wheat Spoon Size (Nabisco)	⅔ cup	102	0
Special K (Kellogg's)	1 cup	110	0

FOOD	PORTION	CALORIES	CHOLESTEROL
Sporting (Kentaur)	1.47 oz	140	0
Sprouts 7 w/ Raisins (Health Valley)	1 oz	90	0
Stoned Wheat Flakes (Health Valley)	1 oz	100	0
Strawberry Squares (Kellogg's)	½ cup	90	0
Sugar Frosted Flakes (Ralston)	¾ cup	110	0
Sugar Sparkled Flakes (Post)	¾ cup	108	0
Super Golden Crisp (Post)	⅞ cup	104	0
Swiss Breakfast Raisin Nut (Health Valley)	1 oz	100	0
Swiss Breakfast Tropical Fruit (Health Valley)	1 oz	100	0
Team (Nabisco)	1 cup	110	0
Total (General Mills)	1 cup	110	0
Total Corn Flakes (General Mills)	1 cup	110	0
Trix (General Mills)	1 cup	110	0
Uncle Sam Cereal (US Mills)	1 oz	110	0
Wheat Bran Millers Flakes (Health Valley)	1 oz	70	0
Wheat Flakes (Erewhon)	1 oz	100	0

FOOD	PORTION	CALORIES	CHOLESTEROL
Wheat Germ (Kretschmer)	¼ cup	110	0
Wheaties (General Mills)	1 cup	110	0
WITH 1% MILK			
Cheerios (General Mills)	1 cup + ½ cup milk	160	5
Crispy Wheats 'n Raisins (General Mills)	¾ cup + ½ cup milk	160	5
Honey Buc Wheat Crisp (General Mills)	¾ cup + ½ cup milk	160	5
Honey Nut Cheerios (General Mills)	1 cup + ½ cup milk	160	5
Total Corn Flakes (General Mills)	1 cup + ½ cup milk	160	3
Total (General Mills)	1 cup + ½ cup milk	160	5
Trix (General Mills)	1½ cup + ½ cup milk	160	3
Wheaties (General Mills)	1 cup + ½ cup milk	160	5
WITH 2% MILK			
Alpha-Bits (Post)	1 cup + ½ cup milk	172	9

FOOD	PORTION	CALORIES	CHOLESTEROL
BooBerry (General Mills)	1 cup + ½ cup milk	170	9
Cinnamon Toast Crunch (General Mills)	1 cup + ½ cup milk	180	9
Cocoa Puffs (General Mills)	1 cup + ½ cup milk	170	9
Frankenberry (General Mills)	1 cup + ½ cup milk	170	9
Fruity Pebbles (Post)	⅞ cup + ½ cup milk	173	9
Honeycomb (Post)	1⅓ cups + ½ cup milk	171	9
Oats, Old Fashioned; as prep (Roman Meal)	⅓ cup + ½ cup milk	160	10
Oats, Quick; as prep (Roman Meal)	⅓ cup + ½ cup milk	160	10
Oats, Wheat, Dates, Raisins, Almonds Cereal; as prep (Roman Meal)	⅓ cup + ½ cup milk	170	5
Oats, Wheat, Honey, Coconut, Almonds Cereal; as prep (Roman Meal)	⅓ cup + ½ cup milk	190	5
Oats, Wheat, Rye Flax Cereal; as prep (Roman Meal)	⅓ cup + ½ cup milk	120	5

FOOD	PORTION	CALORIES	CHOLESTEROL
Original Cereal w/ Wheat, Rye, Bran, Flax; as prep (Roman Meal)	⅓ cup + ½ cup milk	120	5
Pac-Man (General Mills)	1 cup + ½ cup milk	170	9
Shredded Wheat (Sunshine)	1 biscuit + ½ cup milk	150	9
Shredded Wheat Bite Size (Sunshine)	⅔ cup + ½ cup milk	170	9
Total Oatmeal Apple Cinnamon Almond Instant (General Mills)	1.5 oz pkg + ½ cup milk	210	9
Total Oatmeal Apple Cinnamon Instant (General Mills)	1.25 oz pkg + ½ cup milk	190	9
Total Oatmeal Quick (General Mills)	1 oz pkg + ½ cup milk	150	9
Total Oatmeal Regular Flavor Instant (General Mills)	1 oz pkg + ½ cup milk	150	9
WITH SKIM MILK BooBerry (General Mills)	1 cup + ½ cup milk	150	3
Brown Sugar & Honey Body Buddies (General Mills)	1 cup + ½ cup milk	150	3
Cheerios (General Mills)	1 cup + ½ cup milk	150	5

FOOD	PORTION	CALORIES	CHOLESTEROL
Circus Fun (General Mills)	1 cup + ½ cup milk	150	3
Clusters (General Mills)	½ cup + ½ cup milk	140	3
Cocoa Puffs (General Mills)	1 cup + ½ cup milk	150	3
Count Chocula (General Mills)	1 cup + ½ cup milk	150	3
Country Corn Flakes (General Mills)	1 cup + ½ cup milk	150	3
Crispy Wheats 'n Raisins (General Mills)	¾ cup + ½ cup milk	150	3
Frankenberry (General Mills)	1 cup + ½ cup milk	150	3
Fruit & Fiber Harvest Medley (Post)	½ cup + ½ cup milk	131	2
Fruit & Fiber Peach Raisin Almond (Post)	½ cup + ½ cup milk	129	2
Golden Grahams (General Mills)	¾ cup + ½ cup milk	150	3
Grape-Nuts (Post)	¼ cup + ½ cup milk	148	2
Honey Buc Wheat Crisp (General Mills)	¾ cup + ½ cup milk	150	3

FOOD	PORTION	CALORIES	CHOLESTEROL
Honey Nut Cheerios (General Mills)	1 cup + ½ milk	150	3
Ice Cream Cones Chocolate Chip (General Mills)	¾ cup + ½ cup milk	150	3
Ice Cream Cones Vanilla (General Mills)	¾ cup + ½ cup milk	150	3
Kaboom (General Mills)	1 cup + ½ cup milk	150	3
Lucky Charms (General Mills)	1 cup + ½ cup milk	150	3
Muesli (Ralston)	½ cup + ½ cup milk	200	3
Natural Raisin Bran (Post)	½ cup + ½ cup milk	127	2
Natural Sugar & Honey Body Buddies (General Mills)	1 cup + ½ cup milk	150	3
Oat Bran; as prep (Quaker)	⅓ cup + ½ cup milk	140	3
Oatmeal Raisin Crisp (General Mills)	½ cup + ½ cup milk	150	3
Pac-Man (General Mills)	1 cup + ½ cup milk	150	3
Raisin Grape-Nuts (Post)	¼ cup + ½ cup milk	144	2

FOOD	PORTION	CALORIES	CHOLESTEROL
Shredded Wheat (Sunshine)	1 biscuit + ½ cup milk	135	3
Shredded Wheat Bite Size (Sunshine)	⅔ cup + ½ cup milk	200	3
Total (General Mills)	1 cup + ½ cup milk	150	3
Total Corn Flakes (General Mills)	1 cup + ½ cup milk	150	3
Total Oatmeal Apple Cinnamon Almond Instant (General Mills)	1.5 oz pkg + ½ cup milk	190	3
Total Oatmeal Apple Cinnamon Instant (General Mills)	1.25 oz pkg + ½ cup milk	170	3
Total Oatmeal Mixed Nut Instant (General Mills)	1.3 oz pkg + ½ cup milk	180	3
Total Oatmeal Quick (General Mills)	1 oz pkg + ½ cup milk	130	3
Total Oatmeal Regular Flavor Instant (General Mills)	1 oz pkg + ½ cup milk	130	3
Trix (General Mills)	1 cup + ½ cup milk	150	3
Trix (General Mills)	1½ cup + ½ cup milk	150	3

FOOD	PORTION	CALORIES	CHOLESTEROL
Wheaties (General Mills)	1 cup + ½ cup milk	150	3
WITH WHOLE MILK			
Brown Sugar & Honey Body Buddies (General Mills)	1 cup + ½ cup milk	185	17
Circus Fun (General Mills)	1 cup + ½ cup milk	185	17
Clusters (General Mills)	½ cup + ½ cup milk	175	17
Country Corn Flakes (General Mills)	1 cup + ½ cup milk	185	17
Fortified Oat Flakes (Post)	⅔ cup + ½ cup milk	181	17
Golden Grahams (General Mills)	¾ cup + ½ cup milk	185	17
Ice Cream Cones Chocolate Chip (General Mills)	¾ cup + ½ cup milk	185	17
Ice Cream Cones Vanilla (General Mills)	¾ cup + ½ cup milk	185	17
Kaboom (General Mills)	1 cup + ½ cup milk	185	17
Lucky Charms (General Mills)	1 cup + ½ cup milk	185	17

FOOD	PORTION	CALORIES	CHOLESTEROL
Oatmeal Raisin Crisp (General Mills)	½ cup + ½ cup milk	185	17
Shredded Wheat (Sunshine)	1 biscuit + ½ cup milk	165	17
Shredded Wheat Bite Size (Sunshine)	⅔ cup + ½ cup milk	225	17
Sugar Sparkled Flakes (Post)	¾ cup + ½ cup milk	184	17
Total Oatmeal Mixed Nut Instant (General Mills)	1.3 oz pkg + ½ cup milk	215	17
Trix (General Mills)	1 cup + ½ cup milk	185	17

CHAYOTE

FRESH

cooked, cut up	1 cup	38	0
raw; cut up	1 cup	32	0

CHEESE

(*see also* CHEESE DISHES, CHEESE SUBSTITUTE, COTTAGE CHEESE, CREAM CHEESE)

NATURAL

Blue (Kraft)	1 oz	100	30
Blue (Sargento)	1 oz	100	21
Blue Spread (Roka Brand)	1 oz	70	20

FOOD	PORTION	CALORIES	CHOLESTEROL
Brick (Kraft)	1 oz	110	30
Brick (Land O'Lakes)	1 oz	110	25
Brick (Sargento)	1 oz	105	27
Brie (Sargento)	1 oz	95	28
Burger Cheese (Sargento)	1 oz	106	27
Cajun (Sargento)	1 oz	110	28
Camembert (Sargento)	1 oz	85	20
Caraway (Kraft)	1 oz	100	30
Cheddar (Alpine Lace)	1 oz	97	25
Cheddar (Armour)	1 oz	110	30
Cheddar (Kraft)	1 oz	110	30
Cheddar (Land O'Lakes)	1 oz	110	30
Cheddar (Sargento)	1 oz	114	30
Cheddar New York (Sargento)	1 oz	114	30
Cheddar Port Wine w/ Almonds, Cheese Log (Cracker Barrel)	1 oz	90	15
Cheddar Sharp Nut Log (Sargento)	1 oz	97	18

FOOD	PORTION	CALORIES	CHOLESTEROL
Cheddar Sharp w/ Almonds, Cheese Ball (Cracker Barrel)	1 oz	90	15
Cheddar Sharp w/ Almonds, Cheese Log (Cracker Barrel)	1 oz	90	15
Cheddar Shredded (Weight Watchers)	1 oz	80	28
Cheddar Smokey w/ Almonds, Cheese Log (Cracker Barrel)	1 oz	90	15
Cheddar, Lower Salt (Armour)	1 oz	110	30
Cheddar-Jack Light Natural (Dorman's)	1 oz	90	23
Colby (Alpine Lace)	1 oz	85	19
Colby (Kraft)	1 oz	110	30
Colby (Land O'Lakes)	1 oz	110	25
Colby (Sargento)	1 oz	112	27
Colby-Jack (Sargento)	1 oz	109	27
Edam (Holland Farm)	1 oz	97	25
Edam (Kraft)	1 oz	90	20
Edam (Land O'Lakes)	1 oz	110	25
Edam (Sargento)	1 oz	101	25

FOOD	PORTION	CALORIES	CHOLESTEROL
Farmer (Friendship)	4 oz	160	40
Farmer (Holland Farm)	1 oz	102	26
Farmer No Salt Added (Friendship)	4 oz	160	40
Farmers Cheese (May-Bud)	1 oz	90	20
Farmers Cheese (Sargento)	1 oz	102	26
Farmers Cheese (White Clover)	1 oz	90	20
Farmers Cheese (White Clover)	1 oz	81	18
Feta (Sargento)	1 oz	75	25
Feta (White Clover)	1 oz	90	20
Finland Swiss (Sargento)	1 oz	107	26
Fior di Latte (Polly-O)	1 oz	80	20
Fontina (Sargento)	1 oz	110	33
Gorgonzola (Sargento)	1 oz	100	21
Gouda (Holland Farm)	1 oz	103	27
Gouda (Kraft)	1 oz	110	30
Gouda (Land O'Lakes)	1 oz	110	30

FOOD	PORTION	CALORIES	CHOLESTEROL
Gouda (Sargento)	1 oz	101	32
Grated (Polly-O)	1 oz	130	25
Gruyere (Sargento)	1 oz	117	31
Havarti (Casino)	1 oz	120	35
Havarti (Sargento)	1 oz	118	31
Hoop (Friendship)	4 oz	84	8
Italian Style Grated Cheese (Sargento)	1 oz	108	26
Jack Slim Light Natural (Dorman's)	1 oz	90	22
Jarlsberg (Sargento)	1 oz	100	16
Limburger (Sargento)	1 oz	93	26
Limburger Natural Little Gem Size (Mohawk Valley)	1 oz	90	25
Lorraine (Universal Food)	1 oz	100	25
Monterey Jack (Alpine Lace)	1 oz	80	14
Monterey Jack (Armour)	1 oz	110	30
Monterey Jack (Holland Farm)	1 oz	102	27
Monterey Jack (Kraft)	1 oz	110	30

FOOD	PORTION	CALORIES	CHOLESTEROL
Monterey Jack (Land O'Lakes)	1 oz	110	20
Monterey Jack Lower Salt (Armour)	1 oz	110	30
Monterey Jack w/ Jalapeno Peppers (Kraft)	1 oz	110	30
Monterey Jack w/ Peppers Mild (Kraft)	1 oz	110	30
Mozzarella (Alpine Lace)	1 oz	72	15
Mozzarella (M.H. Greenbaum, Inc.)	3½ oz	334	59
Mozzarella Lite Sandwich Slices (Polly-O)	1 oz	70	15
Mozzarella Low-Moisture (Casino)	1 oz	90	25
Mozzarella Low-Moisture Part-Skim (Sargento)	1 oz	79	15
Mozzarella Low-Moisture Whole Milk (Sargento)	1 oz	90	25
Mozzarella Low-Sodium Light (Dorman's)	1 oz	80	15
Mozzarella Part-Skim (Polly-O)	1 oz	80	15
Mozzarella Part-Skim Shredded (Polly-O)	1 oz	80	15
Mozzarella Part-Skim Low-Moisture (Kraft)	1 oz	80	15

FOOD	PORTION	CALORIES	CHOLESTEROL
Mozzarella Part-Skim (Land O'Lakes)	1 oz	80	15
Mozzarella Part-Skim Low-Moisture String Cheese w/ Jalapeno Peppers (Kraft)	1 oz	80	20
Mozzarella Smoked (Polly-O)	1 oz	85	25
Mozzarella Whole Milk (Polly-O)	1 oz	90	20
Mozzarella Whole Milk Sandwich Slices (Polly-O)	1 oz	90	20
Mozzarella Whole Milk Shredded (Polly-O)	1 oz	90	20
Mozzarella w/ Pizza Spices (Sargento)	1 oz	79	15
Muenster (Alpine Lace)	1 oz	104	25
Muenster (Holland Farm)	1 oz	102	27
Muenster (Kraft)	1 oz	110	30
Muenster (Land O'Lakes)	1 oz	100	25
Muenster Red Rind (Sargento)	1 oz	104	27
Nacho (Sargento)	1 oz	106	27
Naturally Slender (Northfield)	1 oz	90	10
Parmesan & Romano Grated (Sargento)	1 oz	111	24

FOOD	PORTION	CALORIES	CHOLESTEROL
Parmesan Fresh (Sargento)	1 oz	111	19
Parmesan Grated (Kraft)	1 oz	130	30
Parmesan Grated (Polly-O)	1 oz	130	20
Parmesan Grated (Sargento)	1 oz	129	22
Parmesan Natural (Kraft)	1 oz	110	20
Port Wine Nut Log (Sargento)	1 oz	97	18
Provolone (Alpine Lace)	1 oz	85	20
Provolone (Kraft)	1 oz	100	25
Provolone (Land O'Lakes)	1 oz	100	20
Provolone (Sargento)	1 oz	100	20
Provolone Low Sodium Light Natural (Dorman's)	1 oz	90	20
Queso Blanco (Sargento)	1 oz	104	27
Queso de Papa (Sargento)	1 oz	114	30
Ricotta Lite (Polly-O)	2 oz	80	10
Ricotta Lite (Sargento)	1 oz	25	14

FOOD	PORTION	CALORIES	CHOLESTEROL
Ricotta Part-Skim (Polly-O)	2 oz	90	20
Ricotta Part-Skim (Sargento)	1 oz	32	10
Ricotta Part-Skim No Salt (Polly-O)	2 oz	90	20
Ricotta Whole Milk (Polly-O)	2 oz	100	35
Ricotta Whole Milk (Sargento)	1 oz	53	15
Ricotta Whole Milk & Whey (Sargento)	1 oz	40	13
Ricotta Whole Milk No Salt (Polly-O)	2 oz	100	35
Romano (Sargento)	1 oz	110	29
Romano Grated (Casino)	1 oz	130	30
Romano Grated (Polly-O)	1 oz	130	30
Romano Natural (Casino)	1 oz	100	30
Scamorze Part-Skim Low-Moisture (Kraft)	1 oz	80	15
Smokestick (Sargento)	1 oz	103	24
String Cheese (Polly-O)	1 oz	90	15
String Cheese (Sargento)	1 oz	79	15

FOOD	PORTION	CALORIES	CHOLESTEROL
String Cheese Smoked (Sargento)	1 oz	79	15
Swiss (Alpine Lace)	1 oz	100	25
Swiss (Kraft)	1 oz	110	25
Swiss (Land O'Lakes)	1 oz	110	25
Swiss (M.H. Greenbaum, Inc.)	1 oz	106	20
Swiss (Sargento)	1 oz	107	26
Swiss Almond Nut Log (Sargento)	1 oz	94	21
Swiss, Aged (Kraft)	1 oz	110	25
Taco (Sargento)	1 oz	109	27
Taco Shredded (Kraft)	1 oz	110	30
Tilsiter (Sargento)	1 oz	96	29
Tybo Red Wax (Sargento)	1 oz	98	23
blue	1 oz	100	21
blue, crumbled	1 cup	477	102
brick	1 oz	105	27
Brie	1 oz	95	28
Camembert	1 oz	85	20
Cheddar	1 oz	114	30
Cheshire	1 oz	110	29

FOOD	PORTION	CALORIES	CHOLESTEROL
Colby	1 oz	112	27
Edam	1 oz	101	25
feta	1 oz	75	25
fontina	1 oz	110	33
Gouda	1 oz	101	32
Gruyere	1 oz	117	31
Limburger	1 oz	93	26
mozzarella	1 oz	80	22
mozzarella	1 lb	1276	356
mozzarella, low-moisture	1 oz	90	25
mozzarella, low-moisture, part-skim	1 oz	79	15
mozzarella, part-skim	1 oz	72	16
Muenster	1 oz	104	27
Parmesan, grated	1 Tbsp	23	4
Parmesan, grated	1 oz	129	22
Parmesan, hard	1 oz	111	19
Port du Salut	1 oz	100	35
provolone	1 oz	100	20
ricotta, part-skim	½ cup	171	38
ricotta, part-skim	1 cup	340	76
ricotta, whole milk	½ cup	216	63
ricotta, whole milk	1 cup	428	124
Romano	1 oz	110	29
Roquefort	1 oz	105	26
Swiss	1 oz	107	26
Tilsit	1 oz	96	29

FOOD	PORTION	CALORIES	CHOLESTEROL
yogurt cheese (home recipe)	1 oz	20	7
PROCESSED			
American (Alpine Lace)	1 oz	80	20
Borden Lite Line American	1 oz	50	10
Borden Lite Line American Sodium Lite	1 oz	70	10
Borden Lite Line Cheddar Sharp, Natural Shredded Reduced Fat Cheese	1 oz	80	15
Cheez 'N Bacon Singles Pasteurized Process Cheese	1 oz	90	20
Cheez Whiz	1 oz	80	20
Cheez Whiz Hot Mexican	1 oz	80	15
Cheez Whiz Mild Mexican	1 oz	80	15
Cheez Whiz Pimento	1 oz	80	15
Cheez Whiz w/ Jalapeno Peppers	1 oz	80	15
Churney Maple Walnut Cheese Fudge	1 oz	118	7
Churney Mint Cheese Fudge w/ Walnuts	1 oz	117	7
Churney Cheese Fudge w/ Walnuts	1 oz	120	7
Churney Diet Snack Cheddar Flavored	1 oz	70	10
Churney Diet Snack Port Wine Flavored	1 oz	70	10
Cracker Barrel Extra Sharp Cheddar Cold Pack Cheese Food	1 oz	90	20

FOOD	PORTION	CALORIES	CHOLESTEROL
Cracker Barrel Port Wine Cheddar Cold Pack Cheese Food	1 oz	90	20
Cracker Barrel Sharp Cheddar Cold Pack Cheese Food	1 oz	90	20
Cracker Barrel w/ Bacon Cold Pack Cheese Food	1 oz	90	20
Deluxe Pasteurized Process American Cheese (slices)	1 oz	110	25
Deluxe Pasteurized Process American Cheese (loaf)	1 oz	110	25
Deluxe Pasteurized Process Pimento Cheese Slices	1 oz	100	25
Deluxe Pasteurized Process Swiss Cheese Slices	1 oz	90	25
Dorman's Light Lo-Chol Low Cholesterol	1 oz	70	3
Fineform	1 oz	70	8
Formagg American Swiss Slices	¾ oz	70	0
Formagg American White Slices	¾ oz	70	0
Formagg American Yellow Slices	¾ oz	70	0
Formagg Cheddar	1 oz	70	0
Formagg Grated Italian Pasta Topping	1 oz	100	0
Formagg Monterey Jack	1 oz	70	0
Formagg Monterey Jack Jalapeno Flavored	1 oz	70	0
Formagg Mozzarella	1 oz	70	0

FOOD	PORTION	CALORIES	CHOLESTEROL
Formagg Pizza Topper	1 oz	70	0
Formagg Provolone	1 oz	70	0
Formagg Ricotta	1 oz	130	0
Formagg Shredded Cheddar	1 oz	70	0
Formagg Shredded Mozzarella	1 oz	70	0
Formagg Shredded Parmesan	1 oz	70	0
Formagg Shredded Provolone	1 oz	70	0
Formagg Shredded Salad Topping	1 oz	70	0
Formagg Shredded Swiss	1 oz	70	0
Formagg Swiss	1 oz	70	0
Gruyere (M.H.Greenbaum, Inc.)	1 oz	94	44
Gruyere, Hot Pepper (M.H. Greenbaum, Inc.)	1 oz	93	44
Harvest Moon Brand Pasteurized Process Cheese	1 oz	50	10
Harvest Moon Brand American Flavored Pasteurized Process Cheese	1 oz	70	15
Kraft American Pasteurized Process Cheese Spread	1 oz	80	20
Kraft American Singles Pasteurized Process Cheese (colored)	1 oz	90	20
Kraft American Singles Pasteurized Process Cheese (white)	1 oz	90	20
Kraft Jalapeno Pasteurized Process Cheese Spread	1 oz	80	20

FOOD	PORTION	CALORIES	CHOLESTEROL
Kraft Jalapeno Pepper Spread	1 oz	70	15
Kraft Jalapeno Singles Pasteurized Process Cheese	1 oz	90	25
Kraft Monterey Jack Singles Pasteurized Process Cheese	1 oz	90	25
Kraft Olives & Pimento Spread	1 oz	60	15
Kraft Pasteurized Process Cheese Spread w/ Bacon	1 oz	80	20
Kraft Pasteurized Process Cheese Spread w/ Garlic	1 oz	80	15
Kraft Pasteurized Process Cheese Food w/ Bacon	1 oz	90	20
Kraft Pasteurized Process Cheese Food w/ Garlic	1 oz	90	20
Kraft Pimento Singles Pasteurized Process Cheese	1 oz	90	20
Kraft Pimento Spread	1 oz	70	15
Kraft Pineapple Spread	1 oz	70	15
Kraft Relish Spread	1 oz	70	15
Kraft Sharp Singles Pasteurized Process Cheese	1 oz	100	25
Kraft Swiss Singles Pasteurized Process Cheese	1 oz	90	25
Lactaid	1 slice (⅔ oz)	62	18
Land O'Lakes, American	1 oz	110	25
Land O'Lakes, American/ Swiss	1 oz	100	25

FOOD	PORTION	CALORIES	CHOLESTEROL
Land O'Lakes, Golden Velvet Cheese Spread	1 oz	80	15
Land O'Lakes, Jalapeno Cheese Food	1 oz	90	20
Land O'Lakes, LaCheddar Cheese Food	1 oz	90	20
Land O'Lakes, Onion Cheese Food	1 oz	90	15
Land O'Lakes, Pepperoni Cheese Food	1 oz	90	20
Land O'Lakes, Salami Cheese Food	1 oz	100	20
Lifetime Swiss	1 oz	60	9
Light N'Lively Singles American Flavor Pasteurized Process Cheese	1 oz	70	15
Light N'Lively Singles Sharp Cheddar Flavored Pasteurized Process Cheese	1 oz	70	15
Light N'Lively Singles Swiss Flavored Pasteurized Process Cheese	1 oz	70	15
Lunch Wagon Pizza Topping Made w/ Vegetable Oil	1 oz	80	0
Lunch Wagon Sandwich Slices Make w/ Vegetable Oil	1 oz	80	5
Michael's Country Gourmet Spread French Onion	1 oz	48	19
Michael's Country Gourmet Spread Garden Vegetable	1 oz	48	19
Michael's Country Gourmet Spread Garlic & Herbs	1 oz	48	19

FOOD	PORTION	CALORIES	CHOLESTEROL
Mohawk Valley Limburger Pasteurized Process Cheese Spread	1 oz	70	20
Old English Sharp Pasteurized Process Cheese Spread	1 oz	90	20
Old English Sharp Pasteurized Process American Cheese (slices)	1 oz	110	30
Old English Sharp Pasteurized Process American Cheese (loaf)	1 oz	110	30
Sargento American Hot Pepper	1 oz	106	27
Sargento American Sharp Spread	1 oz	106	27
Sargento American w/ Pimento	1 oz	106	27
Sargento Imitation Cheddar	1 oz	85	2
Sargento Imitation Mozzarella	1 oz	80	2
Sargento Process Brick	1 oz	95	25
Sargento Process Swiss	1 oz	95	24
Skitoast	1 oz	65	28
Smokelle Pasteurized Process Cheese Food	1 oz	100	20
Squeez-A-Snak Garlic Flavor Pasteurized Process Cheese Spread	1 oz	90	20
Squeez-A-Snak Hickory Smoke Flavor Pasteurized Process Cheese Spread	1 oz	80	20

FOOD	PORTION	CALORIES	CHOLESTEROL
Squeez-A-Snak Pasteurized Process Cheese Spread w/ Bacon	1 oz	90	20
Squeez-A-Snak Sharp Pasteurized Process Cheese Spread	1 oz	80	20
Velveeta Hot Mexican Pasteurized Process Cheese Spread	1 oz	80	20
Velveeta Mild Mexican Pasteurized Process Cheese Spread	1 oz	80	20
Velveeta Pasteurized Process Cheese Spread	1 oz	80	20
Velveeta Pasteurized Process Cheese Spread Slices	1 oz	90	20
Velveeta Pimento Pasteurized Process Cheese Spread	1 oz	80	20
Weight Watchers Swiss Flavor	1 oz	50	8
American	1 oz	106	27
American, cheese food	1 oz	93	18
American, cheese food, cold pack	1 oz	94	18
American, cheese spread	1 oz	82	16
pimento	1 oz	106	27
Swiss	1 oz	95	24
Swiss, cheese food	1 oz	92	23

CHEESE DISHES

FOOD	PORTION	CALORIES	CHOLESTEROL
fondue (home recipe)	½ cup	303	62

FOOD	PORTION	CALORIES	CHOLESTEROL

CHEESE SUBSTITUTE

FOOD	PORTION	CALORIES	CHOLESTEROL
American & Caraway Cheese Subsititute (Delicia)	1 oz	80	0
American Cheese Substitute (Delicia)	1 oz	80	0
American w/ Hot Peppers Cheese Substitute (Delicia)	1 oz	80	0
Cheezola	1 oz	89	1
Count Down (Fisher)	1 oz	89	1
Count Down Smokey Flavor (Fisher)	1 oz	34	1
Golden Image American Flavored Pasteurized Process Cheese	1 oz	90	5
Golden Image Imitation Colby Cheese	1 oz	110	5
Golden Image Imitation Mild Cheddar Cheese	1 oz	110	5
Hickory Smoked American Cheese Substitute (Delicia)	1 oz	80	0

CHERIMOYA

FOOD	PORTION	CALORIES	CHOLESTEROL
FRESH cherimoya	1	515	0

FOOD	PORTION	CALORIES	CHOLESTEROL

CHERRY

CANDIED
cherry	1 cherry	12	0

CANNED
Red Tart Pitted Cherries (White House)	3.5 oz	43	0
cherries, sour, water packed	1 cup	87	0
cherries, sweet, in heavy syrup	½ cup	107	0
maraschino	1	12	0
sour, in heavy syrup	½ cup	116	0
sour, in light syrup	½ cup	94	0
sweet, in water	½ cup	57	0
sweet, juice pack	½ cup	68	0

FRESH
cherries, sweet	10	49	0

FROZEN
cherries, sour, unsweetened	1 cup	72	0
cherries, sweetened	1 cup	232	0

JUICE
Black Cherry (Smucker's)	8 oz	130	0
Mountain Cherry Pure & Light (Dole)	6 oz	87	0

CHESTNUTS

Chinese dried	1 oz	103	0
Chinese; cooked	1 oz	44	0

FOOD	PORTION	CALORIES	CHOLESTEROL
Chinese; roasted	1 oz	68	0
Japanese; cooked	1 oz	16	0
Japanese; roasted	1 oz	57	0
cooked	1 oz	37	0
dried; peeled	1 oz	105	0
roasted	1 oz	70	0
roasted	1 cup	350	0

CHEWING GUM

Hubba Bubba, Original & Fruit	1 stick	23	0
Hubba Bubba, Strawberry, Grape & Raspberry	1 stick	23	0
Wrigley's	1 stick	10	0

CHIA SEEDS

dried	1 oz	134	0

CHICKEN

(*see also* CHICKEN DISHES, CHICKEN SUBSTITUTE, DINNER, HOT DOGS)

CANNED			
Chicken Salad (The Spreadables)	¼ can	100	16
FRESH			
Breast Boneless, Oven Stuffer; cooked (Perdue)	3 oz	141	72
Breast Boneless; cooked (Perdue)	3 oz	141	72
Breast Cutlets Thin-Sliced, Oven Stuffer; cooked (Perdue)	3 oz	141	72

FOOD	PORTION	CALORIES	CHOLESTEROL
Breast Quarters, meat only; cooked (Perdue)	3 oz	169	72
Breast Split, meat only; cooked (Perdue)	3 oz	169	72
Breast Whole, Oven Stuffer, meat only; cooked (Perdue)	3 oz	169	72
Breast Whole, meat only; cooked (Perdue)	3 oz	169	72
Cornish Game Hen Fresh Whole; cooked (Perdue)	3 oz	205	75
Drumsticks, Oven Stuffer, meat only; cooked (Perdue)	3 oz	185	78
Drumsticks, meat only; cooked (Perdue)	3 oz	185	78
Leg Quarters, meat only; cooked (Perdue)	3 oz	199	79
Oven Stuffer Roaster Whole, meat only; cooked (Perdue)	3 oz	205	75
Thighs, Boneless Cutlets, Oven Stuffer; cooked (Perdue)	3 oz	176	76
Thighs, Oven Stuffer, meat only; cooked (Perdue)	3 oz	212	80
Thighs, meat only; cooked (Perdue)	3 oz	212	80

FOOD	PORTION	CALORIES	CHOLESTEROL
Whole, Fresh Young, meat only; cooked (Perdue)	3 oz	205	75
Wing Drumettes, meat only; cooked (Perdue)	3 oz	249	72
Wingettes, Oven Stuffer, meat only; cooked (Perdue)	3 oz	249	72
Wingettes, Oven Stuffer, meat only; cooked (Perdue)	3 oz	249	72
Wings, meat only; cooked (Perdue)	3 oz	249	72
back, meat & skin; flour coated, fried	½ back (2.5 oz)	238	64
back, meat & skin; flour coated, fried	1.5 oz	146	39
back, meat & skin; fried	2.5 oz	238	63
back, meat & skin; fried	½ back (4.2 oz)	397	105
back, meat & skin, raw	½ back (3.5 oz)	316	79
back, meat & skin, raw	2.1 oz	188	47
back, meat & skin; roasted	1 oz	96	28
back, meat & skin; roasted	½ back (1.9 oz)	159	46
back, meat & skin; stewed	½ back (2.1 oz)	158	48
back, meat & skin; stewed	1.3 oz	93	28
back, meat only, raw	1 oz	42	25
back, meat only, raw	½ back (1.8 oz)	70	41

FOOD	PORTION	CALORIES	CHOLESTEROL
back, meat only; fried	½ back (2 oz)	167	54
back, meat only; fried	1.2 oz	101	32
back, meat only; fried	½ back (2 oz)	167	54
back, meat only; roasted	.7 oz	57	21
back, meat only; roasted	½ back (1.4 oz)	96	36
back, meat only; stewed	½ back (1.5 oz)	88	36
back, meat only; stewed	1 oz	45	22
breast, meat only; fried	1.8 oz	97	47
breast, meat only; fried	½ breast (3 oz)	161	78
breast, meat only, raw	½ breast (4 oz)	129	68
breast, meat only, raw	2.5 oz	78	41
breast, meat only; roasted	½ breast (3 oz)	142	73
breast, meat only; roasted	1.8 oz	86	44
breast, meat only; stewed	2 oz	86	44
breast, meat only; stewed	½ breast (3.3 oz)	144	73
breast, meat & skin; roasted	½ breast (3.4 oz)	193	83
breast, meat & skin; roasted	2 oz	115	49
breast, meat & skin; stewed	2.3 oz	121	50
breast, meat & skin; stewed	½ breast (3.9 oz)	202	83

FOOD	PORTION	CALORIES	CHOLESTEROL
breast, meat & skin; batter dipped, fried	½ breast (4.9 oz)	364	119
breast, meat & skin; batter dipped, fried	2.9 oz	218	72
breast, meat & skin; flour coated, fried	2.1 oz	131	53
breast, meat & skin; flour coated, fried	½ breast (3.4 oz)	218	88
breast, meat & skin, raw	3.1 oz	150	55
breast, meat & skin, raw	½ breast (5.1 oz)	250	92
broiler or fryer, flesh & skin; roasted	½ chicken (10.5 oz)	715	263
broiler or fryer, flesh & skin; roasted	6.2 oz	426	157
broiler or fryer, flesh & skin; stewed	½ chicken (11.7 oz)	730	262
broiler or fryer, flesh & skin; stewed	1 lb	437	157
capon, flesh & skin, raw	½ chicken (2.1 lbs)	2257	720
capon, flesh & skin, raw	10.4 oz	695	222
capon, flesh & skin; roasted	6.9 oz	448	169
capon, flesh & skin; roasted	½ chicken (1.4 lbs)	1457	549
capon, flesh, skin, giblets & neck, raw	1 chicken (4.7 lbs)	4987	1882
capon, flesh, skin, giblets & neck; roasted	1 chicken (3.1 lbs)	3211	1458
capon, flesh, skin, giblets & neck; roasted	7.6 oz	494	224

FOOD	PORTION	CALORIES	CHOLESTEROL
dark meat w/ skin; batter dipped, fried	½ chicken (9.8 oz)	828	247
dark meat w/ skin; batter dipped, fried	5.9 oz	497	149
dark meat w/ skin; flour coated, fried	3.9 oz	313	101
dark meat w/ skin; flour coated, fried	½ chicken (6.5 oz)	523	169
dark meat w/ skin, raw	5.6 oz	379	130
dark meat w/ skin, raw	½ chicken (9.3 oz)	630	217
dark meat w/ skin; roasted	½ chicken (5.9 oz)	423	152
dark meat w/ skin; roasted	3.5 oz	256	92
dark meat w/ skin; stewed	3.9 oz	256	90
dark meat w/ skin; stewed	½ chicken (6.5 oz)	428	151
dark meat w/o skin; fried	1 cup	334	135
dark meat w/o skin; fried	3.2 oz	217	88
dark meat w/o skin, raw	3.8 oz	136	87
dark meat w/o skin, raw	½ chicken (6.4 oz)	227	146
dark meat w/o skin; roasted	2.8 oz	166	75
dark meat w/o skin; roasted	1 cup	286	130
dark meat w/o skin; stewed	1 cup	269	123
dark meat w/o skin; stewed	3 oz	165	76
drumstick, meat & skin; batter dipped, fried	1.5 oz	115	37
drumstick, meat & skin; batter dipped, fried	2.6 oz	193	62

FOOD	PORTION	CALORIES	CHOLESTEROL
drumstick, meat & skin; flour coated, fried	1 oz	71	26
drumstick, meat & skin; flour coated, fried	1.7 oz	120	44
drumstick, meat & skin, raw	2.6 oz	117	59
drumstick, meat & skin, raw	1.5 oz	71	35
drumstick, meat & skin; roasted	1.8 oz	112	48
drumstick, meat & skin; roasted	1 oz	67	28
drumstick, meat & skin; stewed	2 oz	116	48
drumstick, meat & skin; stewed	1.2 oz	69	28
drumstick, meat only; fried	1.5 oz	82	40
drumstick, meat only, raw	1.3 oz	44	28
drumstick, meat only, raw	2.2 oz	74	48
drumstick, meat only; roasted	1.5 oz	76	41
drumstick, meat only; stewed	1.6 oz	78	40
drumstick, meat only; stewed	1 oz	47	25
flesh & skin, raw	½ chicken (16.1 oz)	990	347
flesh & skin; flour coated, fried	½ chicken (11 oz)	844	283
flesh & skin; flour coated, fried	1 lb	505	169
flesh & skin; fried	½ chicken (16.4 oz)	1347	404
flesh only; fried	1 cup	307	131

FOOD	PORTION	CALORIES	CHOLESTEROL
flesh only; fried	5.4 oz	340	145
flesh only; roasted	5.1 oz	278	130
flesh only; roasted	1 cup	266	125
flesh only; stewed	1 cup	248	116
flesh only; stewed	5.5 oz	278	130
flesh only, raw	½ chicken (11.5 oz)	392	231
leg, meat & skin; batter dipped, fried	5.5 oz	431	142
leg, meat & skin; batter dipped, fried	3.3 oz	259	85
leg, meat & skin; flour coated, fried	3.9 oz	285	105
leg, meat & skin; flour coated, fried	2.4 oz	170	63
leg, meat & skin, raw	5.6 oz	312	138
leg, meat & skin, raw	3.5 oz	189	83
leg, meat & skin; roasted	4 oz	265	105
leg, meat & skin; roasted	2.4 oz	160	64
leg, meat & skin; stewed	4.4 oz	275	105
leg, meat & skin; stewed	2.6 oz	165	63
leg, meat only, raw	4.6 oz	156	104
leg, meat only, raw	2.7 oz	94	62
leg, meat only; fried	3.3 oz	195	93
leg, meat only; fried	2 oz	116	55
leg, meat only; roasted	3.3 oz	182	89
leg, meat only; roasted	2 oz	109	53
leg, meat only; stewed	3.5 oz	187	90

FOOD	PORTION	CALORIES	CHOLESTEROL
leg, meat only; stewed	2.1 oz	111	53
light meat w/ skin; battered dipped, fried	4 oz	312	94
light meat w/ skin; battered dipped, fried	½ chicken (6.6 oz)	520	157
light meat w/ skin; flour coated, fried	½ chicken (4.7 oz)	320	113
light meat w/ skin; flour coated, fried	2.7 oz	192	68
light meat w/ skin, raw	½ chicken (6.8 oz)	362	130
light meat w/ skin, raw	4.1 oz	216	78
light meat w/ skin; roasted	2.8 oz	175	67
light meat w/ skin; roasted	½ chicken (4.6 oz)	293	111
light meat w/ skin; stewed	½ chicken (5.3 oz)	302	111
light meat w/ skin; stewed	3.2 oz	181	66
light meat w/o skin; fried	2.2 oz	123	57
light meat w/o skin; fried	1 cup	268	125
light meat w/o skin, raw	½ chicken (5.2 oz)	168	85
light meat w/o skin, raw	3.1 oz	100	51
light meat w/o skin; roasted	1 cup	242	118
light meat w/o skin; roasted	2.2 oz	110	54
light meat w/o skin; stewed	2.3 oz	113	54
light meat w/o skin; stewed	1 cup	223	107
neck, meat & skin; batter dipped, fried	1.8 oz	172	47

FOOD	PORTION	CALORIES	CHOLESTEROL
neck, meat & skin; flour coated, fried	1.3 oz	119	34
neck, meat & skin, raw	1.8 oz	148	49
neck, meat & skin; simmered	1.3 oz	95	27
neck, meat only, raw	.7 oz	31	17
neck, meat only; fried	.8 oz	50	23
neck, meat only; simmered	.6 oz	32	14
roaster flesh & skin; roasted	½ chicken (1.1 lbs)	1071	365
roaster, flesh & skin; roasted	7.4 oz	469	160
skin only; roasted	from ½ chicken (2 oz)	254	46
skin only; roasted	1.2 oz	154	28
skin only; stewed	1.6 oz	160	28
skin only; stewed	from ½ chicken (2.5 oz)	261	45
skin only; flour coated, fried	1 oz	166	24
skin only; flour coated, fried	from ½ chicken (2 oz)	281	41
skin only; fried	from ½ chicken (6.7 oz)	748	140
skin only; fried	4 oz	449	84
skin only, raw	1.6 oz	164	51
skin only, raw	from ½ chicken (2.8 oz)	275	86

FOOD	PORTION	CALORIES	CHOLESTEROL
stewing, flesh & skin; stewed	6.2 oz	507	140
stewing, flesh & skin; stewed	½ chicken (9.2 oz)	744	205
thigh, meat only, raw	2.4 oz	82	57
thigh, meat only; fried	1.8 oz	113	53
thigh, meat only; roasted	1.8 oz	109	49
thigh, meat only; stewed	1.9 oz	107	49
thigh, meat & skin, raw	3.3 oz	199	79
thigh, meat & skin, raw	2 oz	120	48
thigh, meat & skin; batter dipped, fried	3 oz	238	80
thigh, meat & skin; batter dipped, fried	1.8 oz	144	48
thigh, meat & skin; flour coated, fried	2.2 oz	162	60
thigh, meat & skin; flour coated, fried	1.3 oz	99	37
thigh, meat & skin; roasted	2.2 oz	153	58
thigh, meat & skin; roasted	1.3 oz	91	34
thigh, meat & skin; stewed	2.4 oz	158	57
thigh, meat & skin; stewed	1.4 oz	95	35
whole w/ giblets & neck	1 chicken (2.3 lbs)	2223	940
whole w/ giblets & neck; batter dipped, fried	1 chicken (2.3 lbs)	2987	1054
whole w/ giblets & neck; batter dipped, fried	1 lb	895	316
whole w/ giblets & neck; flour coated, fried	1 lb	577	238
whole w/ giblets & neck; flour coated, fried	1 chicken (1.6 lbs)	1928	795

FOOD	PORTION	CALORIES	CHOLESTEROL
whole w/ giblets & neck; roasted	1 chicken (1.5 lbs)	1598	730
whole w/ giblets & neck; roasted	1 lb	480	219
whole w/ giblets & neck; stewed	1 lb	487	218
whole w/ giblets & neck; stewed	1 chicken (1.6 lbs)	1625	726
wing, meat & skin, raw	1.7 oz	109	38
wing, meat & skin; batter dipped, fried	1.7 oz	159	39
wing, meat & skin; flour coated, fried	1.1 oz	103	26
wing, meat & skin; roasted	1.2 oz	99	29
wing, meat & skin; stewed	1.4 oz	100	28
wing, meat only, raw	1 oz	36	17
wing, meat only; fried	.7 oz	42	17
wing, meat only; roasted	.7 oz	43	18
wing, meat only; stewed	.8 oz	43	18
FROZEN PREPARED			
Kibun Chicken Pasta Salad w/ dressing	½ pkg	220	15
Kibun Chicken Pasta Salad w/o dressing	½ pkg	150	10
MicroMagic Chicken Sandwich	1 (4.5 oz)	390	35
Microwave Chefwich Chicken Parmigiana Sandwich	1 (5 oz)	380	24
Weaver Breast Fillets	3.5 oz	195	84
Weaver Breast Fillets Strips	3.5 oz	200	84

FOOD	PORTION	CALORIES	CHOLESTEROL
Weaver Chicken Nuggets	4 pieces	240	74
Weaver Mini-Drums Crispy	3 oz	205	51
Weaver Mini-Drums Herbs 'n Spice	3 oz	205	51
Weaver Rondelets Cheese	3 oz	215	33
Weaver Rondelets Homestyle	3 oz	185	46
Weaver Rondelets Italian	3 oz	200	44
Weaver Rondelets Original	3 oz	185	46
Weaver Thigh Fillets Strips	3.5 oz	240	95
Weaver Batter Dipped Breast	3.5 oz	250	84
Weaver Batter Dipped Thighs/ Drums	3.5 oz	245	89
Weaver Batter Dipped Wings	3.5 oz	270	78
Weaver Chicken Croquetts	3.5 oz	245	44
Weaver Crispy Dutch Frye Breasts	3.5 oz	285	84
Weaver Crispy Dutch Frye Thighs/Drums	3.5 oz	295	89
Weaver Crispy Dutch Frye Wings	3.5 oz	360	78
Weaver Crispy Light Fried Chicken	2.9 oz	160	70
READY-TO-USE			
Bologna (Health Valley)	3.5 oz	300	49
Bologna (Weaver)	3.5 oz	240	100
Breast (Mr. Turkey)	1 slice (1 oz)	32	9

FOOD	PORTION	CALORIES	CHOLESTEROL
Breast Deli Slice Browned & Roasted (Wampler Longacre)	1 oz	49	12
Breast Deluxe Oven Roasted (Louis Rich)	1 slice (28 g)	30	13
Breast Hickory Smoked (Weaver)	3.5 oz	125	68
Breast Meat (Wampler Longacre)	1 oz	38	10
Breast Oven Roasted (Oscar Mayer)	1 slice (28 g)	29	15
Breast Oven Roasted (Weaver)	3.5 oz	120	68
Breast Smoked (Louis Rich)	1 slice (28 g)	31	13
Breast Smoked (Oscar Mayer)	1 slice (28 g)	26	15
Chicken (Carl Buddig)	1 oz	50	12
Cutlets, Perdue Done It!	3 oz	180	33
Diced Breast Roll (Wampler Longacre)	1 oz	49	12
Diced White Breast (Wampler Longacre)	1 oz	38	10
Nuggets White Breaded Fully Cooked (Wampler Longacre)	1 oz	71	12
Nuggets, Perdue Done It!	3 oz	179	45
Roll (Dutch Family)	1 oz	61	21
Roll (Wampler Longacre)	1 oz	65	22

FOOD	PORTION	CALORIES	CHOLESTEROL
Roll Sliced (Wampler Longacre)	1 oz	63	19
Salad (Wampler Longacre)	1 oz	65	9
Tenders, Perdue Done It!	3 oz	159	51
White Oven Roasted (Louis Rich)	1 slice (28 g)	39	14
White Meat Roll (Weaver)	3.5 oz	130	43
Wings Hot & Spicy, Perdue Done It!	3 oz	186	82
chicken roll, light meat	1 slice (28 g)	45	14
chicken roll, light meat	1 pkg (6 oz)	271	85
poultry salad sandwich spread	1 Tbsp	109	4
poultry salad sandwich spread	1 oz	238	9

CHICKEN DISHES
(*see also* CHICKEN SUBSTITUTE, DINNER)

HOME RECIPE

FOOD	PORTION	CALORIES	CHOLESTEROL
chicken cacciatore	¾ cup	394	99
chicken paprikash	1½ cups	296	90
chicken & dumplings	¾ cup	256	109
chicken & noodles	¾ cup	191	43
chicken a la king	¾ cup	234	76

FOOD	PORTION	CALORIES	CHOLESTEROL
CHICKEN SUBSTITUTE			
Chick Stiks, frzn (Worthington)	3.5 oz	232	tr
Chick-Ketts, frzn (Worthington)	3.5 oz	199	tr
Chik-Nuggets (Loma Linda)	5 nuggets (3 oz)	228	0
Chik-Patties (Loma Linda)	1 patty (3 oz)	226	0
Meatless Chicken (Loma Linda)	2 slices (2 oz)	93	0
Meatless Chicken Supreme; mix not prep (Loma Linda)	¼ cup	50	0
Meatless Fried Chicken (Loma Linda)	1 piece (2 oz)	180	0
Meatless Fried Chicken w/ Gravy (Loma Linda)	2 piece (3 oz)	140	0
Spicy-Chik Minidrums (Loma Linda)	5 pieces (3 oz)	230	0
CHICKPEAS			
CANNED Chickpeas (Hanover)	½ cup	100	0
Garbanzo Lite 50% Less Salt (S&W)	½ cup	110	0
Garbanzo Premium Large (S&W)	½ cup	110	0
chickpeas	1 cup	285	0

FOOD	PORTION	CALORIES	CHOLESTEROL
DRIED			
Garbanzo (Hurst Brand)	1 cup	288	0
cooked	1 cup	269	0
raw	1 cup	729	0

CHICORY

FRESH			
greens, raw	½ cup	21	0

CHILI

Chili Beans (S&W)	½ cup	130	0
Chili Con Carne (Health Valley)	4 oz	170	0
Chili Makin's Original (S&W)	½ cup	100	0
Lentil Chili (Health Valley)	4 oz	110	0
Mild Vegetarian w/ Beans (Health Valley)	4 oz	120	0
Oscar Mayer Chili Con Carne Concentrate	1 oz	78	14
Spicy Vegetarian w/ Beans (Health Valley)	4 oz	120	0
chili w/ beans	1 cup	286	43
chili w/ beans (home recipe)	1 cup	399	61

CHINESE CABBAGE

(*see* CABBAGE)

FOOD	PORTION	CALORIES	CHOLESTEROL

CHINESE FOOD
(*see* ORIENTAL FOOD)

CHIPS
(*see also* POPCORN, PRETZELS, SNACKS)

FOOD	PORTION	CALORIES	CHOLESTEROL
CORN			
Corn Chips (Health Valley)	1 oz	160	0
Corn Chips (Wise)	1 oz	160	0
Corn Chips BBQ (Lance)	1 pkg (1¾ oz)	280	0
Corn Chips Plain (Lance)	1 pkg (1¾ oz)	260	0
Corn Chips w/ Cheese (Health Valley)	1 oz	160	2
Corn Crunchies (Wise)	1 oz	160	0
Corn Nacho Cheese Flavor Spirals Crispy Corn Twists (Wise)	1 oz	160	0
Corn Toasted Spirals Crispy Corn Twists (Wise)	1 oz	160	0
Fritos	1 oz	150	0
Fritos Bar-B-Q	1 oz	150	0
POTATO			
Eagle	1 oz	150	0
Lay's	1 oz	150	0
Lay's Jalapeno & Cheddar Flavored	1 oz	150	0

FOOD	PORTION	CALORIES	CHOLESTEROL
Potato (Kelly's)	1 oz	150	0
Potato (Lance)	1 pkg (1⅛ oz)	190	0
Potato BBQ (Lance)	1 pkg (1⅛ oz)	190	0
Potato Cajun Style (Lance)	1 pkg (1 oz)	160	0
Potato Chips (Health Valley)	1 oz	160	0
Potato Chips (New York Deli)	1 oz	160	0
Potato Chips Barbecue Flavor Ripple (Wise)	1 oz	150	0
Potato Chips Natural Flavor (Wise)	1 oz	160	0
Potato Chips No Salt Added (Cottage Fries)	1 oz	160	0
Potato Country Chips (Health Valley)	1 oz	160	0
Potato Country Ripple (Health Valley)	1 oz	160	0
Potato Dip Chips (Health Valley)	1 oz	160	0
Potato Ripple (Lance)	1 pkg (1⅛ oz)	190	0
Potato Rippled (Kelly's)	1 oz	150	0
Potato Sour Cream & Onion (Lance)	1 pkg (1⅛ oz)	190	0
Potato, Unsalted (Kelly's)	1 oz	150	0

FOOD	PORTION	CALORIES	CHOLESTEROL
Ripple (Lance)	1 oz	160	0
Ruffles	1 oz	150	0
Ruffles Bar-B-Q Flavored	1 oz	150	0
Ruffles Sour Cream & Onion Artificially Flavored	1 oz	150	0
Sour Cream and Onion Ripple (Lance)	1 oz	170	tr
potato	10 chips	105	0
potato	1 oz	148	0
potato sticks	1 oz pkg	148	0
TORTILLA			
Doritos	1 oz	140	0
Doritos Cool Ranch	1 oz	140	0
Doritos Nacho Cheese Flavored	1 oz	140	0
Tortilla Chips (La Famous)	1 oz	140	0
Tortilla Chips Buenitos (Health Valley)	1 oz	130	0
Tortilla Chips Nacho Cheese Flavor Round Bravos (Wise)	1 oz	150	0
Tortilla Chips No Salt Added (La Famous)	1 oz	140	0
Tortilla Jalapeno Cheese (Lance)	1 pkg (1⅛ oz)	160	0
Tortilla Nacho (Lance)	1 pkg (1⅛ oz)	160	0

FOOD	PORTION	CALORIES	CHOLESTEROL

CHITTERLINGS

FRESH

pork, raw	3 oz	213	135
pork; simmered	3 oz	258	122

CHIVES

DRIED

freeze-dried	1 Tbsp	1	0

FRESH

raw	1 tsp	0	0

CHOCOLATE

(*see also* CANDY, CAROB, COCOA, ICE CREAM TOPPINGS, MILK DRINKS)

BAKING

German Sweet (Bakers)	1 oz	144	tr
Semi-Sweet Chocolate (Bakers)	1 oz	136	tr
Unsweetened (Bakers)	1 oz	142	tr
Unsweetened Baking Chocolate (Hershey)	1 oz	190	5

CHIPS

Chocolate Flavored Chips (Bakers)	¼ cup	196	tr
German Sweet Chocolate Chips (Bakers)	¼ cup	203	tr
Real Semi-Sweet Chocolate Chips (Bakers)	¼ cup	201	tr

FOOD	PORTION	CALORIES	CHOLESTEROL
Semi-Sweet Chocolate Chips, miniature (Hershey)	¼ cup	220	10
Semi-Sweet Chocolate Chips, regular (Hershey)	¼ cup	220	10
MIX			
Hershey Instant Mix	3 Tbsp	80	0
Ovaltine; as prep w/ whole milk	8 oz	227	34
Quik Chocolate Flavor (Nestle)	2 tsp	90	0
chocolate mix; as prep w/ whole milk	9 oz	226	33
chocolate powder	2–3 heaping tsp	75	0
SYRUP			
Estee	1 Tbsp	6	0
Hershey's Chocolate Flavored	2 Tbsp	80	0
chocolate	1 cup	653	0
chocolate; as prep w/ whole milk	9 oz	232	33

CHOCOLATE MILK
(see CHOCOLATE, COCOA, MILK DRINKS)

CISCO

smoked	3 oz	151	27
smoked	1 oz	50	9

FOOD	PORTION	CALORIES	CHOLESTEROL

CITRON

candied	1 oz	89	0

CLAM

CANNED

Quahogs (American Original Foods)	4 oz	66	16
meat only	1 cup	236	107
meat only	3 oz	126	57

FRESH

clam; cooked	20 sm	133	60
clam; cooked	3 oz	126	57
raw	3 oz	63	29
raw	9 lg	133	60
raw	20 sm	133	60

HOME RECIPE

clam sauce	½ cup	274	87
clam; breaded & fried	3 oz	171	52
clam; breaded & fried	20 sm	379	115

COCOA
(see also CHOCOLATE)

MIX

Carnation Hot Cocoa 70 Calorie	3 tsp (21 g)	70	2
Carnation Hot Cocoa Milk Chocolate	1 pkg or 4 heaping tsp (1 oz)	110	2

FOOD	PORTION	CALORIES	CHOLESTEROL
Carnation Hot Cocoa Natural Mint	1 pkg or 4 heaping tsp (1 oz)	110	2
Carnation Hot Cocoa Rich Chocolate	1 pkg or 4 heaping tsp (1 oz)	110	2
Carnation Hot Cocoa Rich Chocolate w/ Marshmallows	1 pkg or 4 heaping tsp (1 oz)	110	2
Carnation Hot Cocoa Sugar Free Mint	1 pkg or 4 heaping tsp (15 g)	50	2
Carnation Hot Cocoa Sugar Free Rich Chocolate	1 pkg or 4 heaping tsp (15 g)	50	2
Hershey's Cocoa	⅓ cup	120	0
PREPARED			
Hills Bros. Hot Cocoa Sugar Free; as prep w/ water	6 oz	60	0
Hills Bros. Hot Cocoa; as prep w/ water	6 oz	110	0
hot cocoa	1 cup	218	33

COCONUT

FOOD	PORTION	CALORIES	CHOLESTEROL
Angel Flake Bag (Bakers)	⅓ cup	116	0
Angel Flake Can (Bakers)	⅓ cup	114	0
Premium Shred (Bakers)	⅓ cup	136	0
coconut water	1 Tbsp	3	0
coconut water	1 cup	46	0
cream, canned	1 Tbsp	36	0

FOOD	PORTION	CALORIES	CHOLESTEROL
cream, canned	1 cup	568	0
dried, creamed	1 oz	194	0
dried, sweetened, flaked	1 cup	351	0
dried, sweetened, flaked	7 oz pkg	944	0
dried, sweetened, flaked, canned	1 cup	341	0
dried, sweetened, shredded	7 oz pkg	997	0
dried, sweetened, shredded	1 cup	466	0
dried, toasted	1 oz	168	0
dried, unsweetened	1 oz	187	0
milk, canned	1 Tbsp	30	0
milk, canned	1 cup	445	0
milk, frozen	1 Tbsp	30	0
milk, frozen	1 cup	486	0
raw	1 piece	159	0

COD

CANNED			
Atlantic	3 oz	89	47
Atlantic	1 can (11 oz)	327	171
DRIED			
Atlantic	3 oz	246	129
FRESH			
Atlantic, raw	3 oz	70	37
Atlantic, raw	1 fillet (8.1 oz)	190	99
Atlantic; cooked	1 fillet (6.3 oz)	189	99

FOOD	PORTION	CALORIES	CHOLESTEROL
Atlantic; cooked	3 oz	89	47
Pacific, raw	1 fillet (4.1 oz)	95	43
Pacific, raw	3 oz	70	31
roe, raw	3½ oz	130	360
FROZEN			
Au Poivre Style Cod (Icelandic)	4 oz	100	49
Au Poivre Style Cod (Icelandic)	6 oz	150	74
Bacon Crumb Flavor Cod (Icelandic)	4 oz	216	57
Bacon Crumb Flavor Cod (Icelandic)	6 oz	324	86
Bake 'N' Serve Light Cod (Icelandic)	4 oz	199	46
Bake 'N' Serve Light Cod (Icelandic)	6 oz	300	70
Blackened Style Cod (Icelandic)	4 oz	126	58
Blackened Style Cod (Icelandic)	6 oz	189	86
Cajun Style Cod (Icelandic)	4 oz	138	53
Cajun Style Cod (Icelandic)	6 oz	208	80
Fish in Sauce Danish Dill Cod (Icelandic)	4 oz	95	47
Fish in Sauce Danish Dill Cod (Icelandic)	6 oz	142	71
Scampi Style Cod (Icelandic)	4 oz	110	44

FOOD	PORTION	CALORIES	CHOLESTEROL
Scampi Style Cod (Icelandic)	6 oz	166	66

COFFEE
(see also COFFEE BEVERAGES, COFFEE SUBSTITUTE)

INSTANT			
powder	1 rounded tsp	4	0
powder w/ chicory	1 rounded tsp	6	0

INSTANT, DECAFFEINATED			
powder	1 rounded tsp	4	0

REGULAR			
coffee	6 oz	4	0

COFFEE BEVERAGES
(see also COFFEE SUBSTITUTE)

FOOD	PORTION	CALORIES	CHOLESTEROL
Cafe Amaretto International Coffee (General Foods)	6 oz	51	tr
Cafe Francais International Coffee (General Foods)	6 oz	55	tr
Cafe Francais Sugar Free International Coffee (General Foods)	6 oz	35	tr
Cafe Irish Creme International Coffee (General Foods)	6 oz	55	tr

FOOD	PORTION	CALORIES	CHOLESTEROL
Cafe Irish Creme Sugar Free International Coffee (General Foods)	6 oz	31	tr
Cafe Vienna International Coffee (General Foods)	6 oz	59	tr
Cafe Vienna Sugar Free International Coffee (General Foods)	6 oz	29	tr
Irish Mocha Mint International Coffee (General Foods)	6 oz	51	tr
Irish Mocha Mint Sugar Free International Coffee (General Foods)	6 oz	28	tr
Orange Cappuccino International Coffee (General Foods)	6 oz	59	tr
Orange Cappuccino Sugar Free International Coffee (General Foods)	6 oz	29	tr
Suisse Mocha International Coffee (General Foods)	6 oz	53	tr
Suisse Mocha Sugar Free International Coffee (General Foods)	6 oz	29	tr

COFFEE SUBSTITUTE

FOOD	PORTION	CALORIES	CHOLESTEROL
Postum Instant Coffee Flavored; as prep	6 oz	11	0
Postum Instant; as prep	6 oz	11	0
as prep w/ milk	6 oz	121	25
powder	1 tsp	9	0

FOOD	PORTION	CALORIES	CHOLESTEROL

COFFEE WHITENERS
(see also MILK SUBSTITUTE)

LIQUID			
Coffee Rich	1 Tbsp	20	0
Coffee-Mate	1 oz	31	0
Grand Union	1 Tbsp	24	0
Mocha Mix	1 Tbsp (½ oz)	19	0
non-dairy, frozen	½ oz	20	0
POWDER			
Coffee-Mate	1 pkg (3 g)	16	0
Coffee-Mate	1 tsp	10	0
non-dairy	1 tsp	11	0

COLD CUTS
(see LUNCHEON MEATS/COLD CUTS)

COLESLAW
(see CABBAGE, SALAD)

COLLARDS

FRESH			
cooked	½ cup	13	0
raw; chopped	1 cup	35	0
FROZEN			
frzn; cooked	½ cup	31	0
frzn; not prep	10 oz	93	0

FOOD	PORTION	CALORIES	CHOLESTEROL
COOKIE			
(*see also* BROWNIE, CAKE, DOUGHNUT, PIE)			
HOME RECIPE			
chocolate chip	1 (.4 oz)	59	5
fortune cookie	1 (½ oz)	66	tr
lemon bar	1 (1 oz)	110	37
molasses	1 (1.1 oz)	138	25
oatmeal w/ raisins	1 (.5 oz)	54	5
peanut butter	1 (.5 oz)	61	5
pumpkin bar	1 (1.2 oz)	151	25
raspberry bar	1 (.8 oz)	76	6
sugar	1 (.4 oz)	36	8
READY-TO-EAT			
Amaranth Graham Crackers (Health Valley)	1.2 oz	110	0
Amaranth Jumbo (Health Valley)	.6 oz	70	0
Animal Crackers (Sunshine)	14	120	0
Apple Oatmeal Bar (Lance)	1 pkg (1.65 oz)	190	5
Apple-Cinnamon (Lance)	1 pkg (1 oz)	120	0
Baked Apple Bar (Sunbelt)	1 pkg (1.31 oz)	130	tr
Blueberry (Lance)	1 pkg (1 oz)	120	0
Bonnie (Lance)	1 pkg (¾ oz)	100	5

FOOD	PORTION	CALORIES	CHOLESTEROL
Butter Flavored (Sunshine)	4	120	5
Chip-A-Roos (Sunshine)	2	130	0
Chips'n Middles (Sunshine)	2	140	0
Choc-O-Lunch (Lance)	1⅝₁₆ oz	180	0
Choc-O-Lunch (Lance)	1 oz	130	0
Choc-O-Mint (Lance)	1¼ oz	180	0
Chocolate Chip (Archway)	1	60	5
Chocolate Chip (Lance)	1 pkg (1 oz)	135	5
Chocolate Chip Fudge (Lance)	1 pkg (1 oz)	130	0
Chocolate Coated Snack Wafer (Estee)	1	120	<5
Chocolate Creme Filled Wafer (Estee)	1	20	0
Chocolate Fudge Sandwich (Sunshine)	2	150	0
Chocolate Snack Wafer (Estee)	1	80	0
Cinnamon Jumbo (Health Valley)	½ oz	70	0
Coated Graham (Lance)	1⅝₁₆ oz	180	0
Cup Custard (Sunshine)	2	130	5

FOOD	PORTION	CALORIES	CHOLESTEROL
Fig Bar (Keebler)	1	71	12
Fig Bar (Lance)	1½ oz	150	0
Fig Bars (Sunshine)	2	90	0
Ginger Snaps (Sunshine)	5	100	0
Gingersnaps (Archway)	1	35	0
Golden Fruit Raisin Biscuits (Sunshine)	2	150	0
Graham Cinnamon (Sunshine)	4	70	0
Graham Honey (Sunshine)	4	60	0
Honey Graham (Health Valley)	1 oz	100	0
Hydrox (Sunshine)	3	160	0
Lemon Coolers (Sunshine)	5	140	0
Mallopuffs (Sunshine)	2	140	0
Malt (Lance)	1¼ oz	190	0
Molasses (Archway)	1	100	10
Nut-O-Lunch (Lance)	1 oz	140	0
Oat Bran Animal Cookies (Health Valley)	1 oz	90	0

FOOD	PORTION	CALORIES	CHOLESTEROL
Oat Bran Fruit Cookies (Health Valley)	1 oz	110	0
Oat Bran Fruit Jumbos (Health Valley)	½ oz	70	0
Oat Bran Graham Crackers (Health Valley)	1.1 oz	100	0
Oat Bran Honey Jumbos (Health Valley)	½ oz	70	0
Oatmeal (Archway)	1	110	5
Oatmeal (Lance)	1 pkg (1 oz)	130	0
Oatmeal (Little Debbie)	1 pkg (2.75 oz)	340	1
Oatmeal Country Style (Sunshine)	2	110	0
Oatmeal Date Filled (Archway)	1	100	5
Oatmeal Peanut Sandwich (Sunshine)	2	140	0
Oatmeal, Apple Filled (Archway)	1	90	5
Peanut Butter & Honey Wafers (Sunbelt)	1 pkg (1.2 oz)	160	tr
Peanut Butter Creme Filled Wafer (Lance)	1 pkg (1¾ oz)	240	0
Peanut Butter Jumbo (Health Valley)	½ oz	70	0
Peanut Butter Wafers (Sunshine)	3	120	0

FOOD	PORTION	CALORIES	CHOLESTEROL
Pecan Crunch (Archway)	1	35	0
Pecan Sandie (Keebler)	1	85	0
Raisin Oatmeal (Archway)	1	35	0
Sandwich Cookies (Estee)	1	44–50	0
Select Assortment (Archway)	1	60	5
Sprinkles (Sunshine)	2	130	0
Strawberry (Lance)	1 pkg (1 oz)	120	0
Strawberry Snack Wafer (Estee)	1	80	0
Sugar Wafers (Sunshine)	3	130	0
Tofu Cookies (Health Valley)	1.2 oz	130	0
Van-O-Lunch (Lance)	1⁵⁄₁₆ oz	180	0
Van-O-Lunch (Lance)	1 oz	140	0
Vanilla Snack Wafer (Estee)	1	80	0
Vanilla Creme Filled Wafer (Estee)	1	20	0
Vanilla Wafers (Sunshine)	6	130	5
Vienna Finger Sandwich (Sunshine)	2	140	0

FOOD	PORTION	CALORIES	CHOLESTEROL
Wheat Free (Health Valley)	1.5 oz	160	0
chocolate oatmeal	1 (½ oz)	66	5
fig bar	1 (½ oz)	49	8
gingersnap	1 (¼ oz)	30	2
graham cracker	4 pieces	108	0
graham cracker, chocolate covered	2 pieces	123	tr
lady finger	1	40	39
macaroon	1 (½ oz)	54	0

CORN

FOOD	PORTION	CALORIES	CHOLESTEROL
CANNED			
Cream Style (Libby)	½ cup	80	0
Cream Style (Owatonna)	½ cup	100	0
Cream Style Premium Homestyle (S&W)	½ cup	105	0
Whole Kernel (Libby)	½ cup	80	0
Whole Kernel (Seneca)	½ cup	80	0
Whole Kernel Natural Pack (Libby)	½ cup	80	0
Whole Kernel Natural Pack (Seneca)	½ cup	80	0
Whole Kernel Premium Homestyle (S&W)	½ cup	90	0

FOOD	PORTION	CALORIES	CHOLESTEROL
Whole Kernel Vacuum Pack (Owatonna)	½ cup	100	0
Whole Kernel in Brine (Owatonna)	½ cup	90	0
corn	½ cup	93	0
corn, sweet	½ cup	66	0
corn, cream style	½ cup	93	0
FRESH			
corn, sweet; cooked	1 ear (2.5 oz)	83	0
sweet kernel, raw	½ cup	66	0
FROZEN			
Cob Corn (Ore Ida)	1 ear (5.3 oz)	180	0
Corn Cob (Birds Eye)	1 ear (4.4 oz)	120	0
Corn Cob Little Ears (Birds Eye)	2 ears (4.6 oz)	126	0
Corn Country Style (Budget Gourmet)	5.57 oz	140	15
Corn on the Cob Natural Ears (Birds Eye)	1 ear (5.7 oz)	156	0
Corn Sweet, in Butter Sauce (Budget Gourmet)	5.5 oz	190	15
Kernels; cooked (Health Valley)	5.8 oz	134	0
White Shoepeg (Hanover)	½ cup	80	0
White Sweet (Hanover)	½ cup	80	0

FOOD	PORTION	CALORIES	CHOLESTEROL
Whole Kernel Tendersweet (Birds Eye)	½ cup	82	tr
Whole Kernel Cut (Birds Eye)	½ cup	82	tr
Yellow Sweet (Hanover)	½ cup	80	0
frzn; not prep	½ cup	67	0
on the cob; cooked	1 ear (2.2 oz)	59	0
on the cob; not prep	1 ear (4.4 oz)	123	0
HOME RECIPE			
fritters	1 (1 oz)	62	12
scalloped	½ cup	258	47

CORN CHIPS
(see CHIPS)

CORNMEAL

FOOD	PORTION	CALORIES	CHOLESTEROL
Albers White	1 oz	100	0
Albers Yellow	1 oz	100	0

CORNSTARCH

FOOD	PORTION	CALORIES	CHOLESTEROL
Argo	1 Tbsp	30	0
Argo	1 cup	460	0
Kingsford's	1 Tbsp	30	0
Kingsford's	1 cup	460	0

CORNISH HENS
(see CHICKEN)

FOOD	PORTION	CALORIES	CHOLESTEROL
COTTAGE CHEESE			
REDUCED CALORIE			
Friendship 'N Fruit	6 oz	100	7
Friendship Lactose Reduced, Lowfat	½ cup	90	5
Friendship Large Curd Pot Style, Lowfat	½ cup	100	9
Friendship, Lowfat	½ cup	90	5
Friendship, Lowfat, No Salt Added	½ cup	90	5
Land O'Lakes, 2% Fat	4 oz	100	10
Light n' Lively, Lowfat, 1%	4 oz	80	15
lowfat, 1%	4 oz	82	5
lowfat, 1%	1 cup	164	10
lowfat, 2%	1 cup	203	19
lowfat, 2%	4 oz	101	9
REGULAR			
Friendship w/ Pineapple	½ cup	140	17
Friendship, California Style	½ cup	120	17
Land O'Lakes	4 oz	120	15
creamed	½ cup	109	16
creamed	1 cup	217	31
creamed, w/ fruit	4 oz	140	13
dry curd	1 cup	123	10
COWPEAS			
CANNED			
common	1 cup	184	0

FOOD	PORTION	CALORIES	CHOLESTEROL
common w/ pork	½ cup	99	8
DRIED			
catjang, raw	1 cup	572	0
catjang; cooked	1 cup	200	0
common, raw	1 cup	562	0
common; cooked	1 cup	198	0
FROZEN			
cowpeas	½ cup	112	0

CRAB

CANNED			
blue	3 oz	84	76
blue	1 cup	133	120
FRESH			
Alaska king, raw	3 oz	71	35
Alaska king, raw	1 leg (6 oz)	144	72
Alaska king, raw	1 leg (4.7 oz)	129	72
Alaska king, raw	3 oz	82	45
blue, raw	3 oz	74	66
blue, raw	1 crab (.7 oz)	18	16
blue; cooked	3 oz	87	85
blue; cooked	1 cup	138	135
dungeness, raw	1 crab	140	97

FOOD	PORTION	CALORIES	CHOLESTEROL
dungeness, raw	3 oz	73	50
queen, raw	3 oz	76	47
FROZEN			
Crab Crisp (King & Prince)	4 oz	310	34
Crab Del Rey (King & Prince)	2 oz	102	31
Crab Del Rey (King & Prince)	3 oz	153	47
Crab Del Rey (King & Prince)	4 oz	205	63
HOME RECIPE			
deviled	½ cup	182	125
imperial	½ cup	162	154
stew	1 cup	208	73
stuffed	¾ cup	129	123
READY-TO-USE			
crab cakes	1 cake (2.1 oz)	93	90

CRABAPPLE

FOOD	PORTION	CALORIES	CHOLESTEROL
FRESH			
raw; sliced	1 cup	83	0

CRACKER CRUMBS

FOOD	PORTION	CALORIES	CHOLESTEROL
Cracker Meal (Lance)	1 oz	100	0
Graham (Sunshine)	1 cup	550	0
cracker meal	1 cup	538	0

FOOD	PORTION	CALORIES	CHOLESTEROL

CRACKERS
(see also CRACKER CRUMBS)

FOOD	PORTION	CALORIES	CHOLESTEROL
6 Calorie Wafer (Estee)	1	6	<5
Bonnie (Lance)	1¾₆ oz	160	5
Captain Wafers (Lance)	2 crackers	30	0
Captain Wafers Very Low Sodium (Lance)	2 crackers	30	0
Captain's Wafers w/ Cream Cheese & Chives (Lance)	1⁵⁄₁₆ oz	170	0
Cheddar American Heritage (Sunshine)	5	80	5
Cheese Wheels (Health Valley)	1 oz	140	3
Cheese n' Crackers (Handi-Snacks)	1 pkg	130	15
Cheese-On-Wheat (Lance)	1⁵⁄₁₆ oz	180	0
Cheez-It (Sunshine)	12	70	0
Dark Finn Crisp Bread (Ryvita)	2	38	0
Dark Rye Crisp Bread (Ryvita)	1	26	0
Dark w/ Caraway Seeds Finn Crisp Bread (Ryvita)	2	38	0

FOOD	PORTION	CALORIES	CHOLESTEROL
Gold-N-Chee Spicy (Lance)	15 crackers	70	tr
Herb No Salt (Health Valley)	1 oz	120	0
Hi Ho (Sunshine)	4	80	0
High Fiber Snackbread (Ryvita)	1	14	0
High Fiber Crisp Bread (Ryvita)	1	23	0
Krispy Saltine (Sunshine)	5	60	0
Krispy Unsalted Tops (Sunshine)	5	60	0
Lanchee (Lance)	1¼ oz	180	5
Light Rye Crisp Bread (Ryvita)	1	26	0
Melba Toast Oblong (Lance)	2 crackers	30	0
Melba Toast Round Garlic (Lance)	2 crackers	20	0
Melba Toast Round Onion (Lance)	2 crackers	20	0
Melba Toast Round Plain (Lance)	2 crackers	20	0
Melba Toast Sesame (Lance)	2 crackers	25	0
Nekot (Lance)	1½ oz	210	5
Nip-Chee (Lance)	15⁄16 oz	180	5

FOOD	PORTION	CALORIES	CHOLESTEROL
Original Wheat Snackbread (Ryvita)	1	20	0
Oyster (Nabisco)	37 pieces	124	0
Oyster & Soup (Sunshine)	16	60	0
Oyster Crackers (Lance)	½ oz	70	0
Parmesan American Heritage (Sunshine)	4	70	0
Party Crackers (Estee)	½ oz	40	0
Peanut Butter Toasty Crackers (Little Debbie)	1 pkg (.93 oz)	140	tr
Peanut Butter Toasty Crackers (Little Debbie)	1 pkg (1.4 oz)	200	tr
Peanut Butter Wheat (Lance)	1⁵⁄₁₆ oz	190	0
Peanut Butter 'n Cheese Crackers (Handi-Snacks)	1 pkg	190	0
Pepato Flavor Tuscany Toast (Tuscany)	1 oz	93	0
Pesto Flavor Tuscany Toast (Tuscany)	1 oz	96	3
Pita Crisps (Tuscany)	1 oz	90	0
Ritz (Nabisco)	9 pieces	149	0
Rye Twins (Lance)	2 crackers	30	0
Rye-Chee (Lance)	1⁷⁄₁₆ oz	190	5

FOOD	PORTION	CALORIES	CHOLESTEROL
Rykrisp (Ralston)	4 pieces	91	0
Saltines (Lance)	2	25	0
Saltines, Slug Pack (Lance)	4 crackers	50	0
Sesame (Health Valley)	1 oz	130	0
Sesame American Heritage (Sunshine)	4	70	0
Sesame Crackers (Estee)	½ oz	40	0
Sesame Pita Crisps (Tuscany)	1 oz	96	0
Sesame Twins (Lance)	2 crackers	40	0
Stoned Wheat (Health Valley)	1 oz	120	0
Tam Tams (Manischewitz)	10	147	0
Tam Tams No Salt (Manischewitz)	5	70	0
Tams Garlic (Manischewitz)	10	153	0
Tams Onion (Manischewitz)	10	150	0
Tams Wheat (Manischewitz)	10	150	0
Thin Wheat Snacks (Lance)	7 crackers	80	0
Toastchee (Lance)	1⅜ oz	190	5

FOOD	PORTION	CALORIES	CHOLESTEROL
Toasted Sesame Rye Crisp Bread (Ryvita)	1	31	0
Toasty (Lance)	1¼ oz	180	0
Tomato-Flavor Tuscany Toast (Tuscany)	1 oz	95	0
Town House (Keebler)	9 crackers	157	tr
Triscuit	7 pieces	143	0
Tuscany Toast (Tuscany)	1 oz	95	0
Unsalted (Estee)	2	30	tr
Waldorf Low Salt (Keebler)	9 crackers	130	0
Wheat American Heritage (Sunshine)	4	60	0
Wheat Twins (Lance)	2 crackers	30	0
Wheat Wafers (Sunshine)	8	80	0
Wheatswafer (Lance)	4 crackers	60	0
Wheatswafer (Lance)	2 crackers	30	0
melba toast	1	20	0
saltine	10 pieces	121	0
SNACK			
Cheese Crackers w/ Peanut Butter (Little Debbie)	1 pkg (1.4 oz)	190	tr

FOOD	PORTION	CALORIES	CHOLESTEROL
Peanut Butter Cheese Crackers (Little Debbie)	1 pkg (.93 oz)	130	tr

CRANBERRY

CANNED

CranOrange (Ocean Spray)	2 oz	100	0
CranRaspberry (Ocean Spray)	2 oz	90	0
Cranberry Sauce Jellied Old Fashioned (S&W)	¼ cup	90	0
Cranberry Sauce Whole Berry Old Fashioned (S&W)	¼ cup	90	0
Jellied Cranberry Sauce (Ocean Spray)	2 oz	90	0
Whole Berry Sauce (Ocean Spray)	2 oz	90	0
cranberry sauce, sweetened	½ cup	209	0

FRESH

| Fresh Cranberries (Ocean Spray) | ¼ cup | 25 | 0 |
| cranberries; chopped | 1 cup | 54 | 0 |

JUICE

| Cranberry (Smucker's) | 8 oz | 130 | 0 |

CRANBERRY BEANS

CANNED

| cranberry beans | ½ cup | 108 | 0 |

FOOD	PORTION	CALORIES	CHOLESTEROL
DRIED			
cooked	½ cup	120	0
raw	½ cup	328	0

CRAYFISH

FRESH			
cooked	3 oz	97	151
raw	3 oz	76	118
raw	8	24	37

CREAM

(*see also* SOUR CREAM, SOUR CREAM SUBSTITUTE, WHIPPED TOPPINGS)

LIQUID			
Half & Half (Land O'Lakes)	1 Tbsp	20	5
Whipping Cream (Land O'Lakes)	1 Tbsp	45	15
Whipping Cream, Gourmet Heavy (Land O'Lakes)	1 Tbsp	60	20
half & half	1 Tbsp	20	6
half & half	1 cup	315	89
heavy whipping	1 Tbsp	52	21
light whipping	1 Tbsp	44	17
light, coffee	1 Tbsp	29	10
medium, 25% fat	1 Tbsp	37	13
WHIPPED			
heavy whipping	1 cup	411	163
light whipping	1 cup	345	132

FOOD	PORTION	CALORIES	CHOLESTEROL

CREAM CHEESE

LIGHT (REDUCED FAT)

FOOD	PORTION	CALORIES	CHOLESTEROL
Formagg Cottage	1 oz	80	0
Formagg Cream Cheese Style	1 oz	80	0
Philadelphia Brand Light Cream Cheese Product	1 oz	60	15

NEUFCHATEL

FOOD	PORTION	CALORIES	CHOLESTEROL
Neufchatel (Kraft)	1 oz	80	25
neufchatel	1 oz	74	22

REGULAR

FOOD	PORTION	CALORIES	CHOLESTEROL
Philadelphia Brand	1 oz	100	30
Philadelphia Brand w/ Pimentos	1 oz	90	30
Philadelphia Brand w/ Chives	1 oz	90	30
cream cheese	1 oz	99	31

SOFT

FOOD	PORTION	CALORIES	CHOLESTEROL
Friendship	1 oz	103	31
Philadelphia Brand	1 oz	100	30
Philadelphia Brand w/ Chives & Onion	1 oz	100	30
Philadelphia Brand w/ Honey	1 oz	100	25
Philadelphia Brand w/ Olives & Pimento	1 oz	90	30
Philadelphia Brand w/ Pineapple	1 oz	90	25

FOOD	PORTION	CALORIES	CHOLESTEROL
Philadelphia Brand w/ Smoked Salmon	1 oz	90	25
Philadelphia Brand w/ Strawberries	1 oz	90	25
WHIPPED			
Philadelphia Brand	1 oz	100	30
Philadelphia Brand w/ Bacon & Horseradish	1 oz	90	20
Philadelphia Brand w/ Blue Cheese	1 oz	100	25
Philadelphia Brand w/ Chives	1 oz	90	25
Philadelphia Brand w/ Onions	1 oz	90	20
Philadelphia Brand w/ Pimentos	1 oz	90	20
Philadelphia Brand w/ Smoked Salmon	1 oz	100	25

CREPES

basic crepe, unfilled (home recipe)	1	75	55

CRESS
(*see also* WATERCRESS)

FRESH			
garden, raw	½ cup	8	0
garden; cooked	½ cup	16	0

FOOD	PORTION	CALORIES	CHOLESTEROL

CROAKER

FRESH

| Atlantic, raw | 3 oz | 89 | 52 |
| Atlantic, raw | 1 fillet (2.8 oz) | 83 | 48 |

HOME RECIPE

| Atlantic; breaded & fried | 1 fillet (3.1 oz) | 192 | 73 |
| Atlantic; breaded & fried | 3 oz | 188 | 71 |

CROISSANT

| Colonial Wheat Croissants (Rainbo) | 1 | 300 | 5 |
| croissant | 1 | 235 | 13 |

CROUTONS

| Croutettes (Kellogg) | 1 cup | 144 | 0 |

CUCUMBER

FRESH

| raw | 1 | 39 | 0 |
| raw; sliced | ½ cup | 7 | 0 |

CURRANTS

DRIED

| currants, Zante | 1 cup | 204 | 0 |

FRESH

| currants | ½ cup | 36 | 0 |

FOOD	PORTION	CALORIES	CHOLESTEROL

CUSK

FRESH

| raw | 3 oz | 74 | 35 |
| raw | 1 fillet (4.3 oz) | 106 | 50 |

CUSTARD

(see also PUDDING)

Custard; as prep w/ skim milk (Delmark)	½ cup	97	6
baked (home recipe)	½ cup	152	139
custard; as prep from mix	½ cup	161	80
zabaione (home recipe)	½ cup	159	409

CUTTLEFISH

FRESH

| raw | 3 oz | 67 | 95 |

DANDELION GREENS

FRESH

| cooked | ½ cup | 17 | 0 |
| raw; chopped | ½ cup | 13 | 0 |

DANISH PASTRY

fruit	1 (2.3 oz)	235	56
plain	1 (2 oz)	220	49
plain ring	1 (12 oz)	1305	292

FOOD	PORTION	CALORIES	CHOLESTEROL

DATES

DRIED

FOOD	PORTION	CALORIES	CHOLESTEROL
Dates, California Deglet Noor	10	240	0
Dates; diced (Bordo)	2 oz	203	0
chopped	1 cup	489	0

DIETING AIDS
(*see* NUTRITIONAL SUPPLEMENTS)

DINNER
(*see also* ITALIAN FOOD, MEXICAN FOOD, PASTA DINNERS, POT PIE, ORIENTAL FOOD)

FROZEN

FOOD	PORTION	CALORIES	CHOLESTEROL
Armour Classics Lite Steak Diane	10 oz	290	90
Banquet All White Meat Fried Chicken Platter	9 oz	430	105
Banquet Beans & Frankfurters Dinner	10 oz	510	34
Banquet Beans & Frankfurters Dinner	10 oz	510	34
Banquet Beef Platter	10 oz	460	70
Banquet Chicken Pattie Platter	7.5 oz	370	
Banquet Chopped Beef Dinner	11 oz	420	76
Banquet Extra Helping Beef Dinner	16 oz	865	120
Banquet Extra Helping Lasagne Dinner	16.5 oz	645	38
Banquet Extra Helping Salisbury Steak Dinner	18 oz	910	171

FOOD	PORTION	CALORIES	CHOLESTEROL
Banquet Extra Helping Salisbury Steak Dinner w/ Mushroom Gravy	18 oz	890	169
Banquet Extra Helping Turkey Dinner	19 oz	750	63
Banquet Family Favorites Chicken & Dumplings Dinner	10 oz	420	43
Banquet Family Favorites Macaroni & Cheese Dinner	10 oz	415	28
Banquet Family Favorites Noodles & Chicken Dinner	10 oz	340	45
Banquet Family Favorites Spaghetti & Meatballs Dinner	10 oz	290	28
Banquet Fish Platter	8.75 oz	445	92
Banquet Ham Platter	10 oz	400	49
Banquet Meat Loaf Dinner	11 oz	440	82
Banquet Pot Pies Beef, Chicken, Turkey	7 oz	520	82–37
Banquet Salisbury Steak Dinner	11 oz	495	76
Banquet Turkey Dinner	10.5 oz	385	37
Banquet Western Dinner	11 oz	630	87
Budget Gourmet Cheese Manicotti w/ Meat Sauce	10 oz	450	50
Budget Gourmet Chicken Cacciatore	11 oz	300	60
Budget Gourmet Chicken & Egg Noodle w/ Broccoli	10 oz	450	130
Budget Gourmet Chicken w/ Fettucini	10 oz	400	100

FOOD	PORTION	CALORIES	CHOLESTEROL
Budget Gourmet Italian Sausage Lasagna	10 oz	420	80
Budget Gourmet Italian Syle Meatballs with Noodles & Peppers	10 oz	310	55
Budget Gourmet Linguini w/ Shrimp	10 oz	330	75
Budget Gourmet Pasta Shells and Beef	10 oz	340	35
Budget Gourmet Pepper Steak w/ Rice	10 oz	300	25
Budget Gourmet Scallops & Shrimp Mariner	11.5 oz	320	70
Budget Gourmet Seafood Newburg	10 oz	350	70
Budget Gourmet Sirloin Salisbury Steak	11.5 oz	410	105
Budget Gourmet Sirloin Tips in Burgundy Sauce	11 oz	310	65
Budget Gourmet Sirloin Tips w/ Country Style Vegetables	10 oz	310	40
Budget Gourmet Sliced Turkey Breast	11.1 oz	290	45
Budget Gourmet Slim Selects Beef Stroganoff	8.75 oz	280	60
Budget Gourmet Slim Selects Cheese Ravioli	10 oz	260	45
Budget Gourmet Slim Selects Chicken Enchilada Suiza	9 oz	270	50
Budget Gourmet Slim Selects Chicken-Au-Gratin	9.1 oz	260	70
Budget Gourmet Slim Selects Fettucini w/ Meat Sauce	10 oz	290	25

FOOD	PORTION	CALORIES	CHOLESTEROL
Budget Gourmet Slim Selects French Recipe Chicken	10 oz	260	60
Budget Gourmet Slim Selects Glazed Turkey	9 oz	270	50
Budget Gourmet Slim Selects Ham & Asparagus-Au-Gratin	9 oz	280	40
Budget Gourmet Slim Selects Lasagne w/ Meat Sauce	10 oz	290	25
Budget Gourmet Slim Selects Linguini w/ Scallops & Clams	9.5 oz	280	60
Budget Gourmet Slim Selects Mandarin Chicken	10 oz	290	25
Budget Gourmet Slim Selects Oriental Beef	10 oz	290	25
Budget Gourmet Slim Selects Sirloin Enchilada Ranchero	9 oz	290	35
Budget Gourmet Slim Selects Sirloin Salisbury Steak	9 oz	280	75
Budget Gourmet Slim Selects Sirloin of Beef in Herb Sauce	10 oz	290	25
Budget Gourmet Swedish Meatballs w/ Noodles	10 oz	600	140
Budget Gourmet Sweet & Sour Chicken w/ Rice	10 oz	350	40
Budget Gourmet Teriyaki Chicken	12 oz	360	55
Budget Gourmet Three Cheese Lasagne	10 oz	400	65
Budget Gourmet Turkey A La King w/ Rice	10 oz	390	75
Budget Gourmet Veal Parmigiana	12 oz	440	165

FOOD	PORTION	CALORIES	CHOLESTEROL
Budget Gourmet Yankee Pot Roast	11 oz	380	70
Lean Cuisine Baked Rigatoni w/ Meat Sauce & Cheese	9¾ oz	260	35
Lean Cuisine Beef & Pork Cannelloni w/ Mornay Sauce	9⅝ oz	270	45
Lean Cuisine Cheese Cannelloni w/ Tomato Sauce	9⅛ oz	270	30
Lean Cuisine Chicken & Vegetables w/ Vermicelli	12¾ oz	270	45
Lean Cuisine Chicken a l'Orange w/ Almond Rice	8 oz	270	50
Lean Cuisine Filet of Fish Divan	12⅜ oz	270	90
Lean Cuisine Filet of Fish Florentine	9 oz	240	100
Lean Cuisine Filet of Fish Jardiniere w/ Souffleed Potatoes	11¼ oz	280	95
Lean Cuisine Glazed Chicken w/ Vegetable Rice	8½ oz	270	60
Lean Cuisine Herbed Lamb w/ Rice	10⅜ oz	270	60
Lean Cuisine Meatball Stew	10 oz	250	80
Lean Cuisine Oriental Beef w/ Vegetables & Rice	8⅝ oz	270	45
Lean Cuisine Salisbury Steak w/ Italian Style Sauce & Vegetables	9½ oz	270	95
Lean Cuisine Sliced Turkey Breast in Mushroom Sauce	8 oz	220	50

FOOD	PORTION	CALORIES	CHOLESTEROL
Lean Cuisine Spaghetti w/ Beef & Mushroom Sauce	11½ oz	280	25
Lean Cuisine Stuffed Cabbage w/ Meat in Tomato Sauce	10¾ oz	220	40
Lean Cuisine Turkey Dijon	9½ oz	280	65
Lean Cuisine Vegetable & Pasta w/ Ham	9⅜ oz	280	45
Sensible Chef Beef Pepper Steak w/ Rice Casserole	9 oz	250	54
Sensible Chef Beef Stroganoff w/ Gravy Casserole	9 oz	240	69
Sensible Chef Beef Tips w/ Vegetable & Noodles Casserole	9 oz	250	51
Sensible Chef Chicken & Dumplings	9 oz	330	59
Sensible Chef Chicken Ala King w/ Rice	9 oz	250	49
Swanson Fried Chicken	1 pkg (10.8 oz)	583	184
chicken fricassee	¾ cup	290	72

DIP

READY-TO-USE			
Acapulco (Ortega)	1 oz	8	0
Avocado Guacamole (Kraft)	2 Tbsp	50	0
Bacon & Horseradish (Kraft)	2 Tbsp	60	0

FOOD	PORTION	CALORIES	CHOLESTEROL
Bacon & Horseradish Premium (Kraft)	2 Tbsp	50	10
Blue Cheese Premium (Kraft)	2 Tbsp	45	10
Clam (Kraft)	2 Tbsp	60	10
Clam Premium (Kraft)	2 Tbsp	45	20
Creamy Cucumber Premium (Kraft)	2 Tbsp	50	10
Creamy Onion Premium (Kraft)	2 Tbsp	45	10
French Onion (Kraft)	2 Tbsp	60	0
French Onion Premium (Kraft)	2 Tbsp	45	10
Garlic (Kraft)	2 Tbsp	60	0
Green Onion (Kraft)	2 Tbsp	60	0
Jalapeno Pepper (Kraft)	2 Tbsp	50	0
Jalapeno Pepper Premium (Kraft)	2 Tbsp	60	15
Nacho Cheese Premium (Kraft)	2 Tbsp	50	10

DOCK

FOOD	PORTION	CALORIES	CHOLESTEROL
FRESH cooked	3½ oz	20	0
raw; chopped	½ cup	15	0

FOOD	PORTION	CALORIES	CHOLESTEROL
DOLPHINFISH			
FRESH			
raw	1 fillet (7.2 oz)	174	149
raw	3 oz	73	62
DOUGH			
Fillo Dough (Athens)	1 oz	74	0
DOUGHNUT (see also DUNKIN' DONUTS)			
Cake (Hostess)	1	115	7
Chocolate Covered (Hostess)	1	129	4
Cinnamon (Hostess)	1	109	6
Cinnamon Apple (Earth Grains)	1	310	25
Devil's Food (Earth Grains)	1	330	20
Donut Sticks (Little Debbie)	1 pkg (1.67 oz)	230	tr
Donut Sticks (Little Debbie)	1 pkg (2.5 oz)	330	tr
Glazed Old Fashioned (Earth Grains)	1	310	20
Krunch (Hostess)	1	101	4
Old Fashioned (Hostess)	1	172	10

FOOD	PORTION	CALORIES	CHOLESTEROL
Powdered Old Fashioned (Earth Grains)	1	290	20
Powdered Sugar (Hostess)	1	112	7
cake type, plain	1 (1.5 oz)	164	19
cake type, sugared	1 (1.6 oz)	184	20
jelly filled	1 (2.3 oz)	226	21
raised, plain	1 (1.5 oz)	174	17

DRESSING
(*see* STUFFING/DRESSING)

DRINK MIXER
(*see also* SODA)

FOOD	PORTION	CALORIES	CHOLESTEROL
Bitter Lemon (Schweppes)	6 oz	78	0
Collins Mixer (Schweppes)	6 oz	70	0
Lemon Sour (Schweppes)	6 oz	75	0
Tonic Water (Schweppes)	6 oz	64	0
Tonic Water Diet (Schweppes)	6 oz	tr	0
whiskey sour mix	2 oz	55	0

DRUM

FRESH

FOOD	PORTION	CALORIES	CHOLESTEROL
freshwater, raw	3 oz	101	54
freshwater, raw	1 fillet (6.9 oz)	236	127

FOOD	PORTION	CALORIES	CHOLESTEROL

DUCK

FRESH

flesh & skin, raw	½ duck (1.4 lbs)	2561	481
flesh & skin, raw	10 oz	1159	218
flesh & skin; roasted	6 oz	583	145
flesh & skin; roasted	½ duck (13.4 oz)	1287	320
flesh, raw	½ duck (10.6 oz)	399	233
flesh, raw	4.8 oz	180	105
flesh; roasted	3.5 oz	201	89
flesh; roasted	½ duck (7.8 oz)	445	198
wild, flesh & skin, raw	8.4 oz	505	191
wild, flesh & skin, raw	9.5 oz	571	216

DUMPLING

HOME RECIPE

apple	1 (10.5 oz)	566	19
dumpling	2 (1 oz)	70	33
pear	1 (10.2 oz)	540	41

EEL

FRESH

cooked	3 oz	200	137
cooked	1 fillet (5.6 oz)	375	257

FOOD	PORTION	CALORIES	CHOLESTEROL
raw	1 fillet (7.2 oz)	375	257
raw	3 oz	156	107
SMOKED American smoked eel	1¾ oz	165	35

EGG
(see also EGG SUBSTITUTE)

CHICKEN			
fried w/ butter	1	83	246
hard cooked	1	79	274
poached	1	79	273
raw	1	79	274
scrambled w/ butter & milk	1	95	248
white only	1	16	0
white only	1 cup	118	0
yolk only	1	63	272
yolks	1 cup	897	3894
DISHES			
Cheese Omelet Sandwich (Microwave Chefwich)	1 (5 oz)	410	130
Ham & Cheese Omelet Sandwich (Microwave Chefwich)	1 (5 oz)	380	150
Sausage & Cheese Omelet Sandwich (Microwave Chefwich)	1 (5 oz)	410	120
Western Style Omelet Sandwich (Microwave Chefwich)	1 (5 oz)	360	84

FOOD	PORTION	CALORIES	CHOLESTEROL
HOME RECIPE			
creamed	½ cup	231	310
deviled	2 halves	145	280
egg foo young	1 (5.1 oz)	150	250
omelet; as prep from 2 eggs, butter, milk	4.5 oz	189	497
salad	½ cup	307	562
OTHER POULTRY			
duck, raw	1	130	619
quail, raw	1	14	76
turkey, raw	1	135	737

EGG SUBSTITUTE

FOOD	PORTION	CALORIES	CHOLESTEROL
Egg Beaters (Fleischmann's)	¼ cup	25	0
Egg Beaters w/ Cheez (Fleischmann's)	¼ cup	130	5
Egg Watchers (Tofutti)	2 oz	50	0
Eggstra (Tillie Lewis)	2 oz	433	58
Scramblers, frzn (Morningstar Farms)	3.5 oz	105	3
frozen	¼ cup	96	1
liquid	1½ oz	40	tr
liquid	1 cup	211	3
powder	0.35 oz	44	57
powder	0.7 oz	88	114

FOOD	PORTION	CALORIES	CHOLESTEROL

EGGNOG

FOOD	PORTION	CALORIES	CHOLESTEROL
Eggnog (Land O'Lakes)	8 oz	300	123
eggnog	1 cup	342	149
eggnog	1 qt	1368	596
eggnog flavor mix; as prep w/ milk	9 oz	260	33

EGGPLANT

FOOD	PORTION	CALORIES	CHOLESTEROL
FRESH			
cubed, cooked	½ cup	13	0
raw; cut up	½ cup	11	0
HOME RECIPE			
Baba Ghannouj	¼ cup	55	0

ELDERBERRIES

FOOD	PORTION	CALORIES	CHOLESTEROL
FRESH			
raw	1 cup	105	0

ENDIVE

FOOD	PORTION	CALORIES	CHOLESTEROL
FRESH			
raw; chopped	½ cup	4	0

ENGLISH MUFFIN

FOOD	PORTION	CALORIES	CHOLESTEROL
Best Foods Regular, Placentia	1	130	0
Roman Meal	1	146	0
Shop 'n Save	1	130	0
Thomas' Sourdough	1	130	0
Thomas' Honey Wheat	1	129	0

FOOD	PORTION	CALORIES	CHOLESTEROL
Thomas' Raisin	1	153	0
Thomas' Regular	1	130	0
HOME RECIPE			
cinnamon raisin	1	186	0
honey bran	1	153	0
plain	1	158	0
whole wheat	1	167	1

FALAFEL

FOOD	PORTION	CALORIES	CHOLESTEROL
HOME RECIPE			
falafel	1 pattie (.5 oz)	57	0
falafel	3 patties (1.8 oz)	170	0

FAST FOODS
(*see individual names*)

FAT
(*see also* BUTTER, BUTTER BLENDS, BUTTER SUBSTITUTE, MARGARINE, OIL)

FOOD	PORTION	CALORIES	CHOLESTEROL
Crisco	1 Tbsp	110	0
Crisco Butter Flavor	1 Tbsp	110	0
beef fat; cooked	1 oz	193	27
beef suet, raw	1 oz	242	19
chicken fat, raw	1 oz	201	19
chicken fat, raw	from ½ chicken (1.8 oz)	327	30

FOOD	PORTION	CALORIES	CHOLESTEROL
duck fat	1 Tbsp	115	13
goose fat	1 Tbsp	115	13
lard	1 cup	1849	195
lard	1 stick	831	57
lard	1 Tbsp	115	12
lard	1 tsp	35	2
mutton tallow, raw	1 Tbsp	116	13
pork backfat	1 oz	230	16
pork fat	1 oz	200	26
pork fat, cured; roasted	1 oz	167	24
pork fat, cured; uncooked	1 oz	164	19
shortening, soybean & cottonseed	1 Tbsp	113	0
shortening, soybean & cottonseed	1 cup	1812	0
shortening, soybean & palm	1 cup	1812	0
shortening, soybean & palm	1 Tbsp	113	0
tallow (beef)	1 Tbsp	115	14
tallow (beef)	1 cup	1849	223
turkey fat	1 Tbsp	115	13

FIGS

CANNED

Kadota Figs Whole Fancy (S&W)	½ cup	100	0

DRIED

cooked	½ cup	140	0
whole	10	477	0

FOOD	PORTION	CALORIES	CHOLESTEROL
FRESH			
fig	1 med	50	0

FILBERTS

dried, blanched	1 oz	191	0
dried, unblanched	1 oz	179	0
dry roasted, unblanched	1 oz	188	0
oil roasted, unblanched	1 oz	187	0

FISH
(see also individual names, FISH SUBSTITUTE)

FROZEN			
breaded fillet; as prep	1 (2 oz)	155	64
sticks; as prep	1 stick (1 oz)	76	31
HOME RECIPE			
fish loaf; cooked	3½ oz	124	99

FISH SUBSTITUTE

Fillets, frzn (Worthington)	3.5 oz	209	tr
Ocean Fillet (Loma Linda)	1 (1.7 oz)	130	0
Ocean Fillet (Loma Linda)	1 (2 oz)	160	0
Ocean Platter; mix not prep (Loma Linda)	¼ cup	50	0
Vege-Scallops (Loma Linda)	6 pieces (2.75 oz)	70	0

FOOD	PORTION	CALORIES	CHOLESTEROL

FLATFISH

FRESH

FOOD	PORTION	CALORIES	CHOLESTEROL
cooked	1 fillet (4.5 oz)	148	86
cooked	3 oz	99	58
raw	3 oz	78	41
raw	1 fillet (5.7 oz)	149	78

FLOUNDER

FROZEN

FOOD	PORTION	CALORIES	CHOLESTEROL
Flounder Primavera (King & Prince)	9 oz	270	90
Flounder Primavera (King & Prince)	6 oz	180	60
Flounder Primavera (King & Prince)	4.5 oz	135	45
Flounder Del Rey (King & Prince)	9 oz	327	105

FLOUR

FOOD	PORTION	CALORIES	CHOLESTEROL
All-Purpose (Gold Medal)	1 cup	400	0
All-Purpose (Red Band)	1 cup	390	0
All-Purpose (White Deer)	1 cup	400	0
Drifted Snow (General Mills)	1 cup	400	0
High Protein Better for Bread (Gold Medal)	1 cup	400	0

FOOD	PORTION	CALORIES	CHOLESTEROL
La Pina (Gold Medal)	1 cup	390	0
Self-Rising (Gold Medal)	1 cup	380	0
Self-Rising (Red Band)	1 cup	380	0
Softasilk (General Mills)	¼ cup	100	0
Unbleached (Gold Medal)	1 cup	400	0
White, Self-Rising (Aunt Jemima)	1 cup	479	0
Whole Wheat (Gold Medal)	1 cup	390	0
Whole Wheat (Red Band)	1 cup	400	0
Whole Wheat Blend (Gold Medal)	1 cup	370	0
Wondra	1 cup	400	0
cottonseed, lowfat	1 oz	94	0
cottonseed, partially defatted	1 Tbsp	18	0
cottonseed, partially defatted	1 cup	337	0
peanut, defatted	1 Tbsp	13	0
peanut, defatted	1 cup	196	0
peanut, defatted	1 oz	92	0
peanut, lowfat	1 oz	120	0
peanut, lowfat	1 cup	257	0
potato	½ cup	316	0
rice	1 cup	479	0
sesame, lowfat	1 oz	95	0

FOOD	PORTION	CALORIES	CHOLESTEROL

FRANKFURTER
(*see* HOT DOG)

FRENCH BEANS

DRIED
cooked	1 cup	228	0
raw	1 cup	631	0

FRENCH FRIES
(*see* POTATOES)

FRENCH TOAST

French toast	1 slice	155	112

FROG LEG

frog leg; as prep w/ seasoned flour & fried (home recipe)	1 (.8 oz)	70	12
frog legs, raw	4 lg (3.5 oz)	73	50

FROSTING
(*see* CAKE)

FRUCTOSE
(*see also* SUGAR, SUGAR SUBSTITUTE)

Fructose (Estee)	1 tsp	12	0

FOOD	PORTION	CALORIES	CHOLESTEROL

FRUIT DRINKS

FROZEN

FOOD	PORTION	CALORIES	CHOLESTEROL
Cranberry Juice Cocktail; as prep (Seneca)	6 oz	110	0
Cranberry-Apple Juice Cocktail; as prep (Seneca)	6 oz	110	0
Grape-Cranberry Juice Cocktail; as prep (Seneca)	6 oz	110	0
Raspberry Cranberry Juice Cocktail; as prep (Seneca)	6 oz	110	0
White Grape Juice; as prep (Seneca)	6 oz	110	0
cranberry juice cocktail; as prep	6 oz glass	102	0
fruit punch; as prep w/ water	1 cup	113	0
lemonade; as prep w/ water	1 cup	100	0
limeade; as prep w/ water	1 cup	102	0

MIX

FOOD	PORTION	CALORIES	CHOLESTEROL
Berry Blend; as prep (Crystal Light)	8 oz	3	0
Black Cherry; as prep (Kool-Aid)	8 oz	98	0
Cherry Sugar Free; as prep (Kool-Aid)	8 oz	3	0
Citrus Blend; as prep (Crystal Light)	8 oz	3	0

FOOD	PORTION	CALORIES	CHOLESTEROL
Grape; as prep (Crystal Light)	8 oz	3	0
Grape; as prep (Kool-Aid)	8 oz	98	0
Lemon-Lime Sugar; as prep (Country Time)	8 oz	5	0
Lemon-Lime Sweetened; as prep (Country Time)	8 oz	82	0
Lemon-Lime; as prep (Crystal Light)	8 oz	4	0
Lemonade Sugar Free; as prep (Kool-Aid)	8 oz	4	0
Lemonade Sugar Free; as prep (Country Time)	8 oz	5	0
Lemonade Sugar Sweetened; as prep (Kool-Aid)	8 oz	78	0
Lemonade Sweetened; as prep (Country Time)	8 oz	82	0
Lemonade Flavor Crystals; as prep (Wyler's)	8 oz	92	0
Lemonade; as prep (Crystal Light)	8 oz	5	0
Lemonade; as prep (Kool-Aid)	8 oz	99	0
Mountain Berry Punch Sugar Sweetened; as prep (Kool-Aid)	8 oz	78	0

FOOD	PORTION	CALORIES	CHOLESTEROL
Orange; as prep (Crystal Light)	8 oz	4	0
Orange; as prep (Kool-Aid)	8 oz	98	0
Rainbow Punch; as prep (Kool-Aid)	8 oz	98	0
Raspberry Sugar Sweetened; as prep (Kool-Aid)	8 oz	79	0
Sunshine Punch; as prep (Kool-Aid)	8 oz	99	0
Tang Orange Sugar Free; as prep (General Foods)	8 oz	5	0
Tang Orange; as prep (General Foods)	8 oz	87	0
Tropical Punch Sugar Free; as prep (Kool-Aid)	8 oz	3	0
Tropical Punch Sugar Sweetened; as prep (Kool-Aid)	8 oz	84	0
Wild Strawberry Artifical Flavor Crystals; as prep (Wyler's)	8 oz	80	0
Wild Strawberry Artifical Flavor Crystals; as prep (Wyler's)	8 oz	80	0
fruit punch; as prep w/ water	9 oz	97	0
lemonade powder; as prep w/ water	9 oz	113	0

FOOD	PORTION	CALORIES	CHOLESTEROL
READY-TO-USE			
Any Flavor (Land O'Lakes)	8 oz	120	0
Apple (SIPPS)	8.45 oz	130	0
Apple Cranberry (Mott's)	10 oz	176	0
Apple Cranberry (Mott's)	9.5 oz	167	0
Apple Raspberry (Mott's)	9.5 oz	150	0
Apple Raspberry (Mott's)	10 oz	158	0
Black Cherry Cooler (Health Valley)	13 oz	144	0
Cran-Blueberry (Ocean Spray)	6 oz	120	0
Cran-Grape (Ocean Spray)	6 oz	130	0
Cran-Orange (Ocean Spray)	6 oz	100	0
Cran-Raspberry (Ocean Spray)	6 oz	110	0
Cran-Raspberry Low Calorie (Ocean Spray)	6 oz	40	0
Cran-Tastic (Ocean Spray)	6 oz	110	0
Cranapple (Ocean Spray)	6 oz	130	0
Cranapple Low Calorie (Ocean Spray)	6 oz	40	0

FOOD	PORTION	CALORIES	CHOLESTEROL
Cranberry Apple Cooler (Health Valley)	13 oz	144	0
Cranberry Juice Cocktail (Ocean Spray)	6 oz	110	0
Cranberry Juice Cocktail (Seneca)	6 oz	110	0
Cranberry Juice Cocktail Low Calorie (Ocean Spray)	6 oz	40	0
Cranberry-Apple Juice Cocktail (Seneca)	6 oz	110	0
Cranicot (Ocean Spray)	6 oz	110	0
Fruit Punch (Mott's)	9.5 oz	150	0
Fruit Punch (Mott's)	10 oz	170	0
Fruit Punch (SIPPS)	8.45 oz	130	0
Grape (SIPPS)	8.45 oz	130	0
Grape Apple (Mott's)	10 oz	167	0
Grape Apple (Mott's)	9.5 oz	158	0
Lemon-Lime Cooler (SIPPS)	8.45 oz	130	0
Lemonade (SIPPS)	8.45 oz	85	0
Lemonade (Shasta)	12 oz	146	0

FOOD	PORTION	CALORIES	CHOLESTEROL
Mauna La'i Hawaiian Guava Fruit Drink (Ocean Spray)	6 oz	100	0
Mauna La'i Hawaiian Guava Passion Fruit Drink (Ocean Spray)	6 oz	100	0
Mixed Berry (SIPPS)	8.45 oz	130	0
Orange (SIPPS)	8.45 oz	130	0
Orange Fruit Juice Blend (Mott's)	10 oz	144	0
Pineapple Grapefruit Juice Cocktail (Ocean Spray)	6 oz	110	0
Pink Grapefruit Juice Cocktail (Ocean Spray)	6 oz	80	0
Raspberry Cranberry Juice Cocktail (Seneca)	6 oz	110	0
Sunny Delight Florida Citrus Punch (Sundor)	6 oz	90	0
Sunshine Punch (SIPPS)	8.45 oz	130	0
Wild Cherry (SIPPS)	8.45 oz	130	0
Wild Cherry Cooler (Health Valley)	13 oz	144	0
cranberry apricot	6 oz	118	0
cranberry apple	6 oz	123	0
cranberry grape	6 oz	103	0

FOOD	PORTION	CALORIES	CHOLESTEROL
cranberry juice cocktail	1 cup	147	0
cranberry juice cocktail	6 oz	108	0
fruit punch	6 oz	87	0
grape	6 oz	94	0
orange	6 oz	94	0
orange & apricot	1 cup	128	0
pineapple & grapefruit	1 cup	117	0
pineapple & orange	1 cup	125	0

FRUIT, MIXED
(*see also individual names*)

FOOD	PORTION	CALORIES	CHOLESTEROL
CANNED			
Fruit Cocktail in Heavy Syrup (S&W)	½ cup	90	0
Fruit Cocktail Natural Lite (S&W)	½ cup	60	0
Fruit Cocktail Natural Style (S&W)	½ cup	90	0
Fruit Salad, chilled (Kraft)	½ cup	50	0
Mixed Fruit Chunky Natural Style (S&W)	½ cup	90	0
fruit cocktail, in heavy syrup	½ cup	93	0
fruit cocktail, in juice	½ cup	56	0
fruit cocktail, in water	½ cup	40	0
fruit salad, in heavy syrup	½ cup	94	0
fruit salad, in juice	½ cup	62	0

FOOD	PORTION	CALORIES	CHOLESTEROL
fruit salad, tropical, in heavy syrup	½ cup	110	0
DRIED			
Fruit 'n Nut Mix (Planters)	1 oz	150	0
mixed	11 oz pkg	712	0
FROZEN			
Mixed Fruit in Syrup (Birds Eye)	½ cup	123	0
JUICE			
Apple Citrus (Tree Top)	6 oz	90	0
Apple Citrus, frzn; as prep (Tree Top)	6 oz	90	0
Apple Cranberry (Mott's)	6 oz	83	0
Apple Cranberry (Mott's)	9.5 oz	147	0
Apple Cranberry (Mott's)	8.45 oz	136	0
Apple Cranberry (Tree Top)	6 oz	100	0
Apple Cranberry, frzn; as prep (Tree Top)	6 oz	100	0
Apple Grape (Mott's)	6 oz	86	0
Apple Grape (Mott's)	8.45 oz	128	0
Apple Grape (Mott's)	9.5 oz	139	0

FOOD	PORTION	CALORIES	CHOLESTEROL
Apple Grape (Tree Top)	6 oz	100	0
Apple Grape, frzn; as prep (Tree Top)	6 oz	100	0
Apple Pear (Tree Top)	6 oz	90	0
Apple Pear, frzn; as prep (Tree Top)	6 oz	90	0
Apple Raspberry (Mott's)	6 oz	83	0
Apple Raspberry (Mott's)	8.45 oz	124	0
Apple Raspberry (Tree Top)	6 oz	80	0
Apple Raspberry, frzn; as prep (Tree Top)	6 oz	80	0
Apricot Pineapple Nectar (S&W)	6 oz	120	0
Orange Banana (Chiquita)	6 oz	90	0
Orange Banana (Smucker's)	8 oz	120	0
Orange Fruit Juice Blend (Mott's)	9.5 oz	139	0
Orange-Grapefruit Juice 100% Pure Unsweetened (Kraft)	6 oz	80	0
Orange-Pineapple Juice 100% Pure Unsweetened (Kraft)	6 oz	80	0
Pineapple-Grapefruit (Dole)	6 oz	90	0

FOOD	PORTION	CALORIES	CHOLESTEROL
Pineapple-Orange (Dole)	6 oz	100	0
Pineapple-Orange Banana (Dole)	6 oz	90	0
Pineapple–Pink Grapefruit (Dole)	6 oz	101	0
orange-grapefruit	1 cup	107	0

FRUIT SNACKS

FOOD	PORTION	CALORIES	CHOLESTEROL
Flavor Tree Cherry Fruit People	1 oz	111	0
Flavor Tree Fruit Bears	1.05 oz	117	0
Flavor Tree Fruit Circus	1.05 oz	117	0
Flavor Tree Fruit Nibbles	½ pkg	118	0
Flavor Tree Fruit People	1 oz	111	0
Flavor Tree Lemon Fruit People	1 oz	111	0
Flavor Tree Orange Fruit People	1 oz	111	0
Flavor Tree Strawberry Fruit Roll	1 roll	67	0
Flavor Tree Strawberry Fruit People	1 oz	111	0
Sunkist Fun Fruit Alphabets	.9 oz	100	0
Sunkist Fun Fruit Animals	.9 oz	100	0
Sunkist Fun Fruit Berry Bunch	.9 oz	100	0
Sunkist Fun Fruit Cherry	.9 oz	100	0
Sunkist Fun Fruit Dinosaurs Strawberry	.9 oz	100	0

FOOD	PORTION	CALORIES	CHOLESTEROL
Sunkist Fun Fruit Fantastic Fruit Punch	.9 oz	100	0
Sunkist Fun Fruit Grape	.9 oz	100	0
Sunkist Fun Fruit Numbers	.9 oz	100	0
Sunkist Fun Fruit Raspberry	.9 oz	100	0
Sunkist Fun Fruit Strawberry	.9 oz	100	0
Sunkist Fun Fruit Tropical Fruit	.9 oz	100	0

GARBANZO
(see CHICKPEAS)

GARLIC

powder	1 tsp	9	0
raw	1 clove	4	0

GEFILTEFISH

READY-TO-USE

sweet recipe	1 piece (1.5 oz)	35	12

GELATIN

DRINKS

Orange Flavored Drinking Gelatin w/ NutraSweet (Knox)	1 envelope	39	0

FOOD	PORTION	CALORIES	CHOLESTEROL
MIX			
Apricot; as prep (Jell-O)	½ cup	80	0
Black Cherry; as prep (Jell-O)	½ cup	81	0
Black Raspberry; as prep (Jell-O)	½ cup	81	0
Blackberry; as prep (Jell-O)	½ cup	81	0
Cherry Sugar Free (Diamond Crystal)	½ cup	8	0
Cherry Sugar Free; as prep (Jell-O)	1 pop	9	0
Cherry w/ NutraSweet; as prep (D-Zerta)	½ cup	8	0
Cherry; as prep (Jell-O)	½ cup	81	0
Concord Grape; as prep (Jell-O)	½ cup	81	0
Gelatin Desserts; as prep (Estee)	½ cup	8	0
Hawaiian Pineapple Sugar Free; as prep (Jell-O)	1 pop	8	0
Lemon Sugar Free; as prep (Jell-O)	1 pop	8	0
Lemon Sugar Free (Diamond Crystal)	½ cup	8	0
Lemon w/ NutraSweet; as prep (D-Zerta)	½ cup	8	0

FOOD	PORTION	CALORIES	CHOLESTEROL
Lemon; as prep (Jell-O)	½ cup	81	0
Lime Sugar Free; as prep (Jell-O)	1 pop	8	0
Lime Sugar Free (Diamond Crystal)	½ cup	8	0
Lime w/ NutraSweet; as prep (D-Zerta)	½ cup	9	0
Lime; as prep (Jell-O)	½ cup	81	0
Mixed Fruit Sugar Free; as prep (Jell-O)	1 pop	8	0
Mixed Fruit; as prep (Jell-O)	½ cup	81	0
Orange Pineapple; as prep (Jell-O)	½ cup	81	0
Orange Sugar Free; as prep (Jell-O)	1 pop	8	0
Orange Sugar Free (Diamond Crystal)	½ cup	8	0
Orange w/ NutraSweet; as prep (D-Zerta)	½ cup	8	0
Orange; as prep (Jell-O)	½ cup	81	0
Peach Sugar Free; as prep (Jell-O)	1 pop	8	0
Peach; as prep (Jell-O)	½ cup	81	0

FOOD	PORTION	CALORIES	CHOLESTEROL
Raspberry Sugar Free; as prep (Jell-O)	1 pop	8	0
Raspberry Sugar Free (Diamond Crystal)	½ cup	8	0
Raspberry w/ NutraSweet; as prep (D-Zerta)	½ cup	8	0
Raspberry; as prep (Jell-O)	½ cup	81	0
Strawberry Banana Sugar Free; as prep (Jell-O)	1 pop	8	0
Strawberry Banana; as prep (Jell-O)	½ cup	81	0
Strawberry Sugar Free; as prep (Jell-O)	1 pop	8	0
Strawberry Sugar Free (Diamond Crystal)	½ cup	8	0
Strawberry w/ NutraSweet; as prep (D-Zerta)	½ cup	8	0
Strawberry; as prep (Jell-O)	½ cup	81	0
Triple Berry Sugar Free; as prep (Jell-O)	1 pop	8	0
Wild Strawberry; as prep (Jell-O)	½ cup	81	0
dry, unsweetened	1 Tbsp	23	0

FOOD	PORTION	CALORIES	CHOLESTEROL
GIBLETS			
capon, raw	4 oz	150	335
capon; simmered	1 cup	238	629
chicken; simmered	1 cup	228	570
chicken; flour coated, fried	1 cup	402	647
chicken, raw	2.6 oz	93	196
duck; simmered	1 cup	238	629
turkey, raw	8.6 oz	314	688
turkey; simmered	1 cup	243	606
GINKGO NUTS			
canned	1 oz	32	0
dried	1 oz	99	0
GIZZARD			
chicken, raw	1.3 oz	41	48
chicken; simmered	1 cup	222	281
turkey, raw	4 oz	133	178
turkey; simmered	1 cup	236	336
GOOSE			
FRESH			
flesh & skin, raw	½ goose (2.9 lb)	4893	1055
flesh & skin, raw	11.2 oz	1187	256
flesh & skin; roasted	6.6 oz	574	172
flesh & skin; roasted	½ goose (1.7 lbs)	2362	708

FOOD	PORTION	CALORIES	CHOLESTEROL
flesh, raw	½ goose (2.3 lbs)	1237	640
flesh, raw	6.5 oz	299	155
flesh; roasted	5 oz	340	138
flesh; roasted	½ goose (1.3 lbs)	1406	569

GOOSEBERRIES

canned, in light syrup	½ cup	93	0
raw	1 cup	67	0

GRANOLA
(*see also* CEREAL)

BARS			
Kudos Chocolate Chip	1.2 oz	180	8
Kudos Nutty Fudge	1.3 oz	190	7
Kudos Peanut Butter	1.3 oz	190	6
New Trail, Chocolate Covered Cocoa Creme	1	200	5
New Trail, Chocolate Covered Peanut Butter	1	200	5
Sunbelt Chewy Granola Chocolate Chip	1 bar (1.25 oz)	150	tr
Sunbelt Chewy Granola Oats & Honey	1 bar (1 oz)	130	tr
Sunbelt Chewy Granola w/ Almonds	1 bar (1 oz)	120	tr
Sunbelt Chewy Granola w/ Chocolate Chip	1 bar (1.75 oz)	220	tr
Sunbelt Chewy Granola w/ Raisins	1 bar (1.25 oz)	150	tr

FOOD	PORTION	CALORIES	CHOLESTEROL
Sunbelt Fudge Dipped Chewy Granola Chocolate Chip	1 bar (1.63 oz)	220	tr
Sunbelt Fudge Dipped Chewy Granola Oats & Honey	1 bar (1.38 oz)	190	tr
Sunbelt Fudge Dipped Chewy Granola w/ Peanuts	1 bar (1.5 oz)	200	tr
Sunbelt Fudge Dipped Chewy Granola w/ Peanuts	1 bar (2.25 oz)	300	tr
Sunbelt Granola Cereal Fruit & Nut	1 bar (1 oz)	120	tr
CEREAL			
Cinnamon & Raisin (Nature Valley)	⅓ cup	120	0
Cinnamon & Raisin w/ skim milk (Nature Valley)	⅓ cup + ½ cup milk	160	3
Coconut & Honey (Nature Valley)	⅓ cup	150	0
Coconut & Honey w/ skim milk (Nature Valley)	⅓ cup + ½ cup milk	190	3
Erewhon Date Nut	1 oz	130	0
Erewhon Honey Almond	1 oz	130	0
Erewhon Maple	1 oz	130	0
Erewhon Spiced Apple	1 oz	130	0
Erewhon Sunflower Crunch	1 oz	130	0
Erewhon w/ Bran	1 oz	130	0
Health Valley Real Granola	1 oz	120	0
Nature Valley Fruit & Nut	⅓ cup	170	3

FOOD	PORTION	CALORIES	CHOLESTEROL
Nature Valley Fruit & Nut w/ skim milk	⅓ cup + ½ cup milk	170	3
Nature Valley Toasted Oat Mixture	⅓ cup	130	0
Nature Valley Toasted Oat Mixture w/ skim milk	⅓ cup + ½ cup milk	170	3
Post Hearty Granola	¼ cup	127	0
Post Hearty Granola w/ Raisins	¼ cup	123	0
Post Hearty Granola w/ whole milk	¼ cup + ½ cup milk	203	17

GRAPEFRUIT

Grapefruit (Tree Top)	6 oz	120	0
Sections Chilled Unsweetened (Kraft)	½ cup	50	0
Sections Natural Style (S&W)	½ cup	40	0
Sections in Light Syrup (S&W)	½ cup	80	0
in juice	½ cup	46	0
in light syrup	½ cup	76	0
in water	½ cup	44	0
FRESH Pink (Ocean Spray)	½ med	50	0
Ruby Red (Chiquita)	½ fruit	40	0

FOOD	PORTION	CALORIES	CHOLESTEROL
White (Ocean Spray)	½ med	45	0
grapefruit	½ fruit	38	0
JUICE			
Grapefruit (Mott's)	9.5 oz	118	0
Grapefruit (Mott's)	10 oz	124	0
Grapefruit Juice (Ocean Spray)	6 oz	70	0
Grapefruit Juice 100% Pure Unsweetened (Kraft)	6 oz	70	0
Pink Premium Grapefruit Juice (Ocean Spray)	6 oz	60	0
Unsweetened (S&W)	6 oz	80	0
fresh	1 cup	96	0
frzn, unsweetened	1 cup	93	0
frzn; as prep	1 cup	102	0
frzn; not prep	6 oz container	302	0

GRAPES

FOOD	PORTION	CALORIES	CHOLESTEROL
CANNED			
Thompson Seedless Premium (S&W)	½ cup	100	0
grapes, in heavy syrup	½ cup	94	0
FRESH			
grapes	10	36	0

FOOD	PORTION	CALORIES	CHOLESTEROL
JUICE			
Concord Unsweetened (S&W)	6 oz	100	0
Grape (Seneca)	6 oz	115	0
Grape, frzn; as prep (Seneca)	6 oz	100	0
Natural Grape, frzn; as prep (Seneca)	6 oz	115	0
frzn, sweetened; as prep	1 cup	128	0
frzn, sweetened; not prep	6 oz container	386	0
grape	1 cup	155	0

GRAVY
(*see also* SAUCE)

CANNED			
au jus	1 cup	38	1
au jus	1 can (10.5 oz)	48	1
beef	1 can (10.2 oz)	155	9
beef	1 cup	124	7
chicken	1 cup	189	5
chicken	1 can (10.5 oz)	236	6
mushroom	1 can (10.5 oz)	150	0
mushroom	1 cup	120	0
turkey	1 cup	122	5

FOOD	PORTION	CALORIES	CHOLESTEROL
turkey	1 can (10.5 oz)	152	6
DRY			
Brown Gravy Mix; as prep (Estee)	¼ cup	14	0
Chicken (Diamond Crystal)	2 oz	30	2
Chicken and Herb Gravy Mix; as prep (Estee)	¼ cup	20	tr
au jus; as prep w/ water	1 cup	19	1
au jus; not prep	1 pkg (.8 oz)	79	4
brown; as prep w/ water	1 cup	9	tr
brown; not prep	1 pkg (.9 oz)	85	2
chicken; as prep w/ water	1 cup	83	3
chicken; not prep	1 pkg (.8 oz)	83	2
mushroom; as prep w/ water	1 cup	70	1
mushroom; not prep	1 pkg (.7 oz)	70	1
onion; as prep w/ water	1 cup	80	1
onion; not prep	1 pkg (.8 oz)	77	tr
pork; as prep w/ water	1 cup	76	3
pork; not prep	1 pkg (.7 oz)	76	2
turkey; as prep w/ water	1 cup	87	3
turkey; not prep	1 pkg (.9 oz)	87	2

FOOD	PORTION	CALORIES	CHOLESTEROL

GREAT NORTHERN BEANS

CANNED

FOOD	PORTION	CALORIES	CHOLESTEROL
Great Northern Beans (Hanover)	½ cup	110	0
great northern	1 cup	300	0
DRIED			
Great Northern (Hurst Brand)	1 cup	277	0
cooked	1 cup	210	0
raw	1 cup	621	0

GREEN BEANS

FOOD	PORTION	CALORIES	CHOLESTEROL
CANNED			
Cut Green Beans (Owatonna)	½ cup	20	0
Cut Premium Blue Lake (S&W)	½ cup	20	0
Cuts (Libby)	½ cup	20	0
Cuts (Seneca)	½ cup	20	0
Cuts Natural Pack (Libby)	½ cup	20	0
Cuts Natural Pack (Seneca)	½ cup	20	0
Dilled (S&W)	½ cup	60	0
French (Libby)	½ cup	20	0

FOOD	PORTION	CALORIES	CHOLESTEROL
French (Seneca)	½ cup	20	0
French Natural Pack (Libby)	½ cup	20	0
French Natural Pack (Seneca)	½ cup	20	0
French Style (Owatonna)	½ cup	20	0
French Style Premium Blue Lake (S&W)	½ cup	20	0
Whole (Libby)	½ cup	20	0
Whole (Seneca)	½ cup	20	0
Whole Fancy Stringless (S&W)	½ cup	20	0
Whole Vertical Pack (S&W)	½ cup	20	0
FROZEN			
Bavarian Style Beans & Spaetzle (Birds Eye)	½ cup	98	14
Cut Beans (Southland)	3 oz	25	0
Cut Green Beans (Hanover)	½ cup	20	0
French (Southland)	3 oz	25	0
French Green Beans w/ Toasted Almonds (Birds Eye)	½ cup	52	0

FOOD	PORTION	CALORIES	CHOLESTEROL
French Style Blue Lake (Hanover)	½ cup	25	0
French; cooked (Health Valley)	4.7 oz	36	0
Green Beans Cut (Birds Eye)	½ cup	25	0
Green Beans French (Birds Eye)	½ cup	26	0
Green Beans Italian (Birds Eye)	½ cup	31	0
Green Beans Whole (Birds Eye)	½ cup	30	0
Italian Cut (Hanover)	½ cup	35	0
Whole (Birds Eye)	½ cup	23	0
Whole Blue Lake (Hanover)	½ cup	30	0

GROUNDCHERRIES

fresh	½ cup	37	0

GROUPER

FRESH

cooked	1 fillet (7.1 oz)	238	95
cooked	3 oz	100	40
raw	3 oz	78	31
raw	1 fillet (9.1 oz)	238	95

FOOD	PORTION	CALORIES	CHOLESTEROL

GUAVA

FRESH
guava | 1 | 45 | 0

HOME RECIPE
guava sauce | ½ cup | 43 | 0

GUINEA HEN

meat, w/o skin, raw	½ bird (9.3 oz)	290	166

HADDOCK

FRESH

cooked	1 fillet (5.3 oz)	168	110
cooked	3 oz	95	63
raw	3 oz	74	49
raw	1 fillet (6.8 oz)	168	111
roe, raw	3½ oz	130	360

SMOKED

smoked	3 oz	99	65
smoked	1 oz	33	21

HALIBUT

FRESH

Atlantic & Pacific, raw	½ fillet (7.2 oz)	223	65
Atlantic & Pacific, raw	3 oz	93	27
Atlantic & Pacific; cooked	3 oz	119	35

FOOD	PORTION	CALORIES	CHOLESTEROL
Atlantic & Pacific; cooked	½ fillet (5.6 oz)	223	65
Greenland, raw	½ fillet (7.2 oz)	380	94
Greenland, raw	3 oz	158	39

HAM
(*see also* HAM DISHES, LUNCHEON MEATS/COLD CUTS, PORK, TURKEY)

FOOD	PORTION	CALORIES	CHOLESTEROL
Armour Golden Star Boneless	1 oz	33	13
Armour Golden Star Canned	1 oz	32	11
Armour Lower Salt Boneless	1 oz	34	13
Armour Lower Salt, 93% Fat Free	1 oz	35	14
Armour Star Boneless	1 oz	41	15
Armour Star Canned	1 oz	34	11
Armour Star Speedy Cut	1 oz	44	15
Armour 1877 Boneless	1 oz	42	15
Carl Buddig	1 oz	50	20
Oscar Mayer Boiled w/ Natural Juices	1 slice (21 g)	23	12
Oscar Mayer Breakfast Ham Water Added	1 slice (43 g)	52	21
Oscar Mayer Chopped w/ Natural Juices	1 slice (28 g)	55	17
Oscar Mayer Cracked Black Pepper	1 slice (21 g)	24	11
Oscar Mayer Ham & Cheese Loaf	1 slice (28 g)	76	18
Oscar Mayer Ham Salad Spread w/ Natural Juices	1 oz	59	10

FOOD	PORTION	CALORIES	CHOLESTEROL
Oscar Mayer Ham and Cheese Spread	1 oz	67	15
Oscar Mayer Honey w/ Natural Juices	1 slice (21 g)	26	11
Oscar Mayer Jubilee Boneless	1 oz	46	15
Oscar Mayer Jubilee Canned w/ Natural Juices	1 oz	31	13
Oscar Mayer Jubilee Slice w/ Water Added	1 oz	29	14
Oscar Mayer Jubilee Steak w/ Water Added	1 slice (2 oz)	59	28
Oscar Mayer Smoked Cooked	1 slice (21 g)	23	12
Oscar Mayer Baked Cooked	1 slice (21 g)	21	10
The Spreadables, Ham Salad	¼ can	100	24
canned; chopped	1 slice (21 g)	50	10
canned; chopped	1 oz	68	14
center slice, lean only, raw	4 oz	220	
chopped	1 slice (21 g)	48	11
chopped	1 oz	65	15
ham (13% fat), canned; roasted	3 oz	192	52
ham (13% fat), canned; unheated	1 oz	54	11
ham patties; uncooked	1 patty (2.3 oz)	206	46
ham salad spread	1 Tbsp	32	6

FOOD	PORTION	CALORIES	CHOLESTEROL
ham salad spread	1 oz	61	10
ham, boneless (11% fat); roasted	3 oz	151	50
ham, boneless, extra lean; roasted	3 oz	140	48
ham, boneless, extra lean; unheated	1 slice (1 oz)	46	15
ham, center slice, lean & fat; unheated	4 oz	229	61
ham, extra lean, canned; roasted	3 oz	142	34
ham, extra lean, canned; unheated	1 oz	41	11
minced	1 slice (21 g)	55	15
minced	1 oz	75	20
patties; grilled	1 patty (2 oz)	203	43
sliced, extra lean (5% fat)	1 slice (28 g)	37	13
sliced, regular (11 % fat)	1 slice (28 g)	52	16
steak, boneless, extra lean; unheated	1 oz	35	13
whole, lean & fat; roasted	3 oz	207	52
whole, lean only; roasted	3 oz	133	47

HAM DISHES

HOME RECIPE

croquettes	1 (3.1 oz)	217	77
salad	½ cup	287	237

FOOD	PORTION	CALORIES	CHOLESTEROL

HAZELNUTS

FOOD	PORTION	CALORIES	CHOLESTEROL
dried, blanched	1 oz	191	0
dried, unblanched	1 oz	179	0
dry roasted, unblanched	1 oz	188	0
oil roasted, unblanched	1 oz	187	0

HEART

FOOD	PORTION	CALORIES	CHOLESTEROL
beef, raw	4 oz	132	158
beef; simmered	3 oz	148	164
chicken, raw	6.1 g	9	8
chicken; simmered	1 cup	268	350
pork, raw	1 heart (7.9 oz)	267	296
pork; braised	1 heart (4.3 oz)	191	285
turkey, raw	1 oz	41	33
turkey; simmered	1 cup	257	327

HERBAL TEA
(*see* TEA/HERBAL TEA)

HERBS/SPICES

FOOD	PORTION	CALORIES	CHOLESTEROL
DRIED			
Bar-B-Q Shaker (Diamond Crystal)	½ tsp	4	0
Chef Seasoning (Diamond Crystal)	1 pkg (.45 oz)	2	0
Chef Shaker (Diamond Crystal)	½ tsp	4	0

FOOD	PORTION	CALORIES	CHOLESTEROL
French Shaker (Diamond Crystal)	½ tsp	4	0
Italian Shaker (Diamond Crystal)	½ tsp	4	0
Mexican Shaker (Diamond Crystal)	½ tsp	4	0
allspice, ground	1 tsp	5	0
anise seed	1 tsp	7	0
basil, ground	1 tsp	4	0
bay leaf, crumbled	1 tsp	2	0
caraway seed	1 tsp	7	0
cardamom, ground	1 tsp	6	0
cayenne	1 tsp	6	0
celery seed	1 tsp	8	0
chervil	1 tsp	1	0
chili powder	1 tsp	8	0
chives, freeze-dried	1 Tbsp	1	0
cinnamon, ground	1 tsp	6	0
cloves, ground	1 tsp	7	0
coriander leaf	1 tsp	2	0
coriander leaf, dried	1 tsp	2	0
coriander seed	1 tsp	5	0
cumin seed	1 tsp	8	0
curry powder	1 tsp	6	0
dill seed	1 tsp	6	0
dill weed, dried	1 tsp	3	0
fennel seed	1 tsp	7	0
fenugreek seed	1 tsp	12	0

FOOD	PORTION	CALORIES	CHOLESTEROL
ginger, ground	1 tsp	6	0
mace, ground	1 tsp	8	0
marjoram, dried	1 tsp	2	0
mustard seed, yellow	1 tsp	15	0
nutmeg, ground	1 tsp	12	0
onion powder	1 tsp	7	0
oregano, ground	1 tsp	5	0
paprika	1 tsp	6	0
parsley	1 Tbsp	1	0
parsley, dried	1 tsp	1	0
parsley, freeze-dried	1 Tbsp	1	0
pepper, black	1 tsp	5	0
pepper, red	1 tsp.	6	0
pepper, white	1 tsp.	7	0
poppy seed	1 tsp	15	0
poultry seasoning	1 tsp	5	0
pumpkin pie spice	1 tsp	6	0
rosemary, dried	1 tsp	4	0
saffron	1 tsp	2	0
sage, ground	1 tsp	2	0
savory, ground	1 tsp	4	0
tarragon, ground	1 tsp	5	0
thyme, ground	1 tsp	4	0
turmeric, ground	1 tsp	8	0
FRESH			
coriander	¼ cup	4	0
ginger root	5 slices	8	0

FOOD	PORTION	CALORIES	CHOLESTEROL
ginger root	½ oz	7	0
parsley, raw; chopped	½ cup	10	0

HERRING

CANNED			
w/ tomato sauce	1.9 oz	97	53
FRESH			
Atlantic, raw	3 oz	134	51
Atlantic, raw	1 fillet (6.5 oz)	291	110
Atlantic; cooked	1 fillet (5 oz)	290	110
Atlantic; cooked	3 oz	172	65
Pacific, raw	1 fillet (6.5 oz)	359	141
Pacific, raw	3 oz	166	65
roe, raw	3½ oz	130	360
READY-TO-USE			
Atlantic, kippered	1 fillet (1.4 oz)	87	33
Atlantic, pickled	½ oz	39	12
kippered, fillet	1 sm piece (.7 oz)	42	17
kippered, fillet	1 med piece (.7 oz)	84	34

FOOD	PORTION	CALORIES	CHOLESTEROL

HICKORY NUTS

dried	1 oz	187	0

HONEYDEW

FRESH

Honey Dew (Chiquita)	1 cup	70	0
honeydew; cubed	1 cup	60	0

HORSERADISH

Gold's Hot	1 Tbsp	4	0
Gold's Red	1 Tbsp	4	0
Gold's White	1 Tbsp	4	0
Kraft Horseradish Mustard	1 Tbsp	4	0
Kraft Horseradish Sauce	1 Tbsp	50	5
Kraft Cream Style Prepared (Kraft)	1 Tbsp	8	0
Kraft Prepared	1 Tbsp	4	0
Sauceworks Horseradish Sauce	1 Tbsp	50	5

HOT CAKES
   (see PANCAKES)

HOT DOG
   (see also MEAT SUBSTITUTE, SAUSAGE, SAUSAGE SUBSTITUTE)

CHICKEN

Chicken Weiners (Health Valley)	3.5 oz	290	53
Wampler Longacre	1 (1.6 oz)	115	54

FOOD	PORTION	CALORIES	CHOLESTEROL
Wampler Longacre	1 (2 oz)	144	54
Weaver	1 (1.6 oz)	115	39
chicken	1 (1.5 oz)	116	45

MEAT

FOOD	PORTION	CALORIES	CHOLESTEROL
Beef Weiners (Health Valley)	3.5 oz	288	53
Beef, Armour Lower Salt Jumbo	1	170	30
Beef, Armour Star Jumbo	1	190	30
Chili Dog Sandwich, frzn (Microwave Chefwich)	1 (5 oz)	400	20
Frankfurters (Hebrew National)	1 (1.6 oz)	140	14
Frankfurters (Hebrew National)	1 (1.8 oz)	160	16
Frankfurters Deli (Hebrew National)	1 (2.3 oz)	200	20
Meat, Armour Lower Salt Jumbo	1	170	30
Meat, Armour Star Jumbo	1	190	30
Oscar Mayer Bacon & Cheddar Cheese	1 (1.6 oz)	143	30
Oscar Mayer Beef Franks	1 (1.6 oz)	144	29
Oscar Mayer Beef w/ Cheddar Franks	1 (1.6 oz)	130	29
Oscar Mayer Bun-Length Franks	1 (2 oz)	186	32
Oscar Mayer Bun-Length Wieners	1 (2 oz)	181	27

FOOD	PORTION	CALORIES	CHOLESTEROL
Oscar Mayer Cheese Hot Dogs	1 (1.6 oz)	145	31
Oscar Mayer German Brand Frankfurters	1 (2.7 oz)	230	30
Oscar Mayer Wieners	1 (1.6 oz)	144	27
Oscar Mayer Wieners Little	1 (.3 oz)	28	5
beef	1 (1¾ oz)	184	27
beef	1 (1.5 oz)	142	27
beef	1 (1.9 oz)	180	35
beef & pork	1 (1¾ oz)	183	29
pork, cheesefurter, smokie	1 (1.5 oz)	141	29
TURKEY			
Cheese Franks (Bil Mar Foods)	1 (1.6 oz)	109	29
Mr. Turkey Franks	1 (1.6 oz)	106	31
Mr. Turkey Franks	1 (½ oz)	79	23
Mr. Turkey Franks	1 (2 oz)	132	39
Turkey Cheese Franks (Louis Rich)	1 (1.6 oz)	108	38
Turkey Franks (Louis Rich)	1 (1.6 oz)	103	42
Turkey Weiners (Health Valley)	3.5 oz	238	53
Wampler Longacre	1 (1.6 oz)	102	37
turkey	1 (1.5 oz)	102	48

HUMMUS

HOME RECIPE			
hummus	⅓ cup	140	0

FOOD	PORTION	CALORIES	CHOLESTEROL
hummus	1 cup	420	0

HYACINTH BEANS

DRIED
cooked	1 cup	228	0
raw	1 cup	723	0

ICE CREAM AND FROZEN DESSERTS
(*see also* ICE CREAM, NON-DAIRY)

FOOD	PORTION	CALORIES	CHOLESTEROL
Berry Blend Pops (Crystal Light)	1 bar	14	0
Berry Punch (Jell-O)	1 pop	31	0
Blueberry Fruit 'N Juice Bars (Dole)	1 bar	90	5
Cherry (Jell-O)	1 pop	32	0
Cherry Fresh Lites (Dole)	1 bar	25	0
Cherry Fruit & Juice Bars (Chiquita)	1 bar (2 oz)	50	0
Cherry Fruit Bars (Jell-O)	1 bar (1.8 oz)	39	0
Cherry Italian Ice (Good Humor)	6 oz	138	0
Cherry Vanilla, Coffee, Peach, or Strawberry Ice Cream (Breyers)	½ cup	135	15–20
Cherry/Orange Ice Stripes (Good Humor)	1.5 oz	35	0
Chocolate (Ben & Jerry's)	4 oz	290	49

FOOD	PORTION	CALORIES	CHOLESTEROL
Chocolate Creamy Lites Bar (Carnation)	1 bar	50	8
Chocolate Fudge Heaven Sundae Bar (Carnation)	1 bar	150	7
Chocolate Malted Bars (Carnation)	1 bar	70	19
Chocolate/Vanilla Cool 'N Creamy Bars (Crystal Light)	1 bar	55	1
Double Chocolate Fudge Cool 'N Creamy Bars (Crystal Light)	1 bar	55	1
Dutch Chocolate (American Glace)	4 oz	48	0
French Vanilla (Ben & Jerry's)	4 oz	267	66
Fruit Flavored Sherbet (Land O'Lakes)	4 oz	130	5
Fruit Punch Fruit Slush (Wyler's)	4 oz	140	0
Fruit Punch SunTops (Dole)	1 bar	40	0
Fruit Punch Pops (Crystal Light)	1 bar	14	0
Grape (Jell-O)	1 pop	31	0
Grape SunTops (Dole)	1 bar	40	0
Grape/Lemon Italian Ice (Good Humor)	6 oz	138	0

FOOD	PORTION	CALORIES	CHOLESTEROL
Grape/Lemon Ice Stripes (Good Humor)	1.5 oz	35	0
Lemon Fresh Lites (Dole)	1 bar	25	0
Lemon White Italian Ice (Good Humor)	6 oz	138	0
Lemon/Cherry w/ Gummy Dinosaur Colossal Fossil (Good Humor)	3 oz	75	0
Lemon/Grape w/ Gummy Dinosaur Colossal Fossil (Good Humor)	3 oz	75	0
Lemon/Lime Swirl (Jell-O)	1 pop	33	0
Lemonade SunTops (Dole)	1 bar	40	0
Mandarin Orange Sorbet (Dole)	4 oz	110	0
Mixed Berry (Jell-O)	1 pop	31	0
Mixed Berry Bars (Jell-O)	1 bar (1.8 oz)	42	0
Orange (Jell-O)	1 pop	31	0
Orange Bars (Jell-O)	1 bar (1.8 oz)	42	0
Orange Pops (Crystal Light)	1 bar	13	tr
Orange Sherbet Push-Up (Good Humor)	3 oz	56	0
Orange/Pineapple Swirl (Jell-O)	1 pop	31	0

FOOD	PORTION	CALORIES	CHOLESTEROL
Orange/Raspberry Italian Ice (Good Humor)	6 oz	138	0
Orange/Vanilla Cool 'N Creamy Bars (Crystal Light)	1 bar	31	tr
Original Cheesecake Bar (Carnation)	1 bar	120	12
Passion-fruit (Vitari)	4 oz	80	0
Peach (Vitari)	4 oz	80	0
Peach Fruit 'N Juice Bars (Dole)	1 bar	90	5
Peach Sorbet (Dole)	4 oz	120	0
Pina Colada Fruit 'N Juice Bars (Dole)	1 bar	90	0
Pineapple Fruit 'N Juice Bars (Dole)	1 bar	70	0
Pineapple Sorbet (Dole)	4 oz	120	0
Pineapple Orange Fresh Lites (Dole)	1 bar	25	0
Pineapple Pops (Crystal Light)	1 bar	13	0
Pink Lemonade Pops (Crystal Light)	1 bar	14	0
Raspberry (Jell-O)	1 pop	29	0
Raspberry Banana Fruit & Juice Bars (Chiquita)	1 bar (2 oz)	50	0

FOOD	PORTION	CALORIES	CHOLESTEROL
Raspberry Bars (Jell-O)	1 bar (1.8 oz)	41	0
Raspberry Fruit 'N Juice Bars (Dole)	1 bar	70	0
Raspberry Pops (Crystal Light)	1 bar	14	0
Raspberry Sorbet (Dole)	4 oz	110	0
Raspberry Berry Swirl Bars (Carnation)	1 bar	70	10
Raspberry Fresh Lites (Dole)	1 bar	25	0
Raspberry Fruit & Juice Bars (Chiquita)	1 bar (2 oz)	50	0
Raspberry Peach Bars (Jell-O)	1 bar (1.8 oz)	40	0
Raspberry/Peach Swirl (Jell-O)	1 pop	29	0
Skinny Dip	4 oz	36	0
Strawberries and Cream (Good Humor)	3 oz	96	0
Strawberry (Jell-O)	1 pop	31	0
Strawberry Banana (Jell-O)	1 pop	31	0
Strawberry Banana Bars (Jell-O)	1 bar (1.8 oz)	39	0
Strawberry Banana Fruit & Juice Bars (Chiquita)	1 bar (2 oz)	50	0
Strawberry Banana Swirl (Jell-O)	1 pop	31	0

FOOD	PORTION	CALORIES	CHOLESTEROL
Strawberry Bars (Jell-O)	1 bar (1.8 oz)	41	0
Strawberry Cheesecake Bars (Carnation)	1 bar	125	10
Strawberry Creamy Lites Bar (Carnation)	1 bar	50	7
Strawberry Finger Bar (Good Humor)	2.5 oz	49	0
Strawberry Fruit 'N Juice Bars (Dole)	1 bar	70	0
Strawberry Pops (Crystal Light)	1 bar	13	0
Strawberry Sorbet (Dole)	4 oz	110	0
Strawberry Tropical Mix (Jell-O)	1 bar (1.8 oz)	40	0
Strawberry Berry Swirl Bar (Carnation)	1 bar	70	9
Strawberry Fruit & Juice Bars (Chiquita)	1 bar (2 oz)	50	0
Tahitian Vanilla (American Glace)	4 oz	48	0
Tasti D-Lite	4 oz	40	5
Tropical Orange SunTops (Dole)	1 bar	40	0
Vanilla Caramel Nut, Heaven Bars (Carnation)	1 bar	225	9
Vanilla Fudge Heaven Sundae Bars (Carnation)	1 bar	150	7
Vanilla Fudge Nut (Carnation)	1 bar	222	9

FOOD	PORTION	CALORIES	CHOLESTEROL
Vanilla Ice Cream (Land O'Lakes)	4 oz	140	30
Vanilla Ice Milk (Land O'Lakes)	4 oz	90	10
Watermelon Italian Ice (Good Humor)	6 oz	138	0
Wild Cherry Pops (Crystal Light)	1 bar	13	0
orange sherbet	⅔ cup	181	9
orange sherbet (home recipe)	½ cup	120	9
orange sherbet	1 cup	270	14
vanilla ice milk	1 cup	184	18
vanilla ice milk, soft serve	1 cup	223	13
vanilla, 10% fat	1 cup	269	59
vanilla, 16% fat	1 cup	349	88
vanilla, French, soft serve	1 cup	377	153

ICE CREAM, NON-DAIRY

FOOD	PORTION	CALORIES	CHOLESTEROL
Mocha Mix Chocolate Chip	½ cup	160	0
Mocha Mix Dutch Chocolate	½ cup	135	0
Mocha Mix Mocha Almond Fudge	½ cup	150	0
Mocha Mix Neapolitan	½ cup	130	0
Mocha Mix Strawberry Swirl	½ cup	140	0
Mocha Mix Toasted Almond	½ cup	150	0
Mocha Mix Vanilla	½ cup	138	0
Mocha Mix Vanilla Chocolate Almond	½ cup	150	0

FOOD	PORTION	CALORIES	CHOLESTEROL
Tofulite	4 oz	150	0
Tofutti Cappuccino Love Drops	4 oz	230	0
Tofutti Chocolate Supreme	4 oz	210	0
Tofutti Chocolate Cuties	4 oz	140	0
Tofutti Chocolate Love Drops	4 oz	220	0
Tofutti Lite lite Applejack Vanilla Twirl	4 oz	90	0
Tofutti Lite lite Cappuccino Vanilla Twirl	4 oz	90	0
Tofutti Lite lite Chocolate Vanilla Twirl	4 oz	90	0
Tofutti Lite lite Chocolate Strawberry Twirl	4 oz	90	0
Tofutti Lite lite Strawberry Vanilla Twirl	4 oz	90	0
Tofutti Lite lite Vanilla Chocolate Strawberry Twirl	4 oz	90	0
Tofutti Soft Serve Hi-Lite Chocolate	4 oz	100	0
Tofutti Soft Serve Hi-Lite Vanilla	4 oz	90	0
Tofutti Soft Serve Regular	4 oz	158	0
Tofutti Vanilla	4 oz	200	0
Tofutti Vanilla Almond Bark	4 oz	230	0
Tofutti Vanilla Cuties	4 oz	130	0
Tofutti Vanilla Love Drops	4 oz	220	0
Tofutti Wildberry	4 oz	210	0

FOOD	PORTION	CALORIES	CHOLESTEROL

ICE CREAM TOPPINGS
   (see also SYRUP)

FOOD	PORTION	CALORIES	CHOLESTEROL
Butterscotch Artifically Flavored Topping (Kraft)	1 Tbsp	60	0
Butterscotch Flavored Topping (Smucker's)	2 Tbsp	140	0
Caramel Topping (Kraft)	1 Tbsp	60	0
Carmel Flavored Topping (Smucker's)	2 Tbsp	140	0
Cherry (Smucker's)	1 Tbsp	53	0
Chocolate Caramel Topping (Kraft)	1 Tbsp	60	0
Chocolate Flavored Syrup Topping (Smucker's)	2 Tbsp	130	0
Chocolate Fudge Magic Shell (Smucker's)	2 Tbsp	190	0
Chocolate Fudge Topping (Smucker's)	2 Tbsp	130	0
Chocolate Magic Shell (Smucker's)	2 Tbsp	190	0
Chocolate Nut Magic Shell (Smucker's)	2 Tbsp	200	0
Chocolate Topping (Kraft)	1 Tbsp	60	0
Hot Caramel Topping (Smucker's)	2 Tbsp	150	0
Hot Fudge Topping (Kraft)	1 Tbsp	70	0

FOOD	PORTION	CALORIES	CHOLESTEROL
Hot Fudge Topping (Smucker's)	2 Tbsp	110	0
Marshmallow (Smucker's)	1 Tbsp	68	0
Marshmallow Creme (Kraft)	1 Tbsp	90	0
Peanut Butter Magic Caramel (Smucker's)	2 Tbsp	150	0
Pecans in Syrup (Smucker's)	2 Tbsp	130	0
Pineapple (Smucker's)	2 Tbsp	130	0
Pineapple (Smucker's)	1 Tbsp	54	0
Pineapple Topping (Kraft)	1 Tbsp	50	0
Red Raspberry Topping (Kraft)	1 Tbsp	50	0
Strawberry (Smucker's)	2 Tbsp	120	0
Strawberry (Smucker's)	1 Tbsp	44	0
Strawberry Topping (Kraft)	1 Tbsp	50	0
Walnut Topping (Kraft)	1 Tbsp	90	0
Walnuts in Syrup (Smucker's)	2 Tbsp	130	0
butterscotch sauce (home recipe)	2 Tbsp	151	40
chocolate sauce (home recipe)	2 Tbsp	108	2
hard sauce (home recipe)	2 Tbsp	142	15

FOOD	PORTION	CALORIES	CHOLESTEROL

ICING
(*see* CAKE)

INSTANT BREAKFAST
(*see* BREAKFAST DRINKS)

ITALIAN FOOD
(*see also* DINNER, PASTA, PASTA DINNERS, PASTA SALAD)

FOOD	PORTION	CALORIES	CHOLESTEROL
FROZEN			
Italian Style International Recipe (Birds Eye)	½ cup	101	0
Italian Style International Rice (Birds Eye)	½ cup	119	0

JAM/JELLY/PRESERVE

FOOD	PORTION	CALORIES	CHOLESTEROL
ALL FRUIT			
All Flavors Simply Fruit Spread (Smucker's)	1 tsp	16	0
Blueberry Fruit Spread (Pritikin Foods)	1 tsp	14	0
Peach Fruit Spread (Pritikin Foods)	1 tsp	14	0
Red Raspberry Fruit Spread (Pritikin Foods)	1 tsp	14	0
Strawberry Fruit Spread (Pritikin Foods)	1 tsp	14	0
REDUCED CALORIE			
All Flavors Slenderella Low Calorie Imitation Jam (Smucker's)	1 tsp	8	0

FOOD	PORTION	CALORIES	CHOLESTEROL
All Flavors Slenderella Low Calorie Imitation Jelly (Smucker's)	1 tsp	8	0
All Flavors, Imitation Jelly, Single Service (Smucker's)	⅜ oz pkg	2	0
All Flavors, Jellies, Single Service (Smucker's)	½ oz pkg	38	0
All Flavors, Preserves, Single Service (Smucker's)	½ oz pkg	38	0
All Flavors, Low Sugar Spreads (Smucker's)	1 tsp	8	0
Grape Jelly Reduced Calorie (Kraft)	1 tsp	5	0
Grape Imitation Jelly (Smucker's)	1 tsp	2	0
Jellies, All Flavors (Estee)	1 tsp	2	0
Preserves, All Flavors (Estee)	1 tsp	2	0
Preserves, All Flavors (Louis Sherry)	1 tsp	2	0
Strawberry Imitation Jelly (Smucker's)	1 tsp	2	0
Strawberry Preserves Reduced Calorie (Kraft)	1 tsp	8	0
REGULAR All Flavors Jelly (Home Brands)	2 tsp	35	0

FOOD	PORTION	CALORIES	CHOLESTEROL
All Flavors Preserves (Smucker's)	1 tsp	18	0
All Flavors Jam (Smucker's)	1 tsp	18	0
Apple Butter (BAMA)	2 tsp	25	0
Apple Butter (White House)	1 oz	50	0
Apple Butter Natural (Smucker's)	1 tsp	12	0
Apple Jelly (BAMA)	2 tsp	30	0
Cider Apple Butter (Smucker's)	1 tsp	12	0
Grape Jelly (BAMA)	2 tsp	30	0
Jam, All Varieties (Kraft)	1 tsp	18	0
Jelly, All Varieties (Kraft)	1 tsp	16	0
Orange Marmalade (Smucker's)	1 tsp	18	0
Peach Butter (Smucker's)	1 tsp	15	0
Peach Preserves (BAMA)	2 tsp	30	0
Preserves, All Varieties (Kraft)	1 tsp	16	0
Preserves, All Flavors (Home Brands)	2 tsp	35	0
Red Plum Jam (BAMA)	2 tsp	30	0

FOOD	PORTION	CALORIES	CHOLESTEROL
Strawberry Preserves (BAMA)	2 tsp	30	0

JAPANESE FOOD
(*see* ORIENTAL FOOD)

JELLY
(*see* JAM/JELLY/PRESERVE)

KALE

FRESH			
cooked; chopped	½ cup	21	0
raw; chopped	½ cup	21	0
FROZEN			
chopped; cooked	½ cup	20	0
frzn; not prep	10 oz pkg	79	0

KETCHUP
(*see* CATSUP)

KIDNEY

beef, raw	4 oz	212	322
beef; simmered	3 oz	122	329
pork, raw	3 oz	84	270
pork; braised	3 oz	128	408

KIDNEY BEANS

CANNED			
Dark Red Kidney Beans (Hanover)	½ cup	110	0

FOOD	PORTION	CALORIES	CHOLESTEROL
Dark Red Lite 50% Less Salt (S&W)	½ cup	120	0
Dark Red Premium (S&W)	½ cup	120	0
Kidney, Dark Red (Trappey's)	½ cup	90	0
Kidney, Jalapeno Light Red (Trappey's)	½ cup	90	0
Kidney, Light Red (Trappey's)	½ cup	90	0
Kidney, Red w/ Chili Gravy (Trappey's)	½ cup	100	0
Light Red Kidney Beans in Sauce (Hanover)	½ cup	120	0
kidney	1 cup	208	0
red	1 cup	216	0
DRIED			
California red, raw	1 cup	609	0
California red; cooked	1 cup	219	0
Kidney (Hurst Brand)	1 cup	254	0
cooked	1 cup	225	0
raw	1 cup	613	0
red, raw	1 cup	619	0
red; cooked	1 cup	225	0
red, royal, raw	1 cup	605	0
red, royal; cooked	1 cup	218	0

FOOD	PORTION	CALORIES	CHOLESTEROL
SPROUTS			
cooked	1 lb	152	0
raw	½ cup	27	0
KIWIFRUIT			
FRESH			
Kiwifruit (California Kiwifruit Commission)	2	90	0
kiwifruit	1 med	46	0
KOHLRABI			
FRESH			
raw; sliced	½ cup	19	0
sliced, cooked	½ cup	24	0
KUMQUATS			
FRESH			
kumquats	1	12	0
LAMB			
(*see also* LAMB DISHES)			
FRESH			
chopped, lean & fat; cooked	½ cup	195	69
ground, lean & fat; cooked	½ cup	153	54
leg, w/o bone, lean & fat; roasted	3 oz	237	83
leg, w/o bone, lean only; roasted	3 oz	158	85
loin chop, w/ bone, lean & fat; broiled	1 (2.5 oz)	255	70

FOOD	PORTION	CALORIES	CHOLESTEROL
loin chop, w/ bone, lean only; broiled	1 (1.7 oz)	92	49
patty, lean & fat; cooked	3 oz	229	80
rib chop, w/ bone, lean & fat; cooked	1 (2.4 oz)	273	66
rib chop, w/ bone, lean only; cooked	1 (1.5 oz)	91	43
shoulder shank, lean & fat; cooked	3.2 oz	306	89
shoulder, lean & fat; roasted	3 oz	287	83
shoulder, w/o bone, lean only; roasted	3 oz	174	85
shoulder, w/o bone, lean & fat; roasted	3 oz	287	83

LAMB DISHES

curry	¾ cup	345	89
lamb & potato casserole	¾ cup	277	89
stew	¾ cup	124	29

LAMB'S-QUARTERS

FRESH			
chopped; cooked	½ cup	29	0

LECITHIN
(*see* SOY)

LEEKS

DRIED			
freeze-dried	1 Tbsp	1	0

FOOD	PORTION	CALORIES	CHOLESTEROL
FRESH			
chopped; cooked	¼ cup	8	0
raw	1 (4.4 oz)	76	0
raw; chopped	¼ cup	16	0
LEMON			
CANDIED			
lemon peel	1 oz	90	0
FRESH			
peel	1 Tbsp	0	0
HOME RECIPE			
lemon sauce	2 Tbsp	57	48
JUICE			
Lemon (Seneca)	1 Tbsp	6	0
fresh	1 Tbsp	4	0
frzn	1 Tbsp	3	0
lemon	1 Tbsp	3	0
LEMON EXTRACT			
Virginia Dare	1 tsp	22	0
LEMONADE (*see* FRUIT DRINKS)			
LENTILS			
Lentils; cooked (Hurst Brand)	1 cup	258	0
Zesty Lentil Pilaf (Health Valley)	4 oz	110	0

FOOD	PORTION	CALORIES	CHOLESTEROL
DRIED			
cooked	1 cup	231	0
raw	1 cup	649	0
SPROUTS			
sprouts	½ cup	40	0

LETTUCE

FOOD	PORTION	CALORIES	CHOLESTEROL
FRESH			
butterhead	2 leaves	2	0
iceberg	1 leaf	3	0
looseleaf; shredded	½ cup	5	0
romaine; shredded	½ cup	4	0

LIMA BEANS

FOOD	PORTION	CALORIES	CHOLESTEROL
CANNED			
Lima Beans (Libby)	½ cup	80	0
Lima Beans (Seneca)	½ cup	80	0
Small Fancy (S&W)	½ cup	80	0
large	1 cup	191	0
lima beans	½ cup	93	0
DRIED			
Baby Lima (Hurst Brand)	1 cup	262	0
baby, raw	1 cup	677	0
baby; cooked	1 cup	229	0
cooked	½ cup	104	0

FOOD	PORTION	CALORIES	CHOLESTEROL
large, raw	1 cup	602	0
large; cooked	1 cup	217	0
FROZEN			
Baby (Birds Eye)	½ cup	127	0
Baby Lima Beans (Hanover)	½ cup	110	0
Fordhook (Birds Eye)	½ cup	100	0
Fordhook Lima Beans (Hanover)	½ cup	100	0
Fordhook, raw	10 oz	301	0
Thin; cooked (Health Valley)	6.3 oz	188	0
lima beans, raw	½ cup	94	0
lima beans; cooked	½ cup	85	0

LIME

JUICE			
fresh	1 Tbsp	4	0
lime juice	1 Tbsp	3	0

LINGCOD

FRESH			
raw	½ fillet (6.8 oz)	164	100
raw	3 oz	72	44

FOOD	PORTION	CALORIES	CHOLESTEROL

LIQUOR/LIQUEUR
(*see also* BEER AND ALE, DRINK MIXER, WINE, WINE COOLERS)

FOOD	PORTION	CALORIES	CHOLESTEROL
annisette	⅔ oz	74	0
apricot brandy	⅔ oz	64	0
benedictine	⅔ oz	69	0
bloody mary	1 cocktail (5 oz)	116	0
bourbon & soda	1 cocktail (4 oz)	105	0
coffee liqueur	1.5 oz	174	0
coffee w/ cream liqueur	1.5 oz	154	0
creme de menthe	1.5 oz	186	0
creme de menthe	⅔ oz	67	0
curacao liqueur	⅔ oz	54	0
daiquiri	2½ oz	87	0
gin	1.5 oz	110	0
gin & tonic	1 cocktail (7.5 oz)	171	0
gin ricky	4 oz	150	0
highball	8 oz	166	0
manhattan	2½ oz	116	0
martini	1 cocktail (2.5 oz)	156	0
mint julep	10 oz	210	0
old-fashioned	2½ oz	127	0
piña colada	1 cocktail (4.5 oz)	262	0
planter's punch	3½ oz	175	0

FOOD	PORTION	CALORIES	CHOLESTEROL
rum	1.5 oz	97	0
screwdriver	1 cocktail (7 oz)	174	0
sherry	2oz	84	0
sloe gin fizz	2½ oz	132	0
tequila sunrise	1 cocktail (5.5 oz)	189	0
tom collins	1 cocktail (7.5 oz)	121	0
vermouth, dry	3½ oz	105	0
vermouth, sweet	3½ oz	167	0
vodka	1.5 oz	97	0
whiskey	1.5 oz	105	0
whiskey sour	1 cocktail (3 oz)	123	0
whiskey sour mix; as prep	1 oz	48	0

LIVER
(see also PÂTÉ)

FOOD	PORTION	CALORIES	CHOLESTEROL
beef, raw	4 oz	161	400
beef; braised	3 oz	137	331
beef; pan-fried	3 oz	184	410
chicken, raw	1.1 oz	40	140
duck, raw	1.5 oz	60	227
pork, raw	3 oz	151	341
pork; braised	3 oz	141	302
turkey, raw	3.6 oz	140	475
turkey; simmered	1 cup	237	876

FOOD	PORTION	CALORIES	CHOLESTEROL
LOBSTER			
FRESH			
northern, raw	1 lobster (5.3 oz)	136	143
northern, raw	3 oz	77	81
northern; cooked	1 cup	142	104
northern; cooked	3 oz	83	61
spiny, raw	3 oz	95	60
spiny, raw	1 lobster (7.3 oz)	233	146
FROZEN			
Gulfstream Tails (King & Prince)	6 oz	170	171
Gulfstream Tails (King & Prince)	7 oz	199	200
Gulfstream Tails (King & Prince)	8 oz	227	227
HOME RECIPE			
newburg	1 cup	485	455
LOGANBERRIES			
FROZEN			
loganberries	1 cup	80	0
LOQUATS			
FRESH			
loquats	1	5	0

FOOD	PORTION	CALORIES	CHOLESTEROL

LOTUS ROOT

FRESH

cooked; sliced	10 slices	59	0
raw; sliced	10 slices	45	0

LOTUS SEEDS

dried	1 oz	94	0

LOX

(*see* SALMON)

LUNCHEON MEATS/COLD CUTS

(*see also* CHICKEN, HAM, MEAT SUBSTITUTE, TURKEY)

Beef (Carl Buddig)	1 oz	40	16
Bologna Beef (Health Valley)	3.5 oz	310	49
Bologna Midget (Hebrew National)	1 oz	60	14
Corned Beef (Carl Buddig)	1 oz	40	16
Oscar Mayer Bar-B-Q Loaf	1 slice (28 g)	48	13
Oscar Mayer Bologna Beef Lebanon	1 link (23 g)	49	16
Oscar Mayer Bologna	1 slice (28 g)	90	19
Oscar Mayer Bologna Beef	1 slice (28 g)	90	18
Oscar Mayer Bologna Beef Garlic Flavored	1 slice (28 g)	89	19

FOOD	PORTION	CALORIES	CHOLESTEROL
Oscar Mayer Bologna w/ Cheese	1 slice (23 g)	74	16
Oscar Mayer Braunschweiger German Brand	1 oz	94	46
Oscar Mayer Braunschweiger Sliced	1 slice (28 g)	96	50
Oscar Mayer Braunschweiger Tube	1 oz	96	43
Oscar Mayer Cotto Salami	1 slice (23 g)	54	18
Oscar Mayer Cotto Salami Beef	1 slice (23 g)	46	18
Oscar Mayer Genoa Salami Beef	1 slice (9 g)	34	9
Oscar Mayer Hard Salami	1 slice (9 g)	34	8
Oscar Mayer Head Cheese	1 slice (28 g)	55	26
Oscar Mayer Honey Loaf	1 slice (28 g)	35	14
Oscar Mayer Jalapeno	1 slice (28 g)	72	10
Oscar Mayer Liver Cheese Pork Fat Wrap	1 slice (38 g)	116	76
Oscar Mayer Luncheon Meat	1 slice (28 g)	98	20
Oscar Mayer Luxury Loaf	1 slice (28 g)	38	13
Oscar Mayer New England Brand Sausage	1 slice (23 g)	31	14
Oscar Mayer Old Fashioned Loaf	1 slice (28 g)	64	15

FOOD	PORTION	CALORIES	CHOLESTEROL
Oscar Mayer Olive Loaf	1 slice (28 g)	62	13
Oscar Mayer Pastrami	1 slice (17 g)	16	7
Oscar Mayer Peppered Loaf	1 slice (28 g)	43	13
Oscar Mayer Pickle & Pimiento Loaf	1 slice (28 g)	63	13
Oscar Mayer Picnic Loaf	1 slice (28 g)	62	13
Oscar Mayer Salami for Beer	1 slice (23 g)	55	16
Oscar Mayer Salami for Beer Beef	1 slice (23 g)	66	17
Oscar Mayer Sandwich Spread	1 oz	67	10
Oscar Mayer Smoked Beef	1 slice (14 g)	14	7
Oscar Mayer Summer Sausage Thuringer Cervelat	1 slice (23 g)	73	19
Oscar Mayer Summer Sausage Thuringer Cervelat Beef	1 slice (23 g)	72	18
Oscar Mayer Corned Beef	1 slice (17 g)	16	5
Pastrami (Carl Buddig)	1 oz	40	16
Pork Breakfast Sliced (Health Valley)	3.5 oz	560	77
Salami (Health Valley)	3.5 oz	400	49

FOOD	PORTION	CALORIES	CHOLESTEROL
Salami Midget (Hebrew National)	1 oz	57	11
barbecue loaf, beef	1 slice (23 g)	40	9
beerwurst	1 slice (23 g)	75	13
beerwurst, beef	1 slice (6 g)	19	3
beerwurst, pork	1 slice (6 g)	14	4
beerwurst, pork	1 slice (23 g)	55	13
berliner, pork & beef	1 slice (23 g)	53	11
blood sausage	1 slice (25 g)	95	30
bologna, beef	1 slice (23 g)	72	13
bologna, beef & pork	1 slice (23 g)	73	13
bologna, Lebanon beef	1 slice (23 g)	52	15
bologna, pork	1 slice (23 g)	57	14
braunschweiger	1 oz	102	44
braunschweiger, pork	1 slice (18 g)	65	28
corned beef loaf	1 slice (28 g)	46	12
Dutch brand loaf, pork & beef	1 slice (28 g)	68	13

FOOD	PORTION	CALORIES	CHOLESTEROL
ham & cheese loaf	1 slice (28 g)	147	33
headcheese, pork	1 slice (28 oz)	60	23
honey loaf, pork & beef	1 slice (28 g)	36	10
honey roll sausage	1 slice (23 g)	42	12
liver cheese, pork	1 slice (38 g)	115	66
liver cheese, pork	1 oz	86	49
liverwurst	1 oz	93	45
liverwurst, pork	1 slice (18 g)	59	28
luncheon meat, beef	1 slice (28 g)	87	18
luncheon meat, beef	1 slice (1 oz)	87	18
luncheon meat, beef, thin sliced	5 slices (21 g)	26	9
luncheon meat, pork & beef	1 slice (28 g)	200	31
luncheon meat, pork, canned	1 slice (21 g)	70	13
luncheon meat, pork, canned	1 oz	95	18
luncheon sausage, pork & beef	1 slice (23 g)	60	15
luxury loaf, pork	1 slice (28 g)	40	10
mortadella, beef & pork	1 slice (15 g)	47	8

FOOD	PORTION	CALORIES	CHOLESTEROL
mother's loaf, pork	1 slice (21 g)	59	9
New England brand sausage, pork & beef	1 slice (23 g)	37	11
olive loaf, pork	1 slice (28 g)	67	11
pastrami, beef	1 slice (1 oz)	99	26
peppered loaf, pork & beef	1 slice (28 g)	42	13
pickle & pimiento loaf, pork	1 slice (28 g)	74	10
picnic loaf, pork & beef	1 slice (28 g)	66	11
salami, cooked, beef	1 slice (23 g)	58	14
salami, cooked, beef & pork	1 slice (23 g)	57	15
salami, hard, pork & beef	1 slice (10 g)	42	8
salami, hard, pork & beef	1 pkg (4 oz)	472	89
sandwich spread, pork & beef	1 Tbsp	35	6
sandwich spread, pork & beef	1 oz	67	11
smoked chopped beef	1 slice (1 oz)	38	13
summer sausage, Thuringer, cervelat	1 slice (23 g)	80	16

FOOD	PORTION	CALORIES	CHOLESTEROL

LUPINS

DRIED

cooked	1 cup	197	0
raw	1 cup	668	0

LYCHEES

FRESH

lychees	1	6	0

MACADAMIA NUTS

dried	1 oz	199	0
oil roasted	1 oz	204	0

MACARONI
(see PASTA)

MACKEREL

CANNED

jack	1 can (12.7 oz)	563	285
jack	1 cup	296	150

FRESH

Atlantic, raw	3 oz	174	60
Atlantic, raw	1 fillet (3.9 oz)	229	78
Atlantic; cooked	1 fillet (3.1 oz)	231	66
Atlantic; cooked	3 oz	223	64
king, raw	½ fillet (6.9 oz)	207	106

FOOD	PORTION	CALORIES	CHOLESTEROL
king, raw	3 oz	89	45
Spanish, raw	3 oz	118	65
Spanish, raw	1 fillet (6.6 oz)	260	142
Spanish; cooked	1 fillet (5.1 oz)	230	107
Spanish; cooked	3 oz	134	62

MALTED MILK

LIQUID			
chocolate	1 cup	233	34
natural flavor	1 cup	236	37
POWDER			
Carnation Chocolate	3 heaping tsp (21 g)	79	1
Carnation Original	3 heaping tsp (21 g)	90	4
Malted Milk Chocolate Instant; as prep w/ whole milk (Kraft)	3 tsp + 1 cup milk	240	25
Malted Milk Natural Instant; as prep w/ whole milk (Kraft)	3 tsp + 1 cup milk	240	25
chocolate	¾ oz	83	1
natural flavor	¾ oz	86	4

MANGO

FRESH			
mango	1	135	0

FOOD	PORTION	CALORIES	CHOLESTEROL

MARGARINE
(see also BUTTER BLENDS, BUTTER SUBSTITUTE)

REDUCED CALORIE

FOOD	PORTION	CALORIES	CHOLESTEROL
Blue Bonnet Diet	1 Tbsp	50	0
Fleischmann's Diet	1 Tbsp	50	0
Fleischmann's Diet w/ Lite Salt	1 Tbsp	50	0
Kraft Spread	1 Tbsp	50	0
Kraft Spread (stick)	1 Tbsp	60	0
Mazola Light Corn Oil Spread	1 Tbsp	50	0
Mazola Light Corn Oil Spread	1 cup	835	0
Mazola, Diet	1 Tbsp	50	0
Mazola, Diet	1 cup	815	0
Parkay Diet Soft	1 Tbsp	50	0
Parkay Light Corn Oil Spread	1 Tbsp	70	0
Parkay Spread	1 Tbsp	60	0
Weight Watchers	1 Tbsp	50	0
corn	1 tsp	17	0
corn	1 cup	801	0
soybean	1 cup	801	0
soybean	1 tsp	17	0
soybean & cottonseed	1 tsp	17	0
soybean & cottonseed	1 cup	801	0
soybean & palm	1 cup	801	0
soybean & palm	1 tsp	17	0
REGULAR			
Blue Bonnet	1 Tbsp	100	0

FOOD	PORTION	CALORIES	CHOLESTEROL
Fleischmann's	1 Tbsp	100	0
Fleischmann's Light Corn Oil Stick	1 Tbsp	80	0
Fleischmann's Sweet, Unsalted	1 Tbsp	100	0
Krona (Lever)	1 Tbsp	100	15
Land O'Lakes, Premium Corn Oil Stick	1 Tbsp	100	0
Land O'Lakes, Regular Stick	1 Tbsp	100	0
Mazola	1 Tbsp	100	0
Mazola	1 cup	1650	0
Mazola, Unsalted	1 Tbsp	100	0
Mazola, Unsalted	1 cup	1635	0
Mother's	1 Tbsp	100	0
Mother's, Unsalted	1 Tbsp	100	0
Nucoa	1 Tbsp	100	0
Nucoa	1 cup	1630	0
Parkay	1 Tbsp	100	0
Shedd's Spread Country Crock Classic Quarters	1 Tbsp	80	0
coconut, safflower, palm	1 tsp	34	0
coconut, safflower, palm	1 stick	815	0
corn	1 stick	815	0
corn	1 tsp	34	0
corn, soybean & cottonseed	1 stick	815	0
corn, soybean & cottonseed	1 tsp	34	0
corn, soybean & cottonseed, unsalted	1 tsp	34	0

FOOD	PORTION	CALORIES	CHOLESTEROL
corn, soybean & cottonseed, unsalted	1 stick	809	0
soybean & palm	1 tsp	34	0
soybean & palm	1 stick	815	0
soybean, hydrogenated	1 stick	815	0
soybean, hydrogenated	1 tsp	34	0
sunflower, soybean & cottonseed	1 stick	815	0
sunflower, soybean & cottonseed	1 tsp	34	0
SOFT			
Blue Bonnet Light Tasty Spread	1 Tbsp	60	0
Blue Bonnet Spread	1 Tbsp	80	0
Blue Bonnet Spread Stick (70% fat)	1 Tbsp	90	0
Blue Bonnet Spread Stick (75% fat)	1 Tbsp	90	0
Blue Bonnet Soft	1 Tbsp	100	0
Fleischmann's	1 Tbsp	100	0
Fleischmann's Light Corn Oil Spread	1 Tbsp	80	0
Fleischmann's Sweet, Unsalted	1 Tbsp	100	0
I Can't Believe It's Not Butter! (Lever)	1 Tbsp	90	0
Land O'Lakes Regular Soft Tub	1 Tbsp	100	0
Mother's, Unsalted	1 Tbsp	100	0
Mother's, Salted	1 Tbsp	100	0

FOOD	PORTION	CALORIES	CHOLESTEROL
Nucoa	1 Tbsp	90	0
Nucoa	1 cup	1415	0
Parkay Corn Oil Soft	1 Tbsp	100	0
Parkay Soft	1 Tbsp	100	0
Promise	1 Tbsp	90	0
Shedd's Spread Country Crock	1 Tbsp	80	0
corn	1 tsp	34	0
corn	1 cup	1626	0
safflower	1 tsp	34	0
safflower	1 cup	1626	0
safflower, cottonseed & peanut	1 cup	1626	0
safflower, cottonseed & peanut	1 tsp	34	0
soybean, salted	1 tsp	34	0
soybean, salted	1 cup	1626	0
soybean, unsalted	1 cup	1626	0
soybean, unsalted	1 tsp	34	0
soybean & cottonseed	1 cup	1626	0
soybean & cottonseed	1 tsp	34	0
soybean & cottonseed, unsalted	1 tsp	34	0
soybean & cottonseed, unsalted	1 cup	1626	0
soybean & palm	1 cup	1626	0
soybean & palm	1 tsp	34	0
soybean & safflower	1 tsp	34	0

FOOD	PORTION	CALORIES	CHOLESTEROL
soybean & safflower	1 cup	1626	0
sunflower & peanut	1 cup	1626	0
sunflower & peanut	1 tsp	34	0
SQUEEZE			
Fleischmann's	1 Tbsp	100	0
Parkay Squeeze	1 Tbsp	100	0
soybean & cottonseed	1 tsp	34	0
WHIPPED			
Blue Bonnet Soft Whipped	1 Tbsp	70	0
Blue Bonnet Whipped Stick	1 Tbsp	70	0
Fleischmann's Lightly Salted	1 Tbsp	70	0
Fleischmann's Unsalted	1 Tbsp	70	0
Miracle Brand	1 Tbsp	60	0
Miracle Brand (stick)	1 Tbsp	70	0
Parkay	1 Tbsp	60	0
Parkay (stick)	1 Tbsp	60	0

MARSHMALLOW

FOOD	PORTION	CALORIES	CHOLESTEROL
Funmallows (Kraft)	1	25	0
Funmallows Miniature (Kraft)	10	18	0
Jet-Puffed (Kraft)	1	25	0
Miniature (Kraft)	10	18	0
miniature	1	2	0

FOOD	PORTION	CALORIES	CHOLESTEROL
MATZO			
Daily Thin Tea (Manischewitz)	1	103	0
Dietetic Thins (Manischewitz)	1	91	0
Egg n' Onion (Manischewitz)	1	112	15
Matzo Cracker Miniatures (Manischewitz)	10–20	90	0
Matzo Farfel (Manischewitz)	1 cup	280	0
Matzo Meal (Manischewitz)	1 cup	514	0
Passover (Manischewitz)	1	129	0
Passover Egg (Manischewitz)	1	132	25
Passover Egg Matzo Crackers (Manischewitz)	10	108	20
Unsalted (Manischewitz)	1	110	0
Wheat Matzo Crackers (Manischewitz)	10	90	0
Whole Wheat w/ Bran (Manischewitz)	1	110	0

MAYONNAISE

(*see also* MAYONNAISE TYPE SALAD DRESSING, RELISH)

REDUCED CALORIE			
Best Foods Light	1 Tbsp	50	5
Best Foods Light	1 cup	760	90

FOOD	PORTION	CALORIES	CHOLESTEROL
Diamond Crystal	1 Tbsp	50	5
Hellman's Light	1 Tbsp	50	5
Hellman's Light	1 cup	760	90
Kraft Light Reduced Calorie Mayonnaise	1 Tbsp	45	5
imitation	1 cup	232	103
imitation	1 Tbsp	15	6
soybean	1 Tbsp	34	4
soybean	1 cup	556	58
REGULAR			
Best Foods Real	1 Tbsp	100	5
Best Foods Real	1 cup	1570	95
Hellman's Real	1 Tbsp	100	5
Kraft Real Mayonnaise	1 Tbsp	100	5
Kraft Sandwich Spread	1 Tbsp	50	5
Mother's	1 Tbsp	100	10
mayonnaise	2 Tbsp	196	16
sandwich spread	1 Tbsp	60	12
soybean	1 Tbsp	99	8
soybean	1 cup	1577	130

MAYONNAISE TYPE SALAD DRESSING
(see also MAYONNAISE, RELISH)

FOOD	PORTION	CALORIES	CHOLESTEROL
Bright Day Dressing	1 Tbsp	60	0
Miracle Whip Salad Dressing	1 Tbsp	70	5
Weight Watchers Reduced Calorie Dressing	1 Tbsp	40	5

FOOD	PORTION	CALORIES	CHOLESTEROL
mayonnaise type salad dressing	1 cup	916	60
mayonnaise type salad dressing	2 Tbsp	114	8
REDUCED CALORIE			
soybean w/o cholesterol	1 cup	1084	0
soybean w/o cholesterol	1 Tbsp	68	0

MEAT SUBSTITUTE

(see also CHICKEN SUBSTITUTE, SAUSAGE SUBSTITUTE, TURKEY SUBSTITUTE)

FOOD	PORTION	CALORIES	CHOLESTEROL
Bolono, frzn (Worthington)	3.5 oz	138	1
Corn Dogs (Loma Linda)	1 (2.5 oz)	250	0
Dinner Cuts (Loma Linda)	2 (3.5 oz)	110	0
Dinner Cuts No Salt Added (Loma Linda)	2 (3.5 oz)	110	0
Fripats, frzn (Worthington)	3.5 oz	294	1
Griddle Steaks (Loma Linda)	1 (1.7 oz)	160	0
Griddle Steaks (Loma Linda)	1 (2 oz)	190	0
Leanies, frzn (Worthington)	3.5 oz	252	2
Meatless Big Franks (Loma Linda)	1 (1.8 oz)	100	0
Meatless Bologna (Loma Linda)	2 slices (2 oz)	150	0

FOOD	PORTION	CALORIES	CHOLESTEROL
Meatless Redi-Burger (Loma Linda)	½" slice (2.4 oz)	130	0
Meatless Roast Beef (Loma Linda)	2 slices (2 oz)	107	0
Meatless Salami (Loma Linda)	2 slices (2 oz)	98	0
Meatless Salami, frzn (Worthington)	3.5 oz	198	1
Meatless Savory Meatballs (Loma Linda)	7 (2.5 oz)	190	0
Meatless Sizzle Burger (Loma Linda)	1 (2.5 oz)	210	0
Meatless Sizzle Franks (Loma Linda)	2 (2.4 oz)	170	0
Meatless Swiss Steak w/ Gravy (Loma Linda)	1 steak (2.6 oz)	140	0
Meatless Vita-Burger Chunks (Loma Linda)	¼ cup	70	0
Meatless Vita-Burger Granules (Loma Linda)	3 Tbsp	70	0
Nuteena (Loma Linda)	½" slice (2.4 oz)	160	0
Okara Pattie, frzn (Natural Touch)	3.5 oz	208	tr
Olive Loaf (Loma Linda)	2 slices (2 oz)	119	0
Patties, frzn (Morningstar Farms)	3.5 oz	240	2
Patty Mix (Loma Linda)	¼ cup	50	0

FOOD	PORTION	CALORIES	CHOLESTEROL
Prime Stakes, canned (Worthington)	3.5 oz	182	2
Prosage Chub, frzn (Worthington)	3.5 oz	245	1
Prosage Links, frzn (Worthington)	3.5 oz	280	2
Prosage Patties, frzn (Worthington)	3.5 oz	279	2
Proteena (Loma Linda)	½" slice (2.5 oz)	140	0
Saucettes, canned (Worthington)	3.5 oz	210	2
Savory Dinner Loaf; mix not prep (Loma Linda)	¼ cup	50	0
Stakelets, frzn (Worthington)	3.5 oz	178	1
Stew Pac (Loma Linda)	2 oz	70	0
Tastee Cuts (Loma Linda)	2 pieces (2.5 oz)	70	0
Tender Bits (Loma Linda)	4 pieces (2 oz)	80	0
Tender Rounds w/ Gravy (Loma Linda)	6 pieces (2.6 oz)	120	0
Tofu Pups (Lightlife)	1 (1.5 oz)	92	0
Vege-Burger (Loma Linda)	½ cup	110	0
Vege-Burger NSA (Loma Linda)	½ cup	140	0
Vegelona (Loma Linda)	½ slice	100	0

FOOD	PORTION	CALORIES	CHOLESTEROL
Wham, frzn (Worthington)	3.5 oz	184	2
simulated sausage	1 link (25 g)	64	0
simulated sausage	1 patty (38 g)	97	0

MELON
(*see also individual names*)

FRESH

Cantalene (Chiquita)	1 cup	60	0
Honey Mist (Chiquita)	1 cup	80	0

FROZEN

melon balls	1 cup	55	0

MEXICAN FOOD
(*see also* CHIPS, DINNER, SNACKS)

CANNED

Jalapeno Sliced (Trappey's)	1 oz	6	0
Jalapeno Whole (Trappey's)	2 med peppers	8	0
Mexican Sauce (Pritikin Foods)	4 oz	50	0
Mexican Style Stewed Tomatoes (S&W)	½ cup	40	0
Picante Sauce (Estee)	2 Tbsp	8	0

FOOD	PORTION	CALORIES	CHOLESTEROL
Taco Sauce (Estee)	2 Tbsp	14	0
tomatoes w/ green chilies	½ cup	18	0
FRESH			
chili peppers, hot, raw	1 pepper	18	0
chili peppers, hot, raw; chopped	½ cup	30	0
tamale	1 (3.9 oz)	155	10
tortilla; baked	1 (.7 oz)	43	0
tortilla; steamed	1 (.7 oz)	43	0
FROZEN			
3 Beef Enchiladas (El Charrito)	1 pkg (11 oz)	560	55
3 Cheese Enchiladas (El Charrito)	1 pkg (11 oz)	470	30
3 Chicken Enchiladas (El Charrito)	1 pkg (11 oz)	440	60
4 Grande Beef Enchiladas (El Charrito)	1 pkg (16.5 oz)	890	65
6 Beef Enchiladas (El Charrito)	1 pkg (16.25 oz)	880	75
6 Beef & Cheese Enchiladas (El Charrito)	1 pkg (16.25 oz)	880	70
6 Cheese Enchiladas (El Charrito)	1 pkg (16.25 oz)	780	45
Beef Enchilada Dinner (El Charrito)	1 pkg (13.75 oz)	620	45
Beef & Bean Burritos (Patio)	5 oz	361	24
Beef & Bean Green Chili (Patio)	5 oz	330	26

FOOD	PORTION	CALORIES	CHOLESTEROL
Beef & Red Bean Chili Burritos (Patio)	5 oz	333	20
Beef Enchilada Dinner (Patio)	13.25 oz	514	28
Burrito Dinner (Patio)	12 oz	517	24
Burrito Grande B&B (El Charrito)	1 pkg (6 oz)	430	25
Burrito Grande Green Chili B&B (El Charrito)	1 pkg (6 oz)	410	20
Burrito Grande Jalapeno (El Charrito)	1 pkg (6 oz)	410	25
Burrito Grande Red Chili B&B (El Charrito)	1 pkg (6 oz)	410	25
Burrito Green Chili B&B (El Charrito)	1 pkg (5 oz)	370	20
Burrito Red Chili B&B (El Charrito)	1 pkg (5 oz)	380	20
Burrito Red Hot B&B (El Charrito)	1 pkg (5 oz)	540	20
Burrito Red Hot Beef (El Charrito)	1 pkg (5 oz)	340	20
Cheese Enchilada Dinner (El Charrito)	1 pkg (13.75 oz)	570	30
Cheese Enchilada Dinner (Patio)	12.25 oz	378	17
Chicken Enchilada Dinner (El Charrito)	1 pkg (13.75 oz)	510	50
Fiesta Dinner (Patio)	12.25 oz	461	28

FOOD	PORTION	CALORIES	CHOLESTEROL
Grande Beef Enchilada Dinner (El Charrito)	1 pkg (21 oz)	950	70
Grande Mexican Style Dinner (El Charrito)	1 pkg (20 oz)	850	65
Grande Satillo Dinner (El Charrito)	1 pkg (20.75 oz)	820	45
Mexican Dinner (Patio)	13.25	533	41
Mexican Style Dinner (El Charrito)	1 pkg (14.25 oz)	690	45
Queso Dinner (El Charrito)	1 pkg (13.25 oz)	490	15
Ranchera Dinner (Patio)	13 oz	468	33
Red Hot Burritos (Patio)	5 oz	352	21
Satillo Dinner (El Charrito)	1 pkg (13.5 oz)	570	30
Tortillas, Corn (El Charrito)	2	95	0
Tortillas, Flour (El Charrito)	2	170	0
HOME RECIPE			
burrito	1 (8 oz)	332	34
enchiladas, eggplant	1	142	7
taco salad	1 cup	292	71
tacos verde blanco y rojo	1 (5.6 oz)	296	38
MIX			
Taco Meat Seasoning, Mild (Ortega)	1 oz	90	0

FOOD	PORTION	CALORIES	CHOLESTEROL
Taco Meat Seasoning, Mild; as prep w/ ground beef (Ortega)	3 oz	180	60
Tortilla, Corn Masa Harina; not prep (Quaker)	1 cup	421	0
Tortilla, Wheat Masa Trigo; not prep (Quaker)	1 cup	458	0

MILK
(see also CHOCOLATE, COCOA, MILK DRINKS)

FOOD	PORTION	CALORIES	CHOLESTEROL
CANNED			
Carnation Evaporated	½ cup	170	37
Carnation Evaporated Lowfat	½ cup	110	18
Carnation Evaporated Skimmed	½ cup	100	5
Pet 99 Evaporated Skimmed	½ cup	100	1
Pet Evaporated	½ cup	170	36
condensed, sweetened	1 oz	123	13
evaporated	1 oz	42	9
evaporated, skim	1 oz	25	1
DRIED			
Carnation Nonfat Dry; as prep w/ water	8 oz	80	4
Carnation Nonfat Dry; as prep w/ water	1 qt	320	16
Flash Instant Nonfat; as prep	8 oz	80	5
buttermilk, sweet cream	1 Tbsp	25	5
instantized	1 cup	244	12

FOOD	PORTION	CALORIES	CHOLESTEROL
nonfat	¼ cup	109	6
whey, sweet	1 cup	512	9
whole	¼ cup	159	31
LIQUID, LOWFAT			
Lowfat Buttermilk (Land O'Lakes)	8 oz	100	10
Lowfat Friendship Buttermilk	8 oz	120	14
Lowfat Lactaid	8 oz	102	10
Lowfat Land O'Lakes, 1%	8 oz	100	10
Lowfat Land O'Lakes, 2%	8 oz	120	20
lowfat, 1%, nonfat milk solids added	1 cup	104	10
lowfat, 1%, protein fortified	1 cup	119	10
lowfat, 1%	1 cup	102	10
lowfat, 2%, protein fortified	1 cup	137	19
lowfat, 2%	1 cup	121	18
lowfat buttermilk	1 cup	99	9
lowfat whey, sweet	1 cup	66	5
LIQUID, REGULAR			
Regular Land O'Lakes	8 oz	150	35
regular filled milk	1 cup	154	4
regular goat milk	1 cup	168	28
regular human milk	1 fl oz	21	4
regular imitation milk	1 cup	150	tr
regular Indian buffalo	1 cup	236	46
regular sheep	1 cup	26	4
regular whole, 3.3% fat	1 cup	150	33

FOOD	PORTION	CALORIES	CHOLESTEROL
regular whole, low sodium	1 cup	149	33
LIQUID, SKIM			
Skim Land O'Lakes	8 oz	90	5
skim	1 cup	86	4
skim, nonfat milk solids added	1 cup	90	5
skim, protein fortified	1 cup	100	5

MILK DRINKS
(see also BREAKFAST DRINKS, CHOCOLATE, COCOA)

FOOD	PORTION	CALORIES	CHOLESTEROL
Chocolate Milk (Land O'Lakes)	8 oz	210	30
Chocolate Milk, 1% (Land O'Lakes)	8 oz	160	5
Chocolate Skim Milk (Land O'Lakes)	8 oz	140	5
chocolate, lowfat, 1%	1 cup	158	7
chocolate, lowfat, 2%	1 cup	179	17
chocolate, whole	1 cup	208	30
strawberry flavor mix; as prep w/ whole milk	9 oz	234	33

MILK SUBSTITUTE
(see also COFFEE WHITENERS)

FOOD	PORTION	CALORIES	CHOLESTEROL
Vitamite (Deihl)	8 oz	100	0

MILKFISH

FOOD	PORTION	CALORIES	CHOLESTEROL
FRESH			
raw	3 oz	126	44

FOOD	PORTION	CALORIES	CHOLESTEROL

MILKSHAKE

FOOD	PORTION	CALORIES	CHOLESTEROL
Chocolate (Micro Magic)	1 shake (11.5 oz)	440	50
Strawberry (Micro Magic)	1 shake (11.5 oz)	440	49
Vanilla (Micro Magic)	1 shake (11.5 oz)	490	56
chocolate thick shake	10.6 oz	356	32
chocolate, fast food	10 oz	360	37
strawberry, fast food	10 oz	319	31
vanilla, fast food	10 oz	314	32
vanilla thick shake	11 oz	350	37

MINERAL WATER/BOTTLED WATER

FOOD	PORTION	CALORIES	CHOLESTEROL
Artesia	7 oz	0	0
Artesia Almund	7 oz	0	0
Artesia Cranberi	7 oz	0	0
Artesia Lemin	7 oz	0	0
Artesia Orange	7 oz	0	0
Crystal Geyser Sparkling Mineral Water	6 oz	0	0
Crystal Geyser Sparkling Mineral Water Cherry Chocolate	6 oz	0	0
Crystal Geyser Sparkling Mineral Water Lemon	6 oz	0	0
Crystal Geyser Sparkling Mineral Water Lime	6 oz	0	0
Crystal Geyser Sparkling Mineral Water Natural Wild Cherry w/ Vitafort	6 oz	0	0

FOOD	PORTION	CALORIES	CHOLESTEROL
Crystal Geyser Sparkling Mineral Water Orange	6 oz	0	0
Diamond Spring Water	1 qt (liter)	0	0
Mountain Valley Water	1 qt (liter)	0	0
Perrier	6.5 oz	0	0
Poland Springs	8 oz	0	0
Vichy (Schweppes)	6 oz	0	0

MISO

miso	½ cup	284	0

MOCHA

Bavarian Mint Mocha Sugar Free; as prep (Hills Bros.)	6 oz	35	0
Bavarian Mint Mocha; as prep (Hills Bros.)	6 oz	50	0
Cafe Mocha; as prep (Hills Bros.)	6 oz	50	0
Cafe Mocha; as prep (MJB Co.)	6 oz	50	0
Cherry Mocha; as prep (MJB Co.)	6 oz	50	0
Fudge Mocha Sugar Free; as prep (MJB Co.)	6 oz	40	0
Mint Mocha Sugar Free; as prep (MJB Co.)	6 oz	35	0
Mint Mocha; as prep (MJB Co.)	6 oz	50	0

FOOD	PORTION	CALORIES	CHOLESTEROL
Swiss Mocha; as prep (Hills Bros.)	6 oz	40	0
Vanilla Mocha Sugar Free; as prep (MJB Co.)	6 oz	40	0

MOLASSES

Grandma's Gold Label	1 Tbsp	70	0
Grandma's Green Label	1 Tbsp	70	0
blackstrap	1 Tbsp	43	0
molasses	1 Tbsp	46	0

MONKFISH

FRESH			
raw	3 oz	64	21

MOTHBEANS

DRIED			
cooked	1 cup	207	0
raw	1 cup	673	0

MOUSSE

Chocolate Mousse No Bake Dessert (Jell-O)	1 pkg (3.5 oz)	415	4
Chocolate Mousse No Bake Dessert; as prep (Jell-O)	½ cup	141	9
Chocolate Fudge Mousse No Bake Dessert (Jell-O)	1 pkg (3.5 oz)	406	4

FOOD	PORTION	CALORIES	CHOLESTEROL
Chocolate Fudge Mousse No Bake Dessert; as prep (Jell-O)	½ cup	138	9

HOME RECIPE

FOOD	PORTION	CALORIES	CHOLESTEROL
crab	¼ cup	364	136
orange	½ cup	87	1

MUFFIN

FROZEN

FOOD	PORTION	CALORIES	CHOLESTEROL
Apple Cinnamon Spice Hearty Fruit Muffins (Sara Lee)	1	220	0
Banana Nut Bran Hearty Fruit Muffins (Sara Lee)	1	230	0
Blueberry Hearty Fruit Muffins (Sara Lee)	1	200	0
Golden Corn Hearty Fruit Muffins (Sara Lee)	1	250	0
Oatmeal 'N Fruit Hearty Fruit Muffins (Sara Lee)	1	230	0
Raisin Bran Hearty Fruit Muffins (Sara Lee)	1	220	0

HOME RECIPE

FOOD	PORTION	CALORIES	CHOLESTEROL
apple	1 (1.6 oz)	137	21
blueberry	1 (1.9 oz)	147	22
bran	1 (1.9 oz)	104	21
corn	1 (1.6 oz)	169	40

FOOD	PORTION	CALORIES	CHOLESTEROL
orange	1 (1.6 oz)	137	33
plain	1 (1.6 oz)	158	25
whole wheat	1 (1.6 oz)	123	31
MIX			
Blueberry Muffin Mix Bakery Style; as prep (Duncan Hines)	1	190	10
Bran & Honey Nut Muffin Mix Bakery Style; as prep (Duncan Hines)	1	200	10
Bran Date Muffin; as prep (Jiffy)	1	110	10
Cinnamon Swirl Muffin Mix Bakery Style; as prep (Duncan Hines)	1	200	10
Corn Muffin; as prep (Jiffy)	1	115	10
READY-TO-EAT			
Oat Bran Blueberry (Health Valley)	2 oz	140	0
Oat Bran Almond/Date (Health Valley)	2 oz	170	0
Oat Bran Raisin (Health Valley)	2 oz	140	0

MULLET

FRESH

striped, raw	3 oz	99	42
striped, raw	1 fillet (4.2 oz)	139	59

FOOD	PORTION	CALORIES	CHOLESTEROL
striped; cooked	1 fillet (3.3 oz)	139	59
striped; cooked	3 oz	127	54

MUNG BEANS

DRIED

cooked	1 cup	213	0
mung beans long rice	1 cup	492	0
raw	1 cup	719	0

SPROUTS

cooked	½ cup	13	0
raw	½ cup	16	0
stir-fried	½ cup	31	0

MUSHROOM

CANNED

Mushrooms (Libby)	¼ cup	35	0
Mushrooms (Seneca)	¼ cup	35	0
mushrooms	½ cup	19	0

DRIED

shitake	4	44	0

FRESH

raw	1	5	0
raw; sliced	½ cup	9	0
shitake; cooked	4	40	0
sliced; cooked	½ cup	21	0

FOOD	PORTION	CALORIES	CHOLESTEROL
FROZEN			
Mushroom Vegetable Crisp (Ore Ida)	2⅔ oz	130	5

MUSSEL

FRESH			
blue, raw	3 oz	73	24
blue, raw	1 cup	129	42
blue; cooked	3 oz	147	48

MUSTARD

READY-TO-USE			
Kosciuszko	1 tbsp	11	0
Kraft Horseradish Mustard	1 Tbsp	4	0
Kraft Pure Prepared	1 Tbsp	4	0
Plochman's Yellow Mustard	1 Tbsp	11	0
Plochman's Dijon Mustard	1 Tbsp	11	0
Plochman's Spicy Brown Mustard	1 Tbsp	11	0
Plochman's Stone Ground Mustard	1 Tbsp	11	0
Sauceworks Hot Mustard Sauce	1 Tbsp	35	5

MUSTARD GREENS

FRESH			
cooked; chopped	½ cup	11	0
raw; chopped	½ cup	7	0

FOOD	PORTION	CALORIES	CHOLESTEROL
FROZEN			
frzn; chopped, cooked	½ cup	14	0
frzn; not prep	½ cup	15	0

NATTO

natto	½ cup	187	0

NAVY BEANS

CANNED			
Navy Beans (Hanover)	½ cup	100	0
navy	1 cup	296	0
DRIED			
Navy (Hurst Brand)	1 cup	277	0
cooked	1 cup	259	0
raw	1 cup	697	0
SPROUTS			
cooked	3½ oz	78	0
raw	½ cup	35	0

NECTARINE

FRESH			
nectarine	1	67	0

NEUFCHATEL CHEESE
(see CREAM CHEESE)

NON-DAIRY CREAMERS
(see COFFEE WHITENERS)

FOOD	PORTION	CALORIES	CHOLESTEROL

NON-DAIRY WHIPPED TOPPINGS
(*see* WHIPPED TOPPINGS)

NOODLES
(*see also* PASTA DINNERS)

FOOD	PORTION	CALORIES	CHOLESTEROL
noodle pudding (home recipe)	½ cup	132	27
CANNED			
chow mein noodles	½ cup	228	3
DRY			
Egg Noodles (Creamette)	2 oz	221	70
Egg Noodles (Skinner)	2 oz	220	55
Egg Noodles Enriched (Ronzoni)	2 oz	211	61
Egg Noodles, uncooked (Mueller's)	2 oz	220	55
Fine, Medium, Wide & Extra Wide (P&R)	2 oz	220	55
Spinach Egg Noodles (Ronzoni)	2 oz	209	61
Spinach Egg Noodles Light 'N Fluffy (Skinner)	2 oz	220	55
egg noodles	½ cup	100	25

NUTRITIONAL SUPPLEMENTS
(*see also* BREAKFAST BAR, BREAKFAST DRINKS)

FOOD	PORTION	CALORIES	CHOLESTEROL
DIET			
Slender Chocolate (Carnation)	10 oz	220	4

FOOD	PORTION	CALORIES	CHOLESTEROL
Slender Chocolate Fudge (Carnation)	10 oz	220	4
Slender Chocolate Malt (Carnation)	10 oz	220	4
Slender Milk Chocolate (Carnation)	10 oz	220	4
Slender Vanilla (Carnation)	10 oz	220	5
Slender Bars Chocolate (Carnation)	2 bars	270	tr
Slender Bars Chocolate Chip (Carnation)	2 bars	270	tr
Slender Bars Chocolate Peanut Butter (Carnation)	2 bars	270	tr
Slender Bars Vanilla (Carnation)	2 bars	270	tr
Slender Instant Chocolate (Carnation)	1 pkg (1.06 oz)	110	3
Slender Instant Chocolate; as prep w/ 2% milk (Carnation)	1 pkg + 6 oz milk	200	15
Slender Instant Dutch Chocolate (Carnation)	1 pkg (1.06 oz)	110	2
Slender Instant Dutch Chocolate; as prep w/ 2% milk (Carnation)	1 pkg + 6 oz milk	200	14
Slender Instant French Vanilla (Carnation)	1 pkg (1.04 oz)	110	3
Slender Instant French Vanilla; as prep w/ 2% milk (Carnation)	1 pkg + 6 oz milk	200	15

FOOD	PORTION	CALORIES	CHOLESTEROL
REGULAR			
Ensure Black Walnut (Ross)	8 oz	254	3
Ensure Coffee (Ross)	8 oz	254	3
Ensure Eggnog (Ross)	8 oz	254	3
Ensure Strawberry (Ross)	8 oz	254	3
Ensure Vanilla (Ross)	8 oz	254	3
Ensure Plus, Coffee (Ross)	8 oz	355	4
Ensure Plus, Eggnog (Ross)	8 oz	355	4
Ensure Plus, Strawberry (Ross)	8 oz	355	4
Ensure Plus, Vanilla (Ross)	8 oz	355	4
Isocal (Mead Johnson)	8 oz	250	3
Isocal HCN (Mead Johnson)	8 oz	473	7
Lonalac (Mead Johnson)	1 oz	20	tr
Malsovit Mealwafers	2	152	0
Meal-on-the-Go Food Bar	1 (3 oz)	340	tr
Nutri-Care Strawberry	1 pkg (1.13 oz)	120	5
Nutri-Care, Strawberry; as prep w/ 1 cup whole milk	1 pkg (1.13 oz)	280	45

FOOD	PORTION	CALORIES	CHOLESTEROL
Nutri-Care, Strawberry; as prep w/ 1 cup 2% milk	1 pkg (1.13 oz)	260	25
Sustacal (Mead Johnson)	8 oz	240	2
Sustacal HC (Mead Johnson)	8 oz	360	4
Sustacal Pudding (Mead Johnson)	5 oz	240	tr

NUTS, MIXED
(see also individual names)

FOOD	PORTION	CALORIES	CHOLESTEROL
Cashews & Peanuts, Honey Roasted (Planters)	1 oz	170	0
Mixed Nuts Deluxe, Oil Roasted (Planters)	1 oz	180	0
Mixed Nuts, Dry Roasted (Planters)	1 oz	170	0
Mixed Nuts, Dry Roasted, Unsalted (Planters)	1 oz	170	0
Mixed Nuts, Oil Roasted (Planters)	1 oz	180	0
Mixed Nuts, Oil Roasted, Unsalted (Planters)	1 oz	180	0
Mixed Nuts w/ Peanuts (Guy's)	1 oz	180	0
Nut Topping (Planters)	1 oz	180	0
Tasty Mix (Guy's)	1 oz	130	0

FOOD	PORTION	CALORIES	CHOLESTEROL
Tavern Nuts (Planters)	1 oz	170	0
mixed, dry roasted, w/ peanuts	1 oz	169	0
mixed, oil roasted, w/ peanuts	1 oz	175	0
mixed, oil roasted, w/o peanuts	1 oz	175	0

OCTOPUS

FRESH			
raw	3 oz	70	41

OIL
(see also FAT)

FOOD	PORTION	CALORIES	CHOLESTEROL
Bertolli Classico	1 Tbsp	120	0
Bertolli Extra Light	1 Tbsp	120	0
Bertolli Extra Virgin	1 Tbsp	120	0
Crisco	1 Tbsp	120	0
Italica	1 Tbsp	120	0
Mazola	1 Tbsp	120	0
Mazola	1 cup	1955	0
Mazola No-Stick	2.5 second spray	6	0
Peanut (Planters)	1 Tbsp	120	0
Pompeian	1 Tbsp	130	0
Popcorn (Planters)	1 Tbsp	120	0
Puritan	1 Tbsp	120	0

FOOD	PORTION	CALORIES	CHOLESTEROL
almond	1 cup	1927	0
almond	1 Tbsp	120	0
apricot kernel	1 cup	1927	0
apricot kernel	1 Tbsp	120	0
cocoa butter	1 Tbsp	120	0
coconut	1 Tbsp	120	0
corn	1 cup	1927	0
corn	1 Tbsp	120	0
cottonseed	1 cup	1927	0
cottonseed	1 Tbsp	120	0
grapeseed	1 Tbsp	120	0
hazelnut	1 cup	1927	0
hazelnut	1 Tbsp	120	0
olive	1 Tbsp	119	0
olive	1 cup	1909	0
palm	1 cup	1927	0
palm	1 Tbsp	120	0
palm kernel	1 Tbsp	120	0
palm kernel	1 cup	1927	0
palm, Babassu	1 Tbsp	120	0
peanut	1 cup	1909	0
peanut	1 Tbsp	119	0
poppyseed	1 Tbsp	120	0
rapeseed	1 Tbsp	120	0
rapeseed	1 cup	1927	0
rice bran	1 Tbsp	120	0
safflower	1 Tbsp	120	0

FOOD	PORTION	CALORIES	CHOLESTEROL
safflower	1 cup	1927	0
sesame	1 Tbsp	120	0
soybean	1 Tbsp	120	0
soybean	1 cup	1927	0
soybean & cottonseed	1 Tbsp	120	0
soybean & cottonseed	1 cup	1927	0
soybean, hydrogenated	1 cup	1927	0
soybean, hydrogenated	1 Tbsp	120	0
sunflower	1 Tbsp	120	0
sunflower	1 cup	1927	0
walnut	1 cup	1927	0
walnut	1 Tbsp	120	0
wheat germ	1 Tbsp	120	0

OKRA

FOOD	PORTION	CALORIES	CHOLESTEROL
Okra Cut (Trappey's)	½ cup	25	0
FRESH			
raw	8 pods	36	0
raw; sliced	½ cup	19	0
sliced; cooked	½ cup	25	0
FROZEN			
Cut Okra (Hanover)	½ cup	25	0
Okra Vegetable Crisp (Ore Ida)	3 oz	160	5
Whole Okra (Hanover)	½ cup	35	0

FOOD	PORTION	CALORIES	CHOLESTEROL
frzn; not prep	10 oz pkg	85	0
okra; sliced, cooked	½ cup	34	0
okra; cooked	10 oz pkg	94	0

OLIVES

Ripe Extra Large (S&W)	1 oz	47	0
Ripe Large (S&W)	1 oz	47	0
Ripe Pitted Extra Large (S&W)	1 oz	47	0
Ripe Pitted Jumbo (S&W)	1 oz	47	0
Ripe Pitted Large (S&W)	1 oz	47	0
Spanish Green (Tee Pee)	2 oz	98	0

ONION

CANNED			
Whole Small (S&W)	½ cup	35	0
onions; chopped	½ cup	21	0
DRIED			
onions	1 Tbsp	16	0
FRESH			
onions; chopped, cooked	½ cup	29	0
raw; chopped	1 Tbsp	3	0
FROZEN			
Chopped (Ore Ida)	2 oz	20	0

FOOD	PORTION	CALORIES	CHOLESTEROL
Chopped (Southland)	2 oz	15	0
Onions Small Whole (Birds Eye)	½ cup	40	0
Onions Small w/ Cream Sauce (Birds Eye)	½ cup	100	tr
Rings (Ore Ida)	2 oz	140	0
chopped; cooked	1 Tbsp	4	0
chopped; cooked	½ cup	30	0
chopped; not prep	1 pkg (10 oz)	83	0
onion rings	9 oz pkg	658	0
onion rings	16 oz pkg	1170	0
onion rings; cooked	2 rings	81	0
whole; not prep	10 oz pkg	101	0

ORANGE

FOOD	PORTION	CALORIES	CHOLESTEROL
CANDIED orange peel	1 oz	90	0
CANNED Mandarin Natural Style (S&W)	½ cup	60	0
Mandarin Oranges in Light Syrup (Dole)	½ cup	76	0
Mandarin Selected Sections in Heavy Syrup (S&W)	½ cup	76	0

FOOD	PORTION	CALORIES	CHOLESTEROL
FRESH			
orange	1	62	0
peel	1 Tbsp	0	0
peel; grated	1 tsp	0	0
JUICE			
Orange (Tree Top)	6 oz	90	0
Orange Juice (Ocean Spray)	6 oz	90	0
Orange Juice 100% Pure Unsweetened (Kraft)	6 oz	90	0
Unsweetened 100% Juice (S&W)	6 oz	83	0
chilled	1 cup	110	0
fresh	1 cup	111	0
frzn; as prep	1 cup	112	0
frzn; not prep	6 oz container	339	0
orange juice	1 cup	104	0

ORANGE EXTRACT

Virginia Dare	1 tsp	22	0

ORGAN MEATS
(*see* BRAINS, GIBLETS, GIZZARD, HEART, KIDNEY, LIVER)

ORIENTAL FOOD
(*see also* DINNER, RICE)

CANNED			
Chun King Divider Pak Beef Chow Mein	7 oz	100	15

FOOD	PORTION	CALORIES	CHOLESTEROL
Chun King Divider Pak Beef Chow Mein	8 oz	110	20
Chun King Divider Pak Beef Pepper Oriental	7 oz	110	15
Chun King Divider Pak Chicken Chow Mein	7 oz	110	15
Chun King Divider Pak Chicken Chow Mein	8 oz	120	10
Chun King Divider Pak Pork Chow Mein Mein	7 oz	120	25
Chun King Divider Pak Shrimp Chow Mein	7 oz	100	30
Chun King Stir-Fry Entree Chow Mein w/ Chicken	6 oz	220	45
Chun King Stir-Fry Entree Chow Mein w/Beef	6 oz	290	50
Chun King Stir-Fry Entree Pepper Steak	6 oz	250	50
Chun King Stir-Fry Entree Sukiyaki	6 oz	290	50
Chun King Stir-Fry Entree Egg Foo Young	5 oz	140	140
chop suey w/ meat	1 cup	144	5
chow mein chicken	1 cup	95	8
chow mein noodles	½ cup	228	3
FROZEN Birds Eye Chinese Style International Recipe	½ cup	68	tr
Birds Eye Chinese Style Stir-Fry Vegetable	½ cup	36	0

FOOD	PORTION	CALORIES	CHOLESTEROL
Birds Eye Chow Mein Style International Recipe	½ cup	89	tr
Birds Eye Japanese Style International Recipe	½ cup	88	tr
Birds Eye Japanese Style Stir-Fry Vegetalbe	½ cup	29	0
Birds Eye Mandarin Style International Recipe	½ cup	86	tr
Budget Gourmet Slim Select Mandarin Chicken	10 oz	290	25
Budget Gourmet Slim Select Oriental Beef	10 oz	290	25
Budget Gourmet Teriyaki Chicken	12 oz	360	55
La Choy Fresh & Lite Almond Chicken	9.75 oz	290	33
La Choy Fresh & Lite Beef Teriyaki	10 oz	280	48
La Choy Fresh & Lite Beef & Broccoli	11 oz	290	54
La Choy Fresh & Lite Imperial Chicken Chow Mein	11 oz	270	45
La Choy Fresh & Lite Pepper Steak	10 oz	290	54
La Choy Fresh & Lite Shrimp w/ Lobster Sauce	10 oz	220	99
La Choy Fresh & Lite Spicy Chicken Oriental	9.75 oz	290	27
La Choy Fresh & Lite Sweet & Sour Chicken	10 oz	280	33
Lean Cuisine Chicken Chow Mein w/ Rice	11¼ oz	250	30

FOOD	PORTION	CALORIES	CHOLESTEROL
Lean Cuisine Shrimp & Chicken Cantonese w/ Noodles	10⅛ oz	260	105
Lean Cuisine Szechwan Beef w/ Noodles & Vegetables	9¼ oz	280	90
HOME RECIPE			
chicken teriyaki	¾ cup	399	92
chop suey w/ pork	1 cup	375	62
chow mein chicken	1 cup	255	78
chow mein pork	1 cup	425	89
chow mein shrimp	1 cup	221	55
egg foo yung	1 (5.1 oz)	150	250
wonton; fried	½ cup	111	31
MIX			
Kikkoman Chow Mein Seasoning	1⅛ oz pkg	98	tr
Kikkoman Teriyaki Baste & Glaze	1 Tbsp	27	0

OYSTER

FOOD	PORTION	CALORIES	CHOLESTEROL
CANNED			
Whole (Bumble Bee)	½ cup (3.5 oz)	100	55
eastern	1 cup	170	136
eastern	3 oz	58	46
FRESH			
eastern, raw	6 med	58	46
eastern, raw	1 cup	170	136
eastern; cooked	6 med	58	46

FOOD	PORTION	CALORIES	CHOLESTEROL
eastern; cooked	3 oz	117	93
FROZEN			
Carnation Jumbo or Extra Select Breaded Oysters (King & Prince)	3.5 oz	130	26
HOME RECIPE			
eastern; breaded & fried	3 oz	167	69
eastern; breaded & fried	6 med	173	72
oysters Rockefeller	3 oysters	66	38
stew	1 cup	278	100

PANCAKE/WAFFLE SYRUP
(see also SYRUP)

FOOD	PORTION	CALORIES	CHOLESTEROL
Alaga Breakfast	2 Tbsp	108	0
Alaga Butter Lite	2 Tbsp	54	0
Alaga Honey Flavor	2 Tbsp	124	0
Alaga Lite	2 Tbsp	54	0
Estee	1 Tbsp	4	0
Golden Griddle (Best Foods)	1 Tbsp	55	0
Golden Griddle (Best Foods)	1 cup	885	0
Karo Pancake Syrup	1 Tbsp	60	0
Light Magic (Whitfield)	2 Tbsp	121	0
Log Cabin Syrup Buttered	1 oz	106	2
Log Cabin Syrup Country Kitchen	1 oz	101	0
Log Cabin Syrup Lite	1 oz	61	0
Log Cabin Syrup Maple Honey	1 oz	106	0

FOOD	PORTION	CALORIES	CHOLESTEROL
Log Cabin Syrup Regular	1 oz	99	0
Tastee	2 Tbsp	121	0
Tastee Maple	2 Tbsp	113	0
Yellow Label (Whitfield)	2 Tbsp	125	0
Yellow Label Butter Flavor (Whitfield)	2 Tbsp	117	0
Yellow Label Maple Flavor (Whitfield)	2 Tbsp	117	0

PANCAKES

FROZEN, READY-TO-USE

Pancake (Morningstar Farms)	3.5 oz	232	4

HOME RECIPE

buckwheat	1 (6" diam)	137	0
buckwheat	1 (4" diam)	68	0
buttermilk	1 (6" diam)	164	54
buttermilk	1 (4" diam)	61	20
plain	1 (6" diam)	164	54
plain	1 (4" diam)	61	20
potato	1 (4" diam)	78	60
zucchini	1 (4" diam)	69	31

FOOD	PORTION	CALORIES	CHOLESTEROL
MIX			
Hungry Jack Extra Lights; as prep (Pillsbury)	3 (4" diam)	210	150
Original Mix; as prep (Aunt Jemima)	3 (4" diam)	200	146
Pancake Mix; as prep (Estee)	3 (3" diam)	100	0
Pancake Mix; not prep (Health Valley)	1 oz	100	0

PAPAYA

FRESH			
Papayas (Produce Marketing Assoc)	½	80	0
papaya	1	117	0
JUICE			
nectar	1 cup	142	0

PARSNIP

FRESH			
cooked; sliced	½ cup	63	0
raw; sliced	½ cup	50	0

PASSION FRUIT

FRESH			
passion fruit	1	18	0

FOOD	PORTION	CALORIES	CHOLESTEROL

PASTA
(see also NOODLES, PASTA DINNERS, PASTA SALAD)

FOOD	PORTION	CALORIES	CHOLESTEROL
DRY			
Acini de Pepe (San Giorgio)	2 oz	210	0
All Shapes (Mueller's)	2 oz	210	0
Alphabets (P&R)	2 oz	210	0
Alphabets (San Giorgio)	2 oz	210	0
Alphabets (Skinner)	2 oz	210	0
Baby Pastina (San Giorgio)	2 oz	210	0
Bows, Medium & Small (P&R)	2 oz	220	55
Capellini (Delmonico)	2 oz	210	0
Capellini (P&R)	2 oz	210	0
Capellini (San Giorgio)	2 oz	210	0
Ditalini (San Giorgio)	2 oz	210	0
Elbow Macaroni (Delmonico)	2 oz	210	0
Elbow Macaroni (San Giorgio)	2 oz	210	0
Elbow Macaroni (Skinner)	2 oz	210	0

FOOD	PORTION	CALORIES	CHOLESTEROL
Elbow Macaroni, Regular & Large (P&R)	2 oz	210	0
Elbow Spaghetti (Delmonico)	2 oz	210	0
Elbows Whole Wheat (Health Valley)	2 oz	170	0
Elbows w/ 4 Vegetables Whole Wheat (Health Valley)	2 oz	170	0
Fettuccini (P&R)	2 oz	210	0
Fettucini (Skinner)	2 oz	210	0
Fetuccini, Egg (P&R)	2 oz	220	55
Fideo Enrollacio (Skinner)	2 oz	210	0
Flakes (San Giorgio)	2 oz	210	0
Fusilli Cut (San Giorgio)	2 oz	210	0
Fusilli Cut (P&R)	2 oz	210	0
Kluski (San Giorgio)	2 oz	220	55
Lasagna (Delmonico)	2 oz	210	0
Lasagna (Skinner)	2 oz	210	0
Lasagna, Jumbo (P&R)	2 oz	210	0

FOOD	PORTION	CALORIES	CHOLESTEROL
Lasagna Spinach Whole Wheat (Health Valley)	2 oz	170	0
Lasagna Whole Wheat (Health Valley)	2 oz	170	0
Lasagne (Mueller's)	2 oz	210	0
Linguini (P&R)	2 oz	210	0
Linguini (San Giorgio)	2 oz	210	0
Linguini (Skinner)	2 oz	210	0
Linguini (Skinner)	2 oz	210	0
Linguini, Egg (Creamette)	2 oz	221	70
Macaroni (Ronzoni)	2 oz	209	0
Manicotti (P&R)	2 oz	210	0
Manicotti (San Giorgio)	2 oz	210	0
Manicotti (Skinner)	2 oz	210	0
Mostaccioli (Delmonico)	2 oz	210	0
Mostaccioli (Skinner)	2 oz	210	0
Mostaccioli Rigati (San Giorgio)	2 oz	210	0
Orzo (San Giorgio)	2 oz	210	0

FOOD	PORTION	CALORIES	CHOLESTEROL
Perciatelli (P&R)	2 oz	210	0
Perciatelli (San Giorgio)	2 oz	210	0
Pot Pie Bows (San Giorgio)	2 oz	220	55
Pot Pie Squares (San Giorgio)	2 oz	220	55
Racing Wheels (San Giorgio)	2 oz	210	0
Ribbon Pasta Whole Wheat (Pritikin Foods)	2 oz	220	0
Rigatoni (Delmonico)	2 oz	210	0
Rigatoni (San Giorgio)	2 oz	210	0
Rigatoni (Skinner)	2 oz	210	0
Rings (P&R)	2 oz	210	0
Rippled Lasagne (San Giorgio)	2 oz	210	0
Ripplets (Skinner)	2 oz	210	0
Rotelle (Creamette)	2 oz	210	0
Rotini (Delmonico)	2 oz	210	0
Rotini (San Giorgio)	2 oz	210	0
Rotini, Rainbow (Creamette)	2 oz	210	0

FOOD	PORTION	CALORIES	CHOLESTEROL
Shell Macaroni (Skinner)	2 oz	210	0
Shells, Large, Medium, Small & Jumbo (P&R)	2 oz	210	0
Shells, Large, Medium, Small & Jumbo (San Giorgio)	2 oz	210	0
Shells, Regular & Jumbo (Delmonico)	2 oz	210	0
Spaghetti (Delmonico)	2 oz	210	0
Spaghetti (San Giorgio)	2 oz	210	0
Spaghetti (Skinner)	2 oz	210	0
Spaghetti, Regular & Thin (P&R)	2 oz	210	0
Spaghetti Wheels (Hanover)	½ cup	90	0
Spaghetti Whole Wheat (Health Valley)	2 oz	170	0
Spaghetti Whole Wheat (Pritikin Foods)	2 oz	220	0
Spaghetti w/ Amaranth Whole Wheat (Health Valley)	2 oz	170	0
Spaghetti w/ Spinach Whole Wheat (Health Valley)	2 oz	170	0
Spaghetti, Egg (Creamette)	2 oz	221	70

FOOD	PORTION	CALORIES	CHOLESTEROL
Spaghetti, Thin (Creamette)	2 oz	210	0
Spaghetti; uncooked (Mueller's)	2 oz	210	0
Spaghettini (Delmonico)	2 oz	210	0
Spaghettini (San Giorgio)	2 oz	210	0
Spinach Macaroni (Ronzoni)	2 oz	203	0
Spinach Macaroni (Ronzoni)	2 oz	206	0
Tubettini (San Giorgio)	2 oz	210	0
Twirls (Skinner)	2 oz	210	0
Twists, Tri Color (Mueller's)	2 oz	210	0
Vermicelli (Delmonico)	2 oz	210	0
Vermicelli (P&R)	2 oz	210	0
Vermicelli (San Giorgio)	2 oz	210	0
Vermicelli (Skinner)	2 oz	210	0
Ziti (Creamette)	2 oz	210	0
Ziti Cut (Delmonico)	2 oz	210	0
Ziti Cut (San Giorgio)	2 oz	210	0

FOOD	PORTION	CALORIES	CHOLESTEROL

PASTA DINNERS
   (*see also* DINNER, PASTA SALAD)

CANNED

FOOD	PORTION	CALORIES	CHOLESTEROL
spaghetti w/ meatballs & tomato sauce	1 cup	258	23
spaghetti w/ tomato sauce & cheese	1 cup	190	15

DRY MIX

FOOD	PORTION	CALORIES	CHOLESTEROL
Kraft American Style Spaghetti Dinner; as prep	1 cup	310	0
Kraft Egg Noodle & Cheese Dinner; as prep	¾ cup	340	50
Kraft Macaroni & Cheese Dinner Family Size; as prep	¾ cup	290	5
Kraft Macaroni & Cheese Dinner; as prep	¾ cup	290	5
Kraft Macaroni & Cheese Deluxe Dinner; as prep	¾ cup	260	20
Kraft Spaghetti w/ Meat Sauce Dinner; as prep	1 cup	360	15
Kraft Spiral Macaroni & Cheese Dinner; as prep	¾ cup	330	10
Kraft Tangy Italian Style Spaghetti Dinner; as prep	1 cup	310	5
Velveeta Shells and Cheese Dinner; as prep	¾ cup	260	25

FROZEN

FOOD	PORTION	CALORIES	CHOLESTEROL
Birds Eye Pasta Primavera Style International Recipe	½ cup	121	3

FOOD	PORTION	CALORIES	CHOLESTEROL
Budget Gourmet Cheese Manicotti w/ Meat Sauce	10 oz	450	50
Budget Gourmet Chicken w/ Fettucini	10 oz	400	100
Budget Gourmet Italian Sausage Lasagne	10 oz	420	80
Budget Gourmet Linguini w/ Shrimp	10 oz	330	75
Budget Gourmet Pasta Alfredo w/ Broccoli	5.5 oz	200	25
Budget Gourmet Pasta Shells & Beef	10 oz	340	35
Budget Gourmet Slim Select Cheese Ravioli	10 oz	260	45
Budget Gourmet Slim Select Fettucini w/ Meat Sauce	10 oz	290	25
Budget Gourmet Slim Select Lasagne w/ Meat Sauce	10 oz	290	25
Budget Gourmet Slim Select Linguini w/ Scallops & Clams	9.5 oz	280	60
Budget Gourmet Three Cheese Lasagna	10 oz	400	65
Lean Cuisine Linguini w/ Clam Sauce	9⅝ oz	260	30
Lean Cuisine Tuna Lasagna w/ Spinach Noodles & Vegetables	9¾ oz	280	25
Lean Cuisine Veal Lasagna	10¼ oz	280	75
Lean Cuisine Veal Primavera	9⅛ oz	250	80
Lean Cuisine Zucchini Lasagna	11 oz	260	20

FOOD	PORTION	CALORIES	CHOLESTEROL
Macaroni & Cheese (Budget Gourmet)	5.3 oz	210	25
OH Boy! Lasagna w/ Meat & Sauce	6 oz	230	35
OH Boy! Spaghetti & Meatballs	7 oz	190	17
Sensible Chef Fettucini Alfredo w/ Chicken Casserole	9 oz	410	56
Sensible Chef Linguini w/ Shrimp & Clams Casserole	9 oz	190	46
Tortellini, Cheese (Budget Gourmet)	5.5 oz	180	15
HOME RECIPE lasagna	1 piece 2½" × 2½" (8.8 oz)	374	107
macaroni & cheese	¾ cup	323	32
manicotti	¾ cup	273	77
noodle pudding	½ cup	132	27
rigatoni w/ sausage sauce	¾ cup	260	59
spaghetti w/ meatballs & cheese	1 cup	407	104
spaghetti w/ meatballs & tomato sauce	1 cup	332	74

PASTA SALAD

FOOD	PORTION	CALORIES	CHOLESTEROL
FROZEN Italian Pasta Salad (Hanover)	½ cup	60	0
Milano Pasta Salad (Hanover)	½ cup	60	0

FOOD	PORTION	CALORIES	CHOLESTEROL
Oriental Pasta Salad (Hanover)	½ cup	80	0
Primavera Pasta Salad (Hanover)	½ cup	50	0

PÂTÉ

CANNED			
goose liver, smoked	1 oz	131	43
goose liver, smoked	1 tbsp	60	20

PEACH

CANNED			
Clingstone Halves (S&W)	½ cup	100	0
Freestone Halves in Heavy Syrup (S&W)	½ cup	100	0
Freestone Sliced in Heavy Syrup (S&W)	½ cup	100	0
Yellow Cling Natural Lite (S&W)	½ cup	50	0
Yellow Cling Natural Style (S&W)	½ cup	90	0
Yellow Cling Sliced Premium in Heavy Syrup (S&W)	½ cup	100	0
Yellow Cling Whole, Spiced, in Heavy Syrup (S&W)	½ cup	90	0
halves in heavy syrup	1 cup	190	0
halves in juice	1 cup	109	0

FOOD	PORTION	CALORIES	CHOLESTEROL
halves in water pack	1 cup	58	0
peaches, spiced, in heavy syrup	1 cup	180	0
DRIED Peaches (Mariani)	¼ cup	140	0
halves	10	311	0
FRESH peach	1	37	0
FROZEN peaches, sweetened, sliced	1 cup	235	0
JUICE Peach (Smucker's)	8 oz	120	0
Pure & Light (Dole)	6 oz	102	0
nectar	1 cup	134	0

PEANUT BUTTER

FOOD	PORTION	CALORIES	CHOLESTEROL
BAMA Creamy Peanut Butter	2 Tbsp	200	0
BAMA Crunchy Peanut Butter	2 Tbsp	200	0
BAMA Jelly & Peanut Butter	2 Tbsp	150	0
Erewhon Chunky Salted	2 Tbsp	190	0
Erewhon Chunky Unsalted	2 Tbsp	190	0
Erewhon Creamy Salted	2 Tbsp	190	0
Erewhon Creamy Unsalted	2 Tbsp	14	0
Estee	1 Tbsp	100	0
Health Valley Chunky	1 Tbsp	83	0

FOOD	PORTION	CALORIES	CHOLESTEROL
Health Valley Chunky No Salt	1 Tbsp	83	0
Health Valley Creamy	1 Tbsp	83	0
Health Valley Creamy No Salt	1 Tbsp	83	0
Home Brand Natural Lightly Salted	2 Tbsp	210	0
Home Brand Natural Unsalted	2 Tbsp	210	0
Home Brand No Sugar Added	2 Tbsp	180	0
Home Brand Real Peanut Butter	2 Tbsp	210	0
Jif Creamy	2 Tbsp	190	0
Jif Crunchy	2 Tbsp	190	0
Reese's Peanut Butter Flavored Chips (Hershey)	¼ cup	230	5
Sexton Salt Free	1 Tbsp	98	0
Skippy Creamy	2 Tbsp	190	0
Skippy Creamy	1 cup	1540	0
Skippy Creamy; w/ 2 slices white bread	1 sandwich	340	0
Skippy Super Chunk	2 Tbsp	190	0
Skippy Super Chunk	1 cup	1540	0
Skippy Super Chunk; w/ 2 slices white bread	1 sandwich	340	0
Smucker's Goober Grape	2 Tbsp	180	0
Smucker's Goober Honey	2 Tbsp	180	0
Smucker's Natural	2 Tbsp	200	0
Smucker's Natural No Salt Added	2 Tbsp	200	0
Teddie Natural Peanut Butter No Salt Added	2 Tbsp	200	0

FOOD	PORTION	CALORIES	CHOLESTEROL
chunk style	1 cup	1520	0
chunk style	2 Tbsp	188	0
peanut butter	1 Tbsp	95	0
peanut butter	1 cup	1526	0
smooth style	2 Tbsp	188	0
smooth style	1 cup	1517	0

PEANUTS

FOOD	PORTION	CALORIES	CHOLESTEROL
Cocktail, Oil Roasted (Planters)	1 oz	170	0
Cocktail, Oil Roasted, Unsalted (Planters)	1 oz	170	0
Dry Roasted (Guy's)	1 oz	170	0
Dry Roasted (Lance)	1⅛ oz	190	0
Dry Roasted (Planters)	1 oz	160	0
Dry Roasted, Honey Roasted (Planters)	1 oz	160	0
Dry Roasted, Unsalted (Planters)	1 oz	170	0
Honey Roasted (Planters)	1 oz	170	0
Honey Toasted P'nuts (Lance)	1⅜ oz	230	0
Honey Toasted P'nuts (Lance)	1¼ oz	210	0
Party Peanuts (Fisher)	1 oz	160	0

FOOD	PORTION	CALORIES	CHOLESTEROL
Peanuts (Beer Nuts)	1 oz	180	0
Redskin, Oil Roasted (Planters)	1 oz	170	0
Redskin, Salted (Lance)	1⅛ oz	190	0
Roasted w/ Shell (Lance)	1¾ oz	190	0
Roasted-in-shell, Salted (Planters)	1 oz	160	0
Roasted-in-shell, Unsalted (Planters)	1 oz	160	0
Salted (Lance)	1⅛ oz	190	0
Salted (Little Debbie)	1 pkg (1.25 oz)	230	tr
Salted, Oil Roasted (Planters)	1 oz	170	0
Spanish, Oil Roasted (Planters)	1 oz	170	0
Spanish, Oil Roasted (Planters)	1 cup	851	0
Spanish, Dry Roasted (Planters)	1 oz	160	0
Spanish, Raw (Planters)	1 oz	150	0
Spanish, Salted (Guy's)	1 oz	170	0
Sweet 'N Crunchy (Planters)	1 oz	140	0

FOOD	PORTION	CALORIES	CHOLESTEROL
boiled	½ cup	102	0
dried	1 oz	161	0
dry roasted	1 cup	855	0
dry roasted	1 oz	164	0
oil roasted	1 oz	165	0
Valencia, oil roasted	1 cup	848	0
Valencia, oil roasted	1 oz	165	0
Virginia, oil roasted	1 oz	161	0
Virginia, oil roasted	1 cup	826	0

PEAR

FOOD	PORTION	CALORIES	CHOLESTEROL
CANNED			
Bartlett Halves in Heavy Syrup (S&W)	½ cup	100	0
Sliced Natural Style (S&W)	½ cup	80	0
halves in light syrup	1 cup	144	0
halves in water pack	1 cup	71	0
pear halves in heavy syrup	1 cup	188	0
pear halves in juice	1 cup	123	0
DRIED			
Pears (Mariani)	¼ cup	150	0
halves	10	459	0
FRESH			
pear	1	98	0
JUICE			
nectar	1 cup	149	0

FOOD	PORTION	CALORIES	CHOLESTEROL

PEAS

CANNED

FOOD	PORTION	CALORIES	CHOLESTEROL
Early June or Sweet (Owatonna)	½ cup	70	0
Peas (Libby)	½ cup	60	0
Peas (Seneca)	½ cup	60	0
Peas Natural Pack (Libby)	½ cup	60	0
Peas Natural Pack (Seneca)	½ cup	60	0
Petit Pois (S&W)	½ cup	70	0
Sweet Peas Perfection (S&W)	½ cup	70	0
Sweet Peas Veri-Green (S&W)	½ cup	70	0
peas, green	½ cup	61	0
DRIED			
Split Peas (Hurst Brand)	1 cup	277	0
Whole Peas (Hurst Brand)	1 cup	272	0
split, raw	1 cup	671	0
split; cooked	1 cup	231	0
FRESH			
peas, edible-podded; cooked	½ cup	34	0
peas, green, raw	½ cup	63	0
peas, green; cooked	½ cup	67	0

FOOD	PORTION	CALORIES	CHOLESTEROL
peas, raw	½ cup	30	0
sprouts	½ cup	77	0
FROZEN			
Green (Birds Eye)	½ cup	77	0
Green; cooked (Health Valley)	5.6 oz	126	0
Peas w/ Cream Sauce (Birds Eye)	½ cup	117	tr
Petite Peas (Hanover)	½ cup	70	0
Snow Peas (Hanover)	½ cup	35	0
Sweet Peas (Hanover)	½ cup	70	0
Tiny Tender (Birds Eye)	½ cup	62	0
edible-podded; not prep	½ cup	30	0
green; not prep	½ cup	55	0
peas, edible-podded; cooked	½ cup	42	0
peas, green; cooked	½ cup	63	0

PECANS

FOOD	PORTION	CALORIES	CHOLESTEROL
Chips, Halves or Pieces (Planters)	1 oz	190	0
dried	1 oz	190	0
dry roasted	1 oz	187	0
halves, dried	1 cup	721	0
oil roasted	1 oz	195	0

FOOD	PORTION	CALORIES	CHOLESTEROL

PECTIN

Certo Fruit Pectin	1 Tbsp	2	0
Sure-Jell Fruit Pectin	¼ pkg	38	0
Sure-Jell Light Fruit Pectin	¼ pkg	33	0

PEPPER

CANNED

chili, hot	1	18	0
green & red, sweet	½ cup	13	0
jalapeno; chopped	½ cup	17	0

DRIED

green, freeze-dried	1 Tbsp	1	0
red, freeze-dried	1 Tbsp	1	0

FRESH

green, raw	1	18	0
red, raw	1	18	0
red; chopped, cooked	½ cup	12	0

FROZEN

Green, Diced (Southland)	2 oz	10	0
Sweet Red & Green, Cut (Southland)	2 oz	15	0
green & red, sweet, chopped; not prep	1 oz pkg	6	0

PERCH

FRESH

cooked	1 fillet (1.6 oz)	54	53

FOOD	PORTION	CALORIES	CHOLESTEROL
cooked	3 oz	99	98
ocean perch, Atlantic, raw	3 oz	80	36
ocean perch, Atlantic, raw	1 fillet (2.2 oz)	60	27
ocean perch, Atlantic; cooked	1 fillet (1.8 oz)	60	27
ocean perch, Atlantic; cooked	3 oz	103	46
raw	3 oz	77	76
raw	1 fillet (2.1 oz)	55	54

PERSIMMONS

persimmons	1	32	0

PICKLE

Bread 'N Butter Slices (Claussen)	1 slice	7	0
Dill Spears (Claussen)	1 spear	4	0
Kosher Halves (Claussen)	1 half	9	0
Kosher Slices (Claussen)	1 slice	1	0
Kosher Whole (Claussen)	1	9	0
No Garlic Dills (Claussen)	1	17	0
Relish (Claussen)	1 Tbsp	14	0

FOOD	PORTION	CALORIES	CHOLESTEROL
PIE			
(*see also* PIE CRUST)			
CANNED FILLING			
pumpkin pie mix	1 cup	282	0
FROZEN			
Apple (Mrs. Smith's)	⅛ of 9⅝″ pie	390	10
Apple Natural Juice (Mrs. Smith's)	1/7 of 9″ pie	420	5
Apple Streusel Natural Juice (Mrs. Smith's)	1/7 of 9″ pie	420	5
Blueberry (Mrs. Smith's)	⅛ of 9⅝″ pie	380	10
Cherry (Mrs. Smith's)	⅛ of 9⅝″ pie	400	10
Cherry Natural Juice (Mrs. Smith's)	1/7 of 9″ pie	410	10
Coconut Custard (Mrs. Smith's)	⅛ of 9⅝″ pie	330	50
Dutch Apple (Mrs. Smith's)	⅛ of 9⅝″ shell	420	2
Peach (Mrs. Smith's)	⅛ of 9⅝″ pie	365	10
Pecan Thaw 'N' Serve (Mrs. Smith's)	⅛ of 9⅝″ shell	510	30
Pumpkin Custard (Mrs. Smith's)	⅛ of 9⅝″ pie	310	30
HOME RECIPE			
apple	1/7 of 9″ pie	402	7
banana cream	1/7 of 9″ pie	354	83

FOOD	PORTION	CALORIES	CHOLESTEROL
blackberry	½ of 9" pie	372	4
blueberry	½ of 9" pie	411	4
butterscotch	½ of 9" pie	417	108
cherry	½ of 9" pie	462	8
chess	½ of 9" pie	682	201
chocolate chiffon	½ of 9" pie	337	94
chocolate meringue	½ of 9" pie	371	83
coconut custard	½ of 9" pie	346	78
custard	½ of 9" pie	324	136
grasshopper	½ of 9" pie	396	179
key lime	½ of 9" pie	393	87
lemon chiffon	½ of 9" pie	381	145
lemon meringue	½ of 9" pie	399	91
mince	½ of 9" pie	441	6
peach	½ of 9" pie	409	8
pecan	½ of 9" pie	566	114

FOOD	PORTION	CALORIES	CHOLESTEROL
pineapple chiffon	1/7 of 9" pie	337	20
pumpkin	1/7 of 9" pie	287	84
raisin	1/7 of 9" pie	545	132
rhubarb	1/7 of 9" pie	414	7
squash	1/7 of 9" pie	311	87
strawberry	1/7 of 9" pie	282	0
MIX			
Banana Cream No Bake Dessert; as prep (Jell-O)	1/8 pie	233	28
Banana Cream; as prep w/ whole milk (Jell-O)	1/6 of 8" pie	107	12
Chocolate Mousse Pie No Bake Dessert; as prep (Jell-O)	1/8 pie	262	30
Chocolate Cream Pie No Bake Dessert; as prep (Jell-O)	1/8 pie	260	29
Coconut Cream; as prep w/ whole milk (Jell-O)	1/6 of 8" pie	115	12
Lemon; as prep (Jell-O)	1/6 of 8" pie	180	94

FOOD	PORTION	CALORIES	CHOLESTEROL
SNACK			
Apple (Hostess)	1	403	19
Berry (Hostess)	1	391	19
Blueberry (Hostess)	1	378	19
Cherry (Hostess)	1	416	19
Lemon (Hostess)	1	416	32
Marshmallow Pies, Banana (Little Debbie)	1 pkg (1.4 oz)	170	tr
Marshmallow Pies, Banana (Little Debbie)	1 pkg (3 oz)	360	tr
Marshmallow Pies, Chocolate (Little Debbie)	1 pkg (1.38 oz)	170	tr
Marshmallow Pies, Chocolate (Little Debbie)	1 pkg (3 oz)	370	tr
Oatmeal Creme Pies (Little Debbie)	1 pkg (1.33 oz)	160	tr
Peach (Hostess)	1	403	19
Pecan Pie (Little Debbie)	1 pkg (1.83 oz)	170	tr
Pecan Pie (Little Debbie)	1 pkg (3 oz)	280	tr
Raisin Creme Pie (Little Debbie)	1 pkg (1.17 oz)	140	tr
Raisin Creme Pie (Little Debbie)	1 pkg (2.5 oz)	290	tr

FOOD	PORTION	CALORIES	CHOLESTEROL

PIE CRUST
(*see also* PIE)

FROZEN

| Pie Shell (Mrs. Smith's) | ⅛ of 9⅝" shell | 130 | 5 |

HOME RECIPE

| piecrust | 1 for 9" pie | 900 | 0 |

PIEROGI

FROZEN

Potato Cheese (Mrs. T's)	1	70	3
Potato Onion (Mrs. T's)	1	50	1
Sauerkraut (Mrs. T's)	1	60	2

HOME RECIPE

| pierogi | ¾ cup | 307 | 49 |

PIGEON PEAS

DRIED

cooked	½ cup	86	0
cooked	1 cup	204	0
raw	1 cup	704	0

PIGNOLIA
(*see* PINE NUTS)

FOOD	PORTION	CALORIES	CHOLESTEROL
PIGS' EARS AND FEET			
ears, frzn, raw	1 ear (4 oz)	263	93
ears, frzn; simmered	1 ear (3.7 oz)	183	99
feet, pickled	1 oz	58	26
feet, pickled	1 lb	923	419
feet, raw	3.3 oz	251	101
feet; simmered	2.5 oz	138	71
PIKE			
FRESH			
northern, raw	3 oz	75	33
northern, raw	½ fillet (6.9 oz)	175	77
northern; cooked	½ fillet (5.4 oz)	176	78
northern; cooked	3 oz	96	43
roe, raw	3½ oz	130	360
walleye red, raw	3 oz	79	73
walleye, raw	1 fillet (5.6 oz)	147	137
PINE NUTS			
pignolia, dried	1 oz	146	0
pignolia, dried	1 Tbsp	51	0
pinyon, dried	1 oz	161	0
PINEAPPLE			
CANDIED			
slices	1 oz	179	0

FOOD	PORTION	CALORIES	CHOLESTEROL
CANNED			
All Cuts in Juice (Dole)	½ cup	70	0
All Cuts in Syrup (Dole)	½ cup	95	0
Hawaiian 100% Sliced (S&W)	2 slices	90	0
Hawaiian 100% Sliced (S&W)	½ cup	70	0
chunks in heavy syrup	1 cup	199	0
chunks in juice	1 cup	150	0
crushed	1 cup	199	0
sliced in water pack	1 slice	19	0
tidbits	1 cup	199	0
tidbits in juice	1 cup	150	0
tidbits in water pack	1 cup	79	0
FRESH			
Chiquita	1 cup	90	0
pineapple; diced	1 cup	77	0
FROZEN			
chunks, sweetened	½ cup	104	0
JUICE			
Pineapple (Dole)	6 oz	100	0
Pineapple (Mott's)	9.5 oz	169	0
Pineapple (Tree Top)	6 oz	100	0
Unsweetened (S&W)	6 oz	100	0

FOOD	PORTION	CALORIES	CHOLESTEROL
frzn; as prep	1 cup	129	0
frzn; not prep	6 oz container	387	0
pineapple juice	1 cup	139	0

PINK BEANS

DRIED
cooked	1 cup	252	0
raw	1 cup	721	0

PINTO BEANS

CANNED
pinto	1 cup	186	0
DRIED Pinto (Hurst Brand)	1 cup	265	0
cooked	1 cup	235	0
raw	1 cup	656	0
FROZEN cooked	3 oz	152	0
raw	10 oz pkg	484	0
SPROUTS cooked	3½ oz	22	0
raw	3½ oz	62	0

PINYON
(*see* PINE NUTS)

FOOD	PORTION	CALORIES	CHOLESTEROL

PISTACHIO

FOOD	PORTION	CALORIES	CHOLESTEROL
Dry Roasted (Planters)	1 oz	170	0
Natural (Planters)	1 oz	170	0
Pistachios (Lance)	1⅛ oz	180	0
Red Pistachios (Planters)	1 oz	170	0
Roasted Shelled Pistachios (Dole)	1 oz	163	0
dried	1 oz	164	0
dried	1 cup	739	0
dry roasted	1 oz	172	0

PIZZA

(*see also* DOMINO'S PIZZA, SHAKEY'S)

FOOD	PORTION	CALORIES	CHOLESTEROL
FROZEN			
Pizza Round (Lamb-Weston)	4.8 oz	370	10
cheese	⅓ of 10" pie	140	23
HOME RECIPE			
cheese & sausage	⅛ of 14" pie	266	35
MIX			
Ragu Mix for Homemade Pizza Crust	¼ crust	170	0
Ragu Mix for Homemade Pizza Crust; as prep pizza recipe	¼ pizza	300	25

FOOD	PORTION	CALORIES	CHOLESTEROL
SAUCE			
Original Quick & Easy (Contadina)	¼ cup	30	0
Pizza Sauce w/ Italian Cheese (Contadina)	¼ cup	30	tr
Pizza Sauce w/ Pepperoni (Contadina)	¼ cup	40	2
Ragu Pizza Quick Sauce Chunky Style	3 Tbsp	45	0
Ragu Pizza Quick Sauce Chunky Style; as prep muffin recipe	2 muffin halves	220	15
Ragu Pizza Quick Sauce Mushrooms	3 Tbsp	40	0
Ragu Pizza Quick Sauce Mushrooms; as prep muffin recipe	2 muffin halves	220	15
Ragu Pizza Quick Sauce Pepperoni	3 Tbsp	50	0
Ragu Pizza Quick Sauce Pepperoni; as prep muffin recipe	2 muffin halves	230	15
Ragu Pizza Quick Sauce Sausage	3 Tbsp	40	0
Ragu Pizza Quick Sauce Sausage; as prep muffin recipe	2 muffin halves	220	15
Ragu Pizza Quick Sauce Traditional	3 Tbsp	40	0
Ragu Pizza Quick Sauce Traditional; as prep muffin recipe	2 muffin halves	220	15

FOOD	PORTION	CALORIES	CHOLESTEROL
Ragu Pizza Sauce Extra Tomatoes	3 Tbsp	25	0
Ragu Pizza Sauce Extra Tomatoes; as prep pizza recipe	¼ pizza	280	25

PIZZA SAUCE
(see PIZZA, SAUCE; SPAGHETTI SAUCE; TOMATO)

PLANTAINS

FRESH			
raw	1 (6.3 oz)	218	0
sliced; cooked	½ cup	89	0

PLUM

CANNED			
Purple Plums Halves Fancy Unpeeled in Extra Heavy Syrup (S&W)	½ cup	135	0
Purple Plums Whole Fancy Unpeeled in Extra Heavy Syrup (S&W)	½ cup	135	0
plums, purple in heavy syrup	3	119	0
plums, purple in juice	3	55	0
FRESH			
plum	1	36	0

FOOD	PORTION	CALORIES	CHOLESTEROL

POI

FRESH
cooked — ½ cup — 134 — 0

POKEBERRY SHOOTS

FRESH
cooked — ½ cup — 16 — 0
raw — ½ cup — 18 — 0

POLLOCK

FRESH

FOOD	PORTION	CALORIES	CHOLESTEROL
Atlantic, raw	½ fillet (6.8 oz)	177	136
Atlantic, raw	3 oz	78	60
walleye, raw	3 oz	68	61
walleye, raw	1 fillet (2.7 oz)	62	55
walleye; cooked	1 fillet (2.1 oz)	68	58
walleye; cooked	3 oz	96	82

POMEGRANATE

FRESH
pomegranates — 1 — 104 — 0

POMPANO

FRESH
Florida, raw — 3 oz — 140 — 43

FOOD	PORTION	CALORIES	CHOLESTEROL
Florida, raw	1 fillet (3.9 oz)	184	56
Florida; cooked	1 fillet (3.1 oz)	185	56
Florida; cooked	3 oz	179	54

POPCORN
(see also CHIPS, PRETZELS, SNACKS)

FOOD	PORTION	CALORIES	CHOLESTEROL
Bachman Popcorn	1 oz	160	0
Jiffy Pop, Microwave Regular; as prep	4 cups	140	0
Jiffy Pop, Microwave Butter Flavor; as prep	4 cups	140	0
Jiffy Pop, Pan Butter Flavor; as prep	4 cups	130	0
Jiffy Pop, Pan Regular; as prep	4 cups	130	0
Lance Cheese Popcorn	1 pkg (⅞ oz)	130	5
Lance Cheese Popcorn	1 oz	150	5
Lance Plain	1 pkg (1 oz)	140	0
air-popped	1 cup	30	0
popped w/ vegetable oil	1 cup	55	0
sugar syrup coated	1 cup	135	0

POPOVER

FOOD	PORTION	CALORIES	CHOLESTEROL
popover (home recipe)	1 (1.4 oz)	98	61

FOOD	PORTION	CALORIES	CHOLESTEROL

PORK

(*see also* BACON, CANADIAN BACON, HAM, LUNCHEON MEATS/COLD CUTS, SAUSAGE)

The values for cooked pork may differ slightly from values for raw pork. When meat is cooked some moisture and fat is lost, changing the nutritive value slightly. As a rule of thumb, it can be assumed that a 4 oz raw portion will equal a 3 oz cooked portion of meat.

FOOD	PORTION	CALORIES	CHOLESTEROL
FRESH			
center loin chop, lean & fat, raw	1 chop (4.4 oz)	341	86
center loin chop, lean & fat; braised	1 chop (2.6 oz)	266	81
center loin chop, lean & fat; broiled	1 chop (3.1 oz)	275	84
center loin chop, lean & fat; roasted	1 chop (3.1 oz)	268	80
center loin chop, lean & fat; pan-fried	1 chop (3.1 oz)	333	92
center loin chop, lean only, raw	1 chop (3.4 oz)	155	62
center loin chop, lean only; braised	1 chop (2.1 oz)	166	68
center loin chop, lean only; broiled	1 chop (2.5 oz)	166	71
center loin chop, lean only; roasted	1 chop (2.4 oz)	180	68
center loin chop, lean only; pan-fried	1 chop (2.4 oz)	178	71
center loin, lean & fat; braised	3 oz	301	91
center loin, lean & fat; broiled	3 oz	269	82

FOOD	PORTION	CALORIES	CHOLESTEROL
center loin, lean & fat; roasted	3 oz	259	78
center loin, lean & fat; pan-fried	3 oz	318	87
center loin, lean only; broiled	3 oz	196	83
center loin, lean only; roasted	3 oz	204	78
center loin, lean only; pan-fried	3 oz	226	91
ham, fresh, shank half, lean & fat; roasted	3 oz	258	78
ham, fresh, shank half, lean only; roasted	3 oz	183	78
ham, fresh, whole, lean & fat; roasted	3 oz	250	79
ham, fresh, whole, lean only; roasted	3 oz	187	80
ham, fresh, rump half, lean & fat; roasted	3 oz	233	81
ham, fresh, rump half, lean only; roasted	3 oz	187	81
leg, loin & shoulder, lean only; roasted	3 oz	198	79
leg, rump half, lean & fat, raw	3 oz	198	57
leg, rump half, lean only, raw	3 oz	87	51
leg, shank half, lean & fat, raw	3 oz	240	57
leg, shank half, lean only, raw	3 oz	117	51
leg, whole, lean & fat, raw	3 oz	222	63
leg, whole, lean only, raw	3 oz	117	57

FOOD	PORTION	CALORIES	CHOLESTEROL
loin blade chop, lean & fat; braised	1 chop (2.4 oz)	275	72
loin blade chop, lean & fat; braised	1 chop (3.1 oz)	321	79
loin blade chop, lean & fat; pan-fried	1 chop (3.1 oz)	368	85
loin blade chop, lean only; broiled	1 chop (2.1 oz)	177	59
loin blade chop, lean only; braised	1 chop (1.8 oz)	156	57
loin blade chop, lean only; roasted	1 chop (2.5 oz)	198	63
loin blade chop, lean only; pan-fried	1 chop (2.2 oz)	175	60
loin center rib chop, lean & fat, raw	1 chop (3.9 oz)	322	71
loin center rib chop, lean only, raw	1 chop (3 oz)	138	47
loin chop, lean & fat, raw	1 chop (4 oz)	345	81
loin chop, lean & fat, raw	1 chop (3.9 oz)	356	79
loin chop, lean & fat; braised	1 chop (2.3 oz)	267	67
loin chop, lean & fat; braised	1 chop (2.5 oz)	261	73
loin chop, lean & fat; pan-fried	1 chop (2.9 oz)	337	72
loin chop, lean & fat; roasted	1 chop (2.8 oz)	274	68
loin chop, lean & fat; roasted	1 chop (2.9 oz)	262	74

FOOD	PORTION	CALORIES	CHOLESTEROL
loin chop, lean only, raw	1 chop (3 oz)	142	55
loin chop, lean only; broiled	1 chop (2.1 oz)	165	60
loin chop, lean only; pan-fried	1 chop (2 oz)	157	49
loin chop, lean only; roasted	1 chop (2.3 oz)	167	54
loin chop, lean & fat; broiled	1 chop (2.7 oz)	295	76
loin chop, lean only; braised	1 chop (1.8 oz)	147	51
loin, blade, lean & fat; braised	3 oz	348	92
loin, blade, lean & fat; broiled	3 oz	334	83
loin, blade, lean & fat; roasted	3 oz	310	76
loin, blade, lean & fat; pan-fried	3 oz	352	81
loin, blade, lean only; braised	3 oz	266	96
loin, blade, lean only; broiled	3 oz	255	85
loin, blade, lean only; roasted	3 oz	238	76
loin, blade, lean only; pan-fried	3 oz	240	82
loin, lean & fat; braised	3 oz	312	87
loin, lean & fat; broiled	3 oz	294	80
loin, lean & fat; roasted	3 oz	271	77
loin, lean only; braised	3 oz	232	90
loin, lean only; broiled	3 oz	218	81
loin, lean only; roasted	3 oz	204	77

FOOD	PORTION	CALORIES	CHOLESTEROL
lungs, raw	3.5 oz	83	314
lungs; braised	3 oz	84	329
pancreas, raw	4 oz	225	218
pancreas; braised	3 oz	186	268
rib chop, lean only; braised	1 chop (1.8 oz)	147	51
rib chop, lean only; broiled	1 chop (2.1 oz)	162	69
rib chop, lean only; pan-fried	1 chop (2 oz)	160	60
rib chop, lean only; roasted	1 chop (2.2 oz)	162	52
rib chop, lean & fat; braised	1 chop (2.2 oz)	246	64
rib chop, lean & fat; broiled	1 chop (2.6 oz)	264	72
rib chop, lean & fat; pan-fried	1 chop (2.9 oz)	343	74
rib chop, lean & fat; roasted	1 chop (2.6 oz)	252	64
salt pork	1 oz	212	25
shoulder arm picnic, lean only, raw	3 oz	120	54
shoulder arm picnic, lean & fat, raw	3 oz	231	60
shoulder blade Boston steak, lean & fat; braised	1 steak (5.6 oz)	594	178
shoulder blade Boston steak, lean & fat, raw	1 steak (9.6 oz)	737	193
shoulder blade Boston steak, lean only, raw	steak (7.4 oz)	346	142

FOOD	PORTION	CALORIES	CHOLESTEROL
shoulder blade Boston steak, lean only; braised	1 steak (4.6 oz)	382	151
shoulder blade Boston steak, lean only; broiled	1 steak (5.3 oz)	413	159
shoulder blade Boston steak, lean only; roasted	1 steak (5.5 oz)	404	155
shoulder blade Boston steak, lean & fat; broiled	1 steak (6.5 oz)	647	190
shoulder blade Boston steak, lean & fat; roasted	1 steak (6.5 oz)	594	179
shoulder whole, lean & fat, raw	3 oz	234	63
shoulder whole, lean only, raw	3 oz	132	57
shoulder, arm picnic, cured, lean & fat; roasted	3 oz	238	49
shoulder, arm picnic, cured, lean only; roasted	3 oz	145	41
shoulder, arm picnic, lean only; braised	3 oz	211	97
shoulder, arm picnic, lean only; roasted	3 oz	194	81
shoulder, arm picnic, lean & fat; braised	3 oz	293	93
shoulder, arm picnic, lean & fat; roasted	3 oz	281	80
shoulder, blade roll, cured, lean & fat; roasted	3 oz	244	57
shoulder, Boston blade, lean only; braised	3 oz	250	99
shoulder, Boston blade, lean only; broiled	3 oz	233	89

FOOD	PORTION	CALORIES	CHOLESTEROL
shoulder, Boston blade, lean only; roasted	3 oz	218	83
shoulder, Boston blade, lean & fat; braised	3 oz	316	95
shoulder, Boston blade, lean & fat; broiled	3 oz	297	87
shoulder, Boston blade, lean & fat; roasted	3 oz	273	82
shoulder, whole, lean & fat; roasted	3 oz	277	81
shoulder, whole, lean only; roated	3 oz	207	82
sirloin chop, lean & fat, raw	1 chop (4.2 oz)	328	83
sirloin chop, lean & fat; braised	1 chop (2.4 oz)	250	75
sirloin chop, lean & fat; broiled	1 chop (2.8 oz)	278	81
sirloin chop, lean & fat; roasted	1 chop (2.8 oz)	244	76
sirloin chop, lean only, raw	1 chop (3.2 oz)	139	58
sirloin chop, lean only; braised	1 chop (1.9 oz)	149	63
sirloin chop, lean only; broiled	1 chop (2.3 oz)	165	67
sirloin chop, lean only; roasted	1 chop (2.5 oz)	175	67
spareribs, lean & fat, raw	3 oz	243	66
spareribs, lean & fat; braised	3 oz	338	103

FOOD	PORTION	CALORIES	CHOLESTEROL
spleen, raw	4 oz	113	410
spleen; braised	3 oz	127	428
tail, raw	4 oz	427	110
tail; simmered	3 oz	336	110
tenderloin, lean only, raw	3 oz	96	54
tenderloin, lean only; roasted	3 oz	141	79
top loin chop, lean & fat, raw	1 chop (4 oz)	360	77
top loin chop, lean only, raw	1 chop (3.1 oz)	142	48

POT PIE

FOOD	PORTION	CALORIES	CHOLESTEROL
Beef (Banquet)	7 oz	500	25
Beef (Morton)	7 oz	430	29
Chicken (Banquet)	7 oz	540	35
Chicken (Morton)	7 oz	415	35
Tuna (Banquet)	7 oz	540	27
Turkey (Banquet)	7 oz	500	37
Turkey (Morton)	7 oz	420	38

HOME RECIPE

FOOD	PORTION	CALORIES	CHOLESTEROL
beef; baked	4¼" diam	558	48

FOOD	PORTION	CALORIES	CHOLESTEROL
chicken	1 (11 oz)	706	118
turkey	1 (10.6 oz)	710	122

POTATO STARCH

Potato Starch (Manischewitz)	1 cup	570	0

POTATOES
(see also CHIPS)

CANNED			
New Potatoes Extra Small (S&W)	½ cup	45	0
Potatoes (Libby)	½ cup	45	0
Potatoes (Seneca)	½ cup	45	0
Scalloped Potatoes Flavored w/ Ham (Lunch Bucket)	1 container (8.25 oz)	250	35
potatoes	½ cup	54	0
FRESH			
Yukon Gold	1 (5.3 oz)	110	0
baked, flesh only	1 (5 oz)	145	0
baked, flesh & skin	1 (6½ oz)	220	0
baked, skin only	skin from 1 potato	115	0
boiled	½ cup	68	0
boiled	1 (4.7 oz)	119	0

FOOD	PORTION	CALORIES	CHOLESTEROL
flesh & skin; microwaved	1 (7 oz)	212	0
flesh only; microwaved	1 (5.5 oz)	156	0
raw, flesh only	1 (3.9 oz)	88	0
raw, skin only	1 (1.3 oz)	22	0
FROZEN			
Bacon & Cheddar Baked Potato Entree (Idaho Original)	11 oz	982	21
Cheddar Browns (Ore Ida)	3 oz	90	10
Cheddared Potatoes (Budget Gourmet)	5.5 oz	230	35
Cheddared Potatoes & Broccoli (Budget Gourmet)	5 oz	130	25
Chicken & Almond Baked Potato Entree (Idaho Original)	11 oz	433	29
Cottage Fries (Ore Ida)	3 oz	120	0
Crinkle Cuts French Fries (Lamb-Weston)	3 oz	130	5
Crinkle Cuts Lites (Ore Ida)	3 oz	90	0
Crinkle Cuts Microwave (Ore Ida)	3.5 oz	180	0
Crispers! (Ore Ida)	3 oz	230	0
Crispy Crowns (Ore Ida)	3 oz	160	0
Crispy Crowns w/ Onion (Ore Ida)	3 oz	170	0

FOOD	PORTION	CALORIES	CHOLESTEROL
Deep Fries Crinkle Cuts (Heinz)	3 oz	150	0
Deep Fries Shoestrings (Heinz)	3 oz	200	0
French Fries (Heinz)	3 oz	160	0
French Fries Golden Crinkles (Ore Ida)	3 oz	120	0
French Fries Golden Fries (Ore Ida)	3 oz	120	0
French Fries Lites (Ore Ida)	3 oz	90	0
French Fries Pixie Crinkles (Ore Ida)	3 oz	140	0
French Fries Shoestrings (Ore Ida)	3 oz	140	0
Fries Country Style Dinner (Ore Ida)	3 oz	110	0
Golden Patties (Ore Ida)	2.5 oz	140	0
Hash Browns Microwave (Ore Ida)	2 oz	180	0
Hash Browns Shredded (Ore Ida)	3 oz	70	0
Hash Browns Southern Style w/ Butter & Onions (Heinz)	3 oz	110	5
Hash Browns Southern Style (Ore Ida)	3 oz	70	0
Home Browns Hash Browns (Lamb-Weston)	1 piece (2.25 oz)	150	10

FOOD	PORTION	CALORIES	CHOLESTEROL
Italian Baked Potato Entree (Idaho Original)	11 oz	443	41
MunchSkins (Lamb-Weston)	3 oz	120	5
Nacho Potatoes (Budget Gourmet)	5 oz	180	30
Natural Cuts Skin-On (Lamb-Weston)	3 oz	120	0
Natural Slices Skin-On (Lamb-Weston)	3 oz	120	5
Natural Trim Fries Skin-On (Lamb-Weston)	3 oz	140	5
New Potatoes In Sour Cream Sauce (Budget Gourmet)	5 oz	120	20
O'Brien Potatoes (Ore Ida)	3 oz	60	0
Primavera Baked Potato Entree (Idaho Original)	11 oz	499	25
Regular Cut French Fries (Lamb-Weston)	3 oz	130	5
Shoestring French Fries (Lamb-Weston)	3 oz	140	5
Shoestrings Lites (Ore Ida)	3 oz	90	0
Steak House Fries (Lamb-Weston)	3 oz	120	5
Stuffed Potatoes w/ Cheddar Cheese (OH Boy!)	6 oz	142	6

FOOD	PORTION	CALORIES	CHOLESTEROL
Stuffed Potatoes w/ Real Bacon (OH Boy!)	6 oz	116	5
Stuffed Potatoes w/ Sour Cream & Chives (OH Boy!)	6 oz	129	2
Tater Puffs (Lamb-Weston)	3 oz	150	10
Tater Tots (Ore Ida)	3 oz	140	0
Tater Tots Microwave (Ore Ida)	2 oz	200	0
Tater Tots w/ Bacon Flavored Vegetable Protein (Ore Ida)	3 oz	140	0
Tater Tots w/ Onion (Ore Ida)	3 oz	140	0
Tater Wedges (Lamb-Weston)	2 pieces (4 oz)	200	10
Three Cheese Potatoes (Budget Gourmet)	5.75 oz	230	30
Wedges Home Style (Ore Ida)	3 oz	100	0
Western Style Baked Potato Entree (Idaho Original)	11 oz	567	33
Whole Small (Ore Ida)	3 oz	70	0
french fried; not prep	10 strips	107	0
french-fried, cottage-cut; cooked	10 strips	109	0
french-fried; cooked	10 strips	111	0
potato puffs; as prep	½ cup	138	0

FOOD	PORTION	CALORIES	CHOLESTEROL
whole; not prep	½ cup	71	0
HOME RECIPE			
au gratin	½ cup	160	29
au gratin w/ cheese	½ cup	178	18
mashed	½ cup	111	2
O'Brien	1 cup	157	7
potato pancakes	1	495	93
scalloped	½ cup	105	14
scalloped	½ cup	127	7
MIX			
Mashed Idaho; as prep (French's)	½ cup	130	12
Mashed Potato Buds; as prep (Betty Crocker)	½ cup	130	17
Mashed; as prep (Hungry Jack)	½ cup	130	17
Potato Pancakes; as prep (Frenchs)	1	80	10
mashed, dehydrated, flakes	½ cup	361	0
mashed, dehydrated, flakes; as prep	½ cup	118	15
mashed, granules; as prep w/ whole milk	½ cup	137	18
mashed, granules not prep	½ cup	80	0
READY-TO-USE			
salad	½ cup	179	86

POUT

FRESH			
ocean, raw	3 oz	67	44

FOOD	PORTION	CALORIES	CHOLESTEROL
ocean, raw	½ fillet (6.2 oz)	140	92

PRESERVE
(see JAM/JELLY/PRESERVE)

PRETZELS
(see also CHIPS, POPCORN, SNACKS)

FOOD	PORTION	CALORIES	CHOLESTEROL
Bachman Pretzel Rods	1 rod (1 oz)	110	0
Estee Unsalted	5	25	0
J&J Soft Pretzels	1 oz	76	0
Lance Pretzel Twist	1½ oz	150	0
Lance Pretzels	1 oz	100	0
Quinlan Artificial Butter Tiny Thins	1 oz	108	0
Quinlan Beers	1 oz	110	0
Quinlan Cheese Tiny Thins	1 oz	109	0
Quinlan Logs	1 oz	103	0
Quinlan Party Thins	1 oz	109	0
Quinlan Philly Style	1 oz	107	0
Quinlan Rods	1 oz	100	0
Quinlan Sour Cheese Tiny Thins	1 oz	100	0
Quinlan Sour Dough Thins Hard	1 oz	100	0
Quinlan Sticks	1 oz	105	0
Quinlan Thins	1 oz	104	0
Quinlan Tiny Thins	1 oz	109	0
Quinlan Tiny Thins No-Salt	1 oz	115	0

FOOD	PORTION	CALORIES	CHOLESTEROL
Quinlan Ultra Thins	1 oz	106	0
thin slim sticks	47 pieces	110	0
twist, tiny	14 pieces	109	0

PRUNE

CANNED
prunes in heavy syrup	5	90	0

DRIED
Prunes, Pitted (Mariani)	¼ cup	140	0
Prunes, Whole (Mariani)	¼ cup	140	0
cooked w/o sugar	½ cup	113	0
prunes	10	201	0

JUICE
Country Style (Mott's)	6 oz	130	0
Prune (Mott's)	6 oz	130	0
Unsweetened (S&W)	6 oz	120	0
prune juice	1 cup	181	0

PUDDING
(*see also* CUSTARD, PUDDING POPS)

HOME RECIPE
bread w/ raisins	½ cup	180	77
corn	½ cup	97	47
corn	⅔ cup	181	230

FOOD	PORTION	CALORIES	CHOLESTEROL
pumpkin	½ cup	170	105
rice w/ raisins	½ cup	246	136
tapioca	½ cup	169	111
MIX			
Banana Creme Instant (Jell-O)	1 pkg (3.5 oz)	360	tr
Butter Pecan Instant (Jell-O)	1 pkg (3.5 oz)	383	tr
Butterscotch (Jell-O)	1 pkg (3.6 oz)	364	0
Butterscotch Instant (Jell-O)	1 pkg (3.5 oz)	358	tr
Butterscotch; as prep (Estee)	½ cup	70	2
Chocolate (Jell-O)	1 pkg (3.5 oz)	346	0
Chocolate Tapioca Americana (Jell-O)	1 pkg (3.5 oz)	378	0
Chocolate Fudge (Jell-O)	1 pkg (3.5 oz)	345	0
Chocolate; as prep (Estee)	½ cup	70	2
Coconut Cream Instant (Jell-O)	1 pkg (3.5 oz)	416	tr
French Vanilla (Jell-O)	1 pkg (3.5 oz)	365	0
French Vanilla Instant (Jell-O)	1 pkg (3.5 oz)	360	tr
Lemon Instant (Jell-O)	1 pkg (3.5 oz)	376	tr
Lemon; as prep (Estee)	½ cup	70	2

FOOD	PORTION	CALORIES	CHOLESTEROL
Milk Chocolate (Jell-O)	1 pkg (3.5 oz)	362	2
Pineapple Cream Instant (Jell-O)	1 pkg (3.5 oz)	363	tr
Pistachio Instant (Jell-O)	1 pkg (3.5 oz)	383	tr
Vanilla Instant (Jell-O)	1 pkg (3.5 oz)	374	tr
Vanilla; as prep (Estee)	½ cup	70	2
MIX WITH 2% MILK			
Butterscotch Instant Sugar Free; as prep (Jell-O)	½ cup	88	9
Chocolate Instant Sugar Free; as prep (Jell-O)	½ cup	96	9
Chocolate Fudge Instant Sugar Free; as prep (Jell-O)	½ cup	100	9
Chocolate Sugar Free; as prep (Jell-O)	½ cup	91	9
Pistachio Instant Sugar Free; as prep (Jell-O)	½ cup	94	9
Vanilla Instant Sugar Free; as prep (Jell-O)	½ cup	90	9
Vanilla Sugar Free; as prep (Jell-O)	½ cup	82	9
MIX WITH SKIM MILK			
Butterscotch (D-Zerta)	½ cup	69	2

FOOD	PORTION	CALORIES	CHOLESTEROL
Butterscotch w/ NutraSweet; as prep (D-Zerta)	½ cup	69	2
Chocolate w/ NutraSweet; as prep (D-Zerta)	½ cup	65	2
Vanilla (D-Zerta)	½ cup	69	2
Vanilla w/ NutraSweet; as prep (D-Zerta)	½ cup	69	2
MIX WITH WHOLE MILK			
Banana Creme Instant; as prep (Jell-O)	½ cup	168	17
Butter Pecan Instant; as prep (Jell-O)	½ cup	174	17
Butterscotch Instant; as prep (Jell-O)	½ cup	168	17
Butterscotch; as prep (Jell-O)	½ cup	171	17
Chocolate Fudge Instant; as prep (Jell-O)	½ cup	174	17
Chocolate Fudge; as prep (Jell-O)	½ cup	164	17
Chocolate Instant; as prep (Jell-O)	½ cup	176	17
Chocolate Tapioca Americana; as prep (Jell-O)	½ cup	173	17
Chocolate; as prep (Jell-O)	½ cup	165	17

FOOD	PORTION	CALORIES	CHOLESTEROL
Coconut Cream Instant; as prep (Jell-O)	½ cup	182	17
French Vanilla Instant; as prep (Jell-O)	½ cup	168	17
French Vanilla; as prep (Jell-O)	½ cup	171	17
Golden Egg Custard Americana; as prep (Jell-O)	1 pkg (3.5 oz)	378	0
Golden Egg Custard Americana; as prep (Jell-O)	½ cup	167	85
Lemon Instant; as prep (Jell-O)	½ cup	172	17
Milk Chocolate Instant; as prep (Jell-O)	½ cup	178	17
Milk Chocolate; as prep (Jell-O)	½ cup	168	17
Pineapple Cream Instant; as prep (Jell-O)	½ cup	168	17
Pistachio Instant; as prep (Jell-O)	½ cup	172	17
Rice Americana; as prep (Jell-O)	½ cup	177	17
Vanilla Instant; as prep (Jell-O)	½ cup	171	17
Vanilla Tapioca Americana; as prep (Jell-O)	½ cup	166	17

FOOD	PORTION	CALORIES	CHOLESTEROL
Vanilla; as prep (Jell-O)	½ cup	162	17
READY-TO-USE			
Banana Snack Pack (Hunt's)	4.25 oz	180	0
Butterscotch Snack Pack (Hunt's)	4.25 oz	180	0
Butterscotch Sugar Free (Diamond Crystal)	½ cup	80	3
Chocolate Marshmallow Snack Pack (Hunt's)	4.25 oz	170	0
Chocolate Snack Pack (Hunt's)	4.25 oz	180	0
Chocolate Fudge Snack Pack (Hunt's)	4.25 oz	170	0
Chocolate Sugar Free (Diamond Crystal)	½ cup	70	3
German Chocolate Snack Pack (Hunt's)	4.25 oz	190	0
Lemon Snack Pack (Hunt's)	4.25 oz	150	0
Rice Snack Pack (Hunt's)	4.25 oz	190	0
Tapicoa Snack Pack (Hunt's)	4.25 oz	120	0
Vanilla Snack Pack (Hunt's)	4.25	180	0
Vanilla Sugar Free (Diamond Crystal)	½ cup	80	3

FOOD	PORTION	CALORIES	CHOLESTEROL

PUDDING POPS

(*see also* ICE CREAM AND FROZEN DESSERTS, PUDDING)

FOOD	PORTION	CALORIES	CHOLESTEROL
Chocolate Covered Chocolate Pudding Pops (Jell-O)	1 pop	130	2
Chocolate Covered Vanilla Pudding Pops (Jell-O)	1 pop	130	2
Chocolate Fudge Pudding Pops (Jell-O)	1 pop	73	1
Chocolate Pudding Pops (Jell-O)	1 pop	80	tr
Chocolate w/ Chocolate Chips Pudding Pops (Jell-O)	1 pop	82	tr
Chocolate/Caramel Swirl Pudding Pops (Jell-O)	1 pop	78	tr
Chocolate/Vanilla Swirl Pudding Pops (Jell-O)	1 pop	77	tr
Double Chocolate Swirl Pudding Pops (Jell-O)	1 pop	74	1
Milk Chocolate Pudding Pops (Jell-O)	1 pop	75	1
Vanilla Pudding Pops (Jell-O)	1 pop	75	tr
Vanilla w/ Chocolate Chips (Jell-O)	1 pop	82	1

FOOD	PORTION	CALORIES	CHOLESTEROL
PUMPKIN			
CANNED			
Pumpkin (Owatonna)	½ cup	40	0
Solid Pack (Libby's)	1 cup	80	0
pumpkin	½ cup	41	0
FRESH			
cooked; mashed	½ cup	24	0
flowers, raw	1	0	0
flowers; cooked	½ cup	10	0
raw; cubed	½ cup	15	0
SEEDS			
seeds, dried	1 oz	154	0
seeds, whole; roasted	1 oz	127	0
PURSLANE			
FRESH			
cooked	½ cup	10	0
raw	1 cup	7	0
QUAHOGS (see CLAM)			
QUICHE			
lorraine (home recipe)	⅙ of 9" pie	379	159
RABBIT			
stewed	3.5 oz	216	65

FOOD	PORTION	CALORIES	CHOLESTEROL

RADISH

DRIED
oriental	½ cup	157	0
seeds, sprouted, raw	½ cup	8	0

FRESH
Chinese; cooked	½ cup	13	0
daikon; cooked	½ cup	13	0
oriental, raw; sliced	½ cup	8	0
raw	10	7	0
white icicle, raw; sliced	½ cup	7	0

RAISINS

California Seedless (Cinderella)	½ cup	250	0
Golden Raisins (Dole)	½ cup	260	0
Raisins (Dole)	½ cup	260	0
raisins	1 cup	434	0
raisins, golden	1 cup	437	0

HOME RECIPE
raisin sauce	2 Tbsp	51	0

RASPBERRIES

CANNED
whole in heavy syrup	½ cup	117	0

FRESH
raspberries	1 cup	61	0

FOOD	PORTION	CALORIES	CHOLESTEROL
FROZEN			
Red Raspberries Whole in Lite Syrup (Birds Eye)	½ cup	99	0
raspberries, sweetened	1 cup	256	0
JUICE			
Pure & Light (Dole)	6 oz	87	0
Red Raspberry (Smucker's)	8 oz	120	0
RELISH			
Sandwich Spred (Hellman's)	1 Tbsp	55	5
chow chow (home recipe)	1 Tbsp	8	0
chutney apple cranberry (home recipe)	1 Tbsp	16	0
cranberry orange	½ cup	246	0
RHUBARB			
FRESH			
rhubarb	1 cup	26	0
RICE *(see also RICE CAKES)*			
BROWN			
Pritikin Pilaf Brown Rice	½ cup	90	0
Pritikin Spanish Brown Rice	½ cup	100	0
S&W Quick Natural Long Grain; cooked	2 oz	63	0

FOOD	PORTION	CALORIES	CHOLESTEROL
bran	1 oz	80	0
FROZEN			
Birds Eye French Style International Rice	½ cup	106	0
Birds Eye Italian Style International Rice	½ cup	119	0
Birds Eye Rice & Peas w/ Mushrooms	⅔ cup	108	0
Birds Eye Spanish Style International Rice	½ cup	111	0
Budget Gourmet Oriental Rice & Vegetables	5.75 oz	210	20
Budget Gourmet Rice Pilaf w/ Green Beans	5.5 oz	240	10
HOME RECIPE			
pilaf	½ cup	84	22
spanish	¾ cup	363	35
MIX, DRY			
Chun King Stir-Fry Entree	.25 oz	20	0
Fried Rice Seasoning Mix (Kikkoman)	1 oz pkg	91	tr
WHITE			
Minute Rice Drumstick; as prep (General Foods)	½ cup	143	10
Minute Rice Fried; as prep (General Foods)	½ cup	164	0
Minute Rice Long Grain & Wild; as prep (General Foods)	½ cup	149	10

FOOD	PORTION	CALORIES	CHOLESTEROL
Minute Rice Rib Roast; as prep (General Foods)	½ cup	152	10
Minute Rice; as prep (General Foods)	⅔ cup	142	5
S&W Long Grain; cooked	2 oz	61	0

RICE CAKES

FOOD	PORTION	CALORIES	CHOLESTEROL
7 Grain Rice Cakes (Pritikin Foods)	1	35	0
Crispy Rice Cakes Sodium Free (Chico-San)	1	35	0
Crispy Rice Cakes Very Low Sodium (Chico-San)	1	35	0
Plain Rice Cakes (Pritikin Foods)	1	35	0
Sesami Rice Cakes (Pritikin Foods)	1	35	0

ROCKFISH

FOOD	PORTION	CALORIES	CHOLESTEROL
FRESH			
Pacific, raw	1 fillet (6.7 oz)	180	66
Pacific, raw	3 oz	80	29
Pacific; cooked	3 oz	103	38
Pacific; cooked	1 fillet (5.2 oz)	180	66

FOOD	PORTION	CALORIES	CHOLESTEROL

ROE
(*see also individual fish names*)

FRESH
raw	1 oz	39	105
raw	3 oz	119	318

ROLL
(*see also* BISCUIT, CROISSANT, ENGLISH MUFFIN, MUFFIN, POPOVER, SCONE)

HOME RECIPE			
sweet roll	1 (1.8 oz)	143	18
READY-TO-EAT			
Dark Bread (Hollywood)	1	40	0
Dinner (Roman Meal)	1	45	0
Hamburger Bun (Roman Meal)	1	113	0
Hamburger Bun (Shop 'n Save)	1	120	0
Hotdog Bun (Roman Meal)	1	104	0
Light Pan Dinner Rolls Special Formula (Hollywood)	1	60	0
Light Sliced Rolls Special Formula (Hollywood)	1	80	0
Potato Rolls (Martin's)	1	130	0

FOOD	PORTION	CALORIES	CHOLESTEROL

ROUGHY

FRESH

| orange, raw | 3 oz | 107 | 17 |

RUTABAGA

FRESH

| cooked; mashed | ½ cup | 41 | 0 |
| raw; cubed | ½ cup | 25 | 0 |

SABLEFISH

FRESH

| raw | 3 oz | 166 | 42 |
| raw | ½ fillet (6.8 oz) | 377 | 95 |

SMOKED

| sablefish | 1 oz | 72 | 18 |
| sablefish | 3 oz | 218 | 55 |

SALAD
(*see also* PASTA SALAD)

HOME RECIPE

chef	1½ cups	386	244
coleslaw	½ cup	59	0
popeye	½ cup	204	75
taco salad	1 cup	292	71
tossed	1 cup	32	0
waldorf	½ cup	79	8

FOOD	PORTION	CALORIES	CHOLESTEROL

SALAD DRESSING

Salad dressings contain very small amounts of cholesterol in a one tablespoon portion. Some manufacturers' laboratory analysis information on cholesterol consider amounts less than 5 mg in a serving as either none or trace (tr). If you use portions larger than shown below, you may be getting a few milligrams of cholesterol.

FOOD	PORTION	CALORIES	CHOLESTEROL
HOME RECIPE			
french	2 Tbsp	177	0
vinegar & oil	1 Tbsp	72	0
vinegar & oil	2 Tbsp	140	0
MIXES			
Bleu Cheese & Herbs (Good Seasons)	1 pkg	4	tr
Bleu Cheese & Herbs; as prep (Good Seasons)	1 Tbsp	72	tr
Buttermilk Farm Style; as prep (Good Seasons)	1 Tbsp	58	5
Cheese Garlic; as prep (Good Seasons)	1 Tbsp	72	tr
Cheese Italian; as prep (Good Seasons)	1 Tbsp	72	tr
Classic Herb; as prep (Good Seasons)	1 Tbsp	83	0
Garlic & Herbs; as prep (Good Seasons)	1 Tbsp	84	0
Italian Lite; as prep (Good Seasons)	1 Tbsp	27	0
Italian Mild; as prep (Good Seasons)	1 Tbsp	73	0
Italian No Oil; as prep (Good Seasons)	1 Tbsp	7	0

FOOD	PORTION	CALORIES	CHOLESTEROL
Italian; as prep (Good Seasons)	1 Tbsp	71	0
Lemon & Herbs; as prep (Good Seasons)	1 Tbsp	83	0
Zesty Italian Lite; as prep (Good Seasons)	1 Tbsp	31	0
Zesty Italian; as prep (Good Seasons)	1 Tbsp	71	0
READY-TO-USE			
Bacon & Buttermilk (Kraft)	1 Tbsp	80	0
Bacon & Tomato (Kraft)	1 Tbsp	70	0
Blue Cheese (Diamond Crystal)	1 Tbsp	20	5
Blue Cheese (Roka Brand)	1 Tbsp	60	10
Blue Cheese Chunky (Kraft)	1 Tbsp	70	0
Blue Cheese Lite (Wish-Bone)	1 Tbsp	38	tr
Buttermilk Creamy (Kraft)	1 Tbsp	80	0
Buttermilk & Chives Creamy (Kraft)	1 Tbsp	80	5
Buttermilk Lite (Wish-Bone)	1 Tbsp	53	1
Caesar Golden (Kraft)	1 Tbsp	70	0
Ceasar (Wish-Bone)	1 Tbsp	78	1

FOOD	PORTION	CALORIES	CHOLESTEROL
Coleslaw (Kraft)	1 Tbsp	70	10
Creamy Italian (Pritikin Foods)	1 Tbsp	12	0
Cucumber Creamy (Kraft)	1 Tbsp	70	0
Dijon Classic Creamy (Wish-Bone)	1 Tbsp	62	4
Dijon Classic Vinaigrette (Wish-Bone)	1 Tbsp	61	tr
Famous Chef Style (Ott's)	1 Tbsp	40	tr
French (Catalina)	1 Tbsp	70	0
French (Kraft)	1 Tbsp	60	0
French (Pritikin Foods)	1 Tbsp	10	0
French Deluxe (Wish-Bone)	1 Tbsp	59	0
French Lite (Wish-Bone)	1 Tbsp	31	0
Garlic Creamy (Kraft)	1 Tbsp	50	10
Garlic Creamy (Wish-Bone)	1 Tbsp	74	0
Garlic French (Wish-Bone)	1 Tbsp	56	0
Home Style (Diamond Crystal)	1 Tbsp	20	5
Italian (Presto)	1 Tbsp	70	0

FOOD	PORTION	CALORIES	CHOLESTEROL
Italian (Pritikin Foods)	1 Tbsp	6	0
Italian Chef Style (Ott's)	1 Tbsp	80	tr
Italian Creamy (Wish-Bone)	1 Tbsp	56	tr
Italian Creamy w/ Real Sour Cream (Kraft)	1 Tbsp	60	0
Italian Herbal Classics (Wish-Bone)	1 Tbsp	70	0
Italian Oil-Free (Kraft)	1 Tbsp	4	0
Italian Robusto (Wish-Bone)	1 Tbsp	70	0
Oil & Vinegar (Kraft)	1 Tbsp	70	0
Onion & Chive (Wish-Bone)	1 Tbsp	37	0
Onion & Chives Creamy (Kraft)	1 Tbsp	70	0
Ranch (Pritikin Foods)	1 Tbsp	18	0
Ranch Lite (Wish-Bone)	1 Tbsp	42	0
Rancher's Choice Creamy (Kraft)	1 Tbsp	80	5
Red Wine Vinaigrette (Wish-Bone)	1 Tbsp.	50	0
Red Wine Vinegar & Oil (Kraft)	1 Tbsp	50	0

FOOD	PORTION	CALORIES	CHOLESTEROL
Romano & Parmesan Creamy (Wish-Bone)	1 Tbsp	89	6
Russian (Kraft)	1 Tbsp	60	0
Russian (Pritikin Foods)	1 Tbsp	12	0
Russian (Wish-Bone)	1 Tbsp	47	0
Russian Lite (Wish-Bone)	1 Tbsp	22	0
Thousand Island & Bacon (Kraft)	1 Tbsp	60	0
Thousand Island (Diamond Crystal)	1 Tbsp	20	5
Thousand Island (Kraft)	1 Tbsp	60	5
Thousand Island (Wish-Bone)	1 Tbsp	69	4
Thousand Island Lite (Wish-Bone)	1 Tbsp	40	9
Vinaigrette (Pritikin Foods)	1 Tbsp	10	0
Zesty Italian (Kraft)	1 Tbsp	70	0
Zesty Tomato (Pritikin Foods)	1 Tbsp	18	0

READY-TO-USE REDUCED CALORIE

FOOD	PORTION	CALORIES	CHOLESTEROL
Bacon & Tomato Reduced Calorie (Kraft)	1 Tbsp	30	0

FOOD	PORTION	CALORIES	CHOLESTEROL
Bacon Creamy Reduced Calorie (Kraft)	1 Tbsp	30	0
Bacon & Tomato (Estee)	1 Tbsp	8	3
Bleu Cheese (Walden Farms)	1 Tbsp	27	5
Bleu Cheese Natural (Magic Mountain)	1 Tbsp	5	tr
Blue Cheese (Estee)	1 Tbsp	8	10
Blue Cheese Chunky Reduced Calorie (Kraft)	1 Tbsp	30	0
Blue Cheese Reduced Calorie (Roka Brand)	1 Tbsp	14	5
Buttermilk Creamy (Estee)	1 Tbsp	6	5
Buttermilk Creamy Reduced Calorie (Kraft)	1 Tbsp	30	0
Creamy Italian w/ Parmesan (Walden Farms)	1 Tbsp	35	4
Cucumber Creamy Reduced Calorie (Kraft)	1 Tbsp	30	0
Dijon Creamy (Estee)	1 Tbsp	8	30
French (Walden Farms)	1 Tbsp	33	2
French Reduced Calorie (Kraft)	1 Tbsp	25	0

FOOD	PORTION	CALORIES	CHOLESTEROL
French Style Natural (Magic Mountain)	1 Tbsp	4	0
Garlic Creamy w/ Red Wine Vinegar (Estee)	1 Tbsp	2	0
Herb & Spice No Oil (Magic Mountain)	1 Tbsp	2	0
Italian (Walden Farms)	1 Tbsp	9	0
Italian Creamy (Estee)	1 Tbsp	4	5
Italian Creamy Reduced Calorie (Kraft)	1 Tbsp	25	0
Italian French (Estee)	1 Tbsp	4	5
Italian No Sugar Added (Walden Farms)	1 Tbsp	6	0
Italian Reduced Calorie (Kraft)	1 Tbsp	6	0
Italian Sodium Free (Walden Farms)	1 Tbsp	9	0
Northern Italian Natural (Magic Mountain)	1 Tbsp	2	0
Ranch (Walden Farms)	1 Tbsp	35	8
Rancher's Choice Creamy Reduced Calorie (Kraft)	1 Tbsp	30	5
Reduced Calorie (Catalina)	1 Tbsp	16	0
Russian Reduced Calorie (Kraft)	1 Tbsp	30	0

FOOD	PORTION	CALORIES	CHOLESTEROL
Thousand Island (Estee)	1 Tbsp	6	5
Thousand Island (Walden Farms)	1 Tbsp	24	8
Thousand Island Reduced Calorie (Kraft)	1 Tbsp	30	5
French	1 Tbsp	22	1
Italian	1 Tbsp	16	1
Russian	1 Tbsp	23	1
Thousand Island	1 Tbsp	24	2

SALMON

CANNED			
Pink (Bumble Bee)	3 oz	137	45
Pink Skinless (Bumble Bee)	3.25 oz	120	45
Red (Bumble Bee)	3 oz	154	56
chum w/ bone	3 oz	120	33
chum w/ bone	1 can (13.9 oz)	521	144
sockeye w/ bone	3 oz	130	37
sockeye w/ bone	1 can (12.9 oz)	566	161
FRESH			
Salmon Steak (Health Valley)	3.5 oz	220	0
atlantic, raw	3 oz	121	47

FOOD	PORTION	CALORIES	CHOLESTEROL
atlantic, raw	½ fillet (6.9 oz)	281	109
chinook, raw	½ fillet (6.9 oz)	356	131
chinook, raw	3 oz	153	56
chum, raw	3 oz	102	63
chum, raw	½ fillet (6.9 oz)	237	147
coho, raw	½ fillet (6.9 oz)	289	77
coho, raw	3 oz	124	33
coho; cooked	3 oz	157	42
coho; cooked	½ fillet (5.4 oz)	286	76
pink, raw	½ fillet (5.6 oz)	185	83
pink, raw	3 oz	99	44
sockeye, raw	½ fillet (6.9 oz)	333	123
sockeye, raw	3 oz	143	53
sockeye; cooked	3 oz	183	74
sockeye; cooked	½ fillet (5.4 oz)	334	135
HOME RECIPE salmon cake	3.4 oz	241	104
salmon casserole	¾ cup	416	91
salmon rice loaf	6.2 oz	299	133
SMOKED chinook	1 oz	33	7
chinook	3 oz	99	20

FOOD	PORTION	CALORIES	CHOLESTEROL
SALSIFY			
FRESH			
cooked; sliced	½ cup	46	0
raw; sliced	½ cup	55	0
SALT/SEASONED SALT			
(*see also* SALT SUBSTITUTE)			
Garlic Salt (Morton)	1 tsp	3	0
Kosher Salt (Morton)	1 tsp	0	0
Lite Salt Mixture (Morton)	1 tsp	tr	0
Nature's Seasons Seasoning Blend (Morton)	1 tsp	3	0
Salt Iodized (Morton)	1 tsp	tr	0
Salt Non-Iodized (Morton)	1 tsp	0	0
Seasoned Salt (Morton)	1 tsp	4	0
SALT SUBSTITUTE			
Nu-Salt	1 pkg (1 g)	0	0
Salt-It Salt Substitute (Estee)	½ tsp	0	0
Salt Substitute (Morton)	1 tsp	tr	0
Seasoned Salt Substitute (Morton)	1 tsp	2	0

FOOD	PORTION	CALORIES	CHOLESTEROL

SAPODILLA

FRESH

sapodilla	1	140	0

SARDINE

CANNED

Atlantic in oil w/ bone	1 can (3.2 oz)	192	131
Atlantic in oil w/ bone	2 oz	50	34
Pacfic in brine & mustard	1 large (.7 oz)	39	24
Pacific w/ tomato sauce w/ bone	1 can (13 oz)	658	225
Pacific w/ tomato sauce w/ bone	1 oz	68	23

SAUCE

(*see also* GRAVY, PIZZA, SPAGHETTI SAUCE, TOMATO)

DRY

Bar-B-Q Sauce Mix (Diamond Crystal)	2 oz	35	tr
Brown Sauce Mix (Diamond Crystal)	2 oz	15	2
Cheese Sauce Mix (Diamond Crystal)	2 oz	50	2
Cream Sauce Mix (Diamond Crystal)	2 oz	40	3
Italian Sauce Mix (Diamond Crystal)	3 oz	50	0

FOOD	PORTION	CALORIES	CHOLESTEROL
Marinade for Meat (Kikkoman)	1 oz pkg	64	0
Sweet & Sour Sauce Mix (Kikkoman)	2⅛ oz pkg	228	0
Sweet 'n Sour Entree Mix (Chun King)	3.8 oz	370	0
Teriyaki Sauce Mix (Kikkoman)	1½ oz pkg	125	0
bearnaise; as prep w/ milk & butter	1 cup	701	189
bearnaise; not prep	1 pkg (9 oz)	90	tr
cheese; as prep w/ milk	1 cup	307	53
cheese; not prep	1 pkg (1.2 oz)	158	18
curry; as prep w/ milk	1 cup	270	35
curry; not prep	1 pkg (1.2 oz)	151	tr
hollandaise w/ butterfat; as prep w/ water	1 cup	237	51
hollandaise w/ butterfat; not prep	1 pkg (1.2 oz)	187	40
hollandaise w/ oil; as prep w/ water	1 cup	703	189
hollandaise w/ oil; not prep	1 pkg (.9 oz)	93	tr
mushroom; as prep w/ milk	1 cup	228	34
mushroom; not prep	1 pkg (1 oz)	99	0
sour cream; as prep w/ milk	1 cup	509	91
sour cream; not prep	1 pkg (1.2 oz)	180	28

FOOD	PORTION	CALORIES	CHOLESTEROL
stroganoff; as prep w/ milk & water	1 cup	271	38
stroganoff; not prep	1 pkg (1.6 oz)	161	12
sweet & sour; as prep w/ water & vinegar	1 cup	294	0
sweet & sour; not prep	1 pkg (2 oz)	220	0
teriyaki; as prep w/ water	1 cup	131	0
teriyaki; not prep	1 pkg (1.6 oz)	130	0
white; as prep w/ milk	1 cup	241	34
white; not prep	1 pkg (1.7 oz)	230	tr
HOME RECEIPE			
hollandaise	2 Tbsp	130	16
JARRED			
A-1 Steak Sauce (Heublein)	1 Tbsp	14	0
Barbecue (Maull's)	3.5 oz	123	1
Barbecue Beer Flavor, Non-Alcoholic (Maull's)	3.5 oz	128	1
Barbecue Sauce (Estee)	1 Tbsp	18	0
Barbecue Sauce (Kraft)	2 Tbsp	40	0
Barbecue Sauce (Ott's)	1 Tbsp	14	tr

FOOD	PORTION	CALORIES	CHOLESTEROL
Barbecue Sauce Garlic Flavored (Kraft)	2 Tbsp	40	0
Barbecue Sauce Hickory Smoke (Open Pit)	1 Tbsp	25	0
Barbecue Sauce Hickory Smoke Flavor (Kraft)	2 Tbsp	40	0
Barbecue Sauce Hickory Smoke Flavored Onion Bits (Kraft)	2 Tbsp	50	0
Barbecue Sauce Hot (Kraft)	2 Tbsp	40	0
Barbecue Sauce Hot Hickory Smoke Flavored (Kraft)	2 Tbsp	40	0
Barbecue Sauce Italian Seasoning (Kraft)	2 Tbsp	45	0
Barbecue Sauce Kansas City Style (Kraft)	2 Tbsp	45	0
Barbecue Sauce Mesquite Smoke (Kraft)	2 Tbsp	45	0
Barbecue Sauce Onion Bits (Kraft)	2 Tbsp	50	0
Barbecue Sauce Original (Bull's Eye)	2 Tbsp	50	0
Barbecue Sauce Smoky (Ott's)	1 Tbsp	14	tr

FOOD	PORTION	CALORIES	CHOLESTEROL
Barbecue Sauce Thick 'n Tangy Hickory (Open Pit)	1 Tbsp	25	0
Barbecue Sauce Thick'n Spicy Chunky (Kraft)	2 Tbsp	50	0
Barbecue Sauce Thick'n Spicy Hickory Smoked (Kraft)	2 Tbsp	50	0
Barbecue Sauce Thick'n Spicy Kansas City Style (Kraft)	2 Tbsp	60	0
Barbecue Sauce Thick'n Spicy Original (Kraft)	2 Tbsp	50	0
Barbecue Sauce Thick'n Spicy w/ Honey (Kraft)	2 Tbsp	60	0
Barbecue Smoky (Maull's)	3.5 oz	124	1
Barbecue Sweet-N-Mild (Maull's)	3.5 oz	167	1
Barbecue Sweet-N-Smoky (Maull's)	3.5 oz	160	1
Barbecue w/ Onion Bits (Maull's)	3.5 oz	126	1
Cocktail (Sauceworks)	1 Tbsp	12	0
Cocktail Sauce (Estee)	1 Tbsp	10	0
Rib Sauce (Gold's)	1 oz	60	0

FOOD	PORTION	CALORIES	CHOLESTEROL
Steak Sauce (Estee)	½ oz	15	0
Stir-Fry Sauce (Kikkoman)	1 tsp	6	0
Sweet & Sour Sauce (Kikkoman)	1 Tbsp	18	0
Sweet 'N Sour (Sauceworks)	1 Tbsp	20	0
Sweet 'n Sour (Contadina)	½ cup	150	0
Tartar Sauce (Best Foods)	1 Tbsp	70	5
Tartar Sauce (Bright Day)	1 Tbsp	50	0
Tartar Sauce (Hellman's)	1 Tbsp	70	5
Tartar Sauce (Kraft)	1 Tbsp	70	5
Tartar Sauce (Sauceworks)	1 Tbsp	70	5
Tartar Sauce Natural Lemon & Herb Flavor (Sauceworks)	1 Tbsp	70	5
Teriyaki Sauce (Kikkoman)	1 Tbsp	15	tr
Tobasco (McIlhenny)	¼ tsp	tr	0
Worchestershire (Lea & Perrins)	1 Tbsp	59	0
barbecue	1 cup	188	0
teriyaki	1 Tbsp	15	0
teriyaki	1 oz	30	0

FOOD	PORTION	CALORIES	CHOLESTEROL

SAUERKRAUT

CANNED

FOOD	PORTION	CALORIES	CHOLESTEROL
Sauerkraut (Claussen)	½ cup	17	0
Sauerkraut (Libby)	½ cup	20	0
Sauerkraut (Seneca)	½ cup	20	0
canned	½ cup	22	0

JUICE

FOOD	PORTION	CALORIES	CHOLESTEROL
Sauerkraut Juice (S&W)	5 oz	14	0

SAUSAGE

(*see also* HOT DOG, SAUSAGE SUBSTITUTE)

FOOD	PORTION	CALORIES	CHOLESTEROL
Breakfast Sausage, Turkey (Bil Mar Foods)	1 oz	58	16
Knockwurst (Health Valley)	3.5 oz	280	56
Knockwurst (Hebrew National)	1 (3 oz)	260	26
Oscar Mayer Bratwurst Smoked	1 (2.7 oz)	237	40
Oscar Mayer Italian Smoked Cooked Cured	1 (2.6 oz)	264	39
Oscar Mayer Kielbasa	1 oz	83	14
Oscar Mayer Little Friers Pork; cooked	1 (.7 oz)	82	17
Oscar Mayer Polish	1 (2.7 oz)	229	31
Oscar Mayer Smoked	1 oz	83	15

FOOD	PORTION	CALORIES	CHOLESTEROL
Oscar Mayer Smokies, Beef	1 (1.5 oz)	123	27
Oscar Mayer Smokies, Cheese	1 (1.5 oz)	127	29
Oscar Mayer Smokies Links	1 (1.5 oz)	124	28
Oscar Mayer Smokies, Little	1 (.3 oz)	28	6
Polish Kielbasa (Mr. Turkey)	3 oz	177	44
Pork Breakfast Patties (Jones)	1 (2 oz)	136	42
Pork Brown & Serve Links (Jones)	1 (.8 oz)	55	17
Pork Brown & Serve Patties (Jones)	1 (2 oz)	136	42
Pork, Light Breakfast Links (Jones)	1 (.8 oz)	55	17
Pork, Light Breakfast Links (Jones)	1 (2 oz)	136	42
Smoked Sausage (Bil Mar Foods)	3 oz	142	57
bratwurst, pork; cooked	1 link (85 g)	256	51
bratwurst, pork; cooked	1 oz	85	17
bratwurst, pork & beef	1 link (70 g)	226	44
bratwurst, pork & beef	1 oz	92	18
country-style, pork; cooked	1 patty (1 oz)	100	22
country-style, pork; cooked	1 link (½ oz)	48	11
Italian, pork, raw	1 link (2.3 oz)	315	69

FOOD	PORTION	CALORIES	CHOLESTEROL
Italian, pork, raw	1 link (4 oz)	391	86
Italian, pork; cooked	1 link (67 g)	216	52
Italian, pork; cooked	1 link (83 g)	268	65
kielbasa	1 oz	88	19
kielbasa, pork	1 slice (26 g)	81	17
knockwurst, pork & beef	1 link (68 g)	209	39
knockwurst, pork & beef	1 oz	87	16
Polish, pork	1 link (8 oz)	739	158
Polish, pork	1 oz	92	20
pork, country-style, raw	1 patty (2 oz)	238	39
pork, country-style, raw	1 link (1 oz)	118	19
pork, raw	1 patty (2 oz)	238	39
pork, raw	1 link (1 oz)	118	19
pork; cooked	1 patty (1 oz)	100	22
pork; cooked	1 link (½ oz)	48	11
smoked, beef; cooked	1 sausage (1.4 oz)	134	29
smoked, pork	1 link (2⅓ oz)	256	46

FOOD	PORTION	CALORIES	CHOLESTEROL
smoked, pork	1 sm link (½ oz)	62	11
smoked, pork & beef	1 link (2⅓ oz)	229	48
smoked, pork & beef	1 sm link (½ oz)	54	11
Vienna, canned, beef & pork	1 sausage (½ oz)	45	8

SAUSAGE SUBSTITUTE

FOOD	PORTION	CALORIES	CHOLESTEROL
Grillers, frzn (Morningstar Farms)	3.5 oz	290	2
Linketts (Loma Linda)	2 (2.6 oz)	150	0
Links, frzn (Morningstar Farms)	3.5 oz	237	1
Little Links (Loma Linda)	2 (1.6 oz)	80	0

SCALLOP

FRESH

FOOD	PORTION	CALORIES	CHOLESTEROL
raw	3 oz	75	28
raw	2 lg	26	10
raw	5 sm	26	10

FROZEN

FOOD	PORTION	CALORIES	CHOLESTEROL
Lightly Breaded Scallops (King & Prince)	3.5 oz	120	14

HOME RECIPE

FOOD	PORTION	CALORIES	CHOLESTEROL
breaded & fried	2 lg	67	19

FOOD	PORTION	CALORIES	CHOLESTEROL

SCONE

HOME RECIPE

apricot scone	1	232	34
scone	1 (1.4 oz)	130	56

SCROD

FROZEN

Ready-to-Bake Scrod (King & Prince)	5 oz	252	32
Ready-to-Bake Scrod (King & Prince)	8 oz	403	52

SEA BASS
(*see* BASS)

SEATROUT
(*see* TROUT)

SEASONING

Herb Seasoning (American Heart Association)	¼ tsp	tr	0
Instead of Salt All Purpose (Health Valley)	¾ tsp	11	0
Instead of Salt Chicken (Health Valley)	¾ tsp	8	0
Instead of Salt Fish (Health Valley)	¾ tsp	11	0
Instead of Salt Steak & Hamburger (Health Valley)	½ tsp	6	0

FOOD	PORTION	CALORIES	CHOLESTEROL
Instead of Salt Vegetable (Health Valley)	1 tsp	13	0
Lemon Herb Seasoning (American Heart Association)	¼ tsp	tr	0
Original Herb Seasoning (American Heart Association)	¼ tsp	tr	0
Savorex (Loma Linda)	1 tsp	16	0

SEEDS
(see individual names)

SESAME

FOOD	PORTION	CALORIES	CHOLESTEROL
Sesame Nut Mix Oil Roasted (Planters)	1 oz	160	0
Sesame Nut Mix Dry Roasted (Planters)	1 oz	160	0
seeds	1 tsp	16	0
seeds, dried	1 Tbsp	52	0
seeds, dried	1 cup	825	0
seeds, roasted & toasted	1 oz	161	0
sesame butter	1 Tbsp	95	0
tahini, from roasted & toasted kernels	1 Tbsp	89	0
tahini, from unroasted kernels	1 Tbsp	85	0

SHAD

	PORTION	CALORIES	CHOLESTEROL
FRESH			
roe, raw	3½ oz	130	360

FOOD	PORTION	CALORIES	CHOLESTEROL

SHALLOT

DRIED
freeze-dried | 1 Tbsp | 3 | 0

FRESH
chopped | 1 Tbsp | 7 | 0

SHARK

FRESH
raw | 3 oz | 111 | 43

HOME RECIPE
batter-dipped & fried | 3 oz | 194 | 50

SHELLFISH
(*see individual names*, SHELLFISH SUBSTITUTE)

SHELLFISH SUBSTITUTE

FOOD	PORTION	CALORIES	CHOLESTEROL
Crab Delights (Louis Kemp)	2 oz	60	10
Kibun Sea Pasta w/ Shrimp w/ dressing	½ pkg	210	30
Kibun Sea Pasta w/ Shrimp w/o dressing	½ pkg	140	30
Kibun Sea Pasta w/ dressing	½ pkg	220	10
Kibun Sea Pasta w/o dressing	½ pkg	110	10
Kibun Sea Stix Salad Style	4 oz	110	20
Kibun Sea Stix Whole Leg	4 oz	110	20
Kibun Sea Tails	4 oz	110	15
SeaLegs Imitation Lobster Meat	3 oz	80	10

FOOD	PORTION	CALORIES	CHOLESTEROL
crab, imitation	3 oz	87	17
scallop, imitation	3 oz	84	18
shrimp, imitation	3 oz	86	31
surimi	1 oz	28	8
surimi	3 oz	84	25

SHELLIE BEANS

CANNED

shellie beans	½ cup	37	0

SHRIMP

CANNED

canned	1 cup	154	222
canned	3 oz	102	147

FRESH

cooked	4 lg	22	43
cooked	3 oz	84	166
raw	3 oz	90	130
raw	4 lg	30	43

FROZEN

Cooked in the Shell (King & Prince)	4 oz	70	91
Cooked in the Shell (King & Prince)	3.5 oz	65	77
Gourmet Hand Breaded Shrimp Butterfly (King & Prince)	3.5 oz	150	56
Gourmet Hand Breaded Shrimp Round (King & Prince)	3.5 oz	150	56

FOOD	PORTION	CALORIES	CHOLESTEROL
Shrimp Del Ray (King & Prince)	3 oz	85	38
Shrimp Del Ray (King & Prince)	1.5 oz	43	19
Shrimp a la Monterey (King & Prince)	3.5 oz	190	65
Shrimp a la Monterey (King & Prince)	2 oz	107	37
Supreme Hand Breaded Shrimp Butterfly (King & Prince)	3.5 oz	130	55
Supreme Hand Breaded Shrimp Round (King & Prince)	3.5 oz	140	65
Western Style Breaded Shrimp (King & Prince)	3.5 oz	115	70
HOME RECIPE			
jambalaya	¾ cup	188	50
shrimp; breaded & fried	3 oz	206	150
shrimp; breaded & fried	4 lg	73	53
stew	1 cup	207	79
READY-TO-USE			
Fried Shrimp (American Original Foods)	4 oz	253	27

SMELT

FRESH			
rainbow, raw	3 oz	83	60
rainbow; cooked	3 oz	106	76

FOOD	PORTION	CALORIES	CHOLESTEROL

SNACKS
(see also CHIPS; FRUIT SNACKS; NUTS, MIXED; POPCORN; PRETZELS)

FOOD	PORTION	CALORIES	CHOLESTEROL
Cheddar Lites (Health Valley)	.2 oz	40	tr
Cheddar Lites w/ Green Onion (Health Valley)	.2 oz	40	0
Cheese Balls (Lance)	1 pkg (1⅛ oz)	190	5
Cheese Balls (Lance)	1 oz	160	5
Cheetos Crunchy Cheese Flavored	1 oz	160	tr
Cheetos Puffed Balls Cheese Flavored	1 oz	160	tr
Cheetos Puffs Cheese Flavored	1 oz	160	tr
Cornnuts, Barbecue	1 oz	110	0
Cornnuts, Nacho Cheese	1 oz	110	0
Cornnuts, Original	1 oz	120	0
Cornnuts, Unsalted	1 oz	120	0
Crunchy Cheese Twists (Lance)	1 pkg (1½ oz)	230	0
Crunchy Cheese Twists (Lance)	1 oz	150	tr
Funyuns (Frito-Lay)	1 oz	140	0
Gold-N-Chee (Lance)	1⅜ oz	180	5
Gold-N-Chee (Lance)	1 oz	130	0
Munchos	1 oz	150	0

FOOD	PORTION	CALORIES	CHOLESTEROL
Pork Skins (Lance)	½ oz	80	20
Pork Skins Regular (Lance)	½ oz	80	20
Tostada Nacho (Lance)	1 oz	140	tr
Tostada Regular (Lance)	1 oz	150	0
Wheat Snax (Estee)	1 oz	110	0

SNAIL
(see WHELK)

SNAP BEANS

CANNED			
seasoned	½ cup	18	0
snap beans	½ cup	18	0
FRESH			
cooked	½ cup	22	0
raw	½ cup	17	0
FROZEN			
snap beans	½ cup	18	0

SNAPPER

FRESH			
cooked	1 fillet (6 oz)	217	80
cooked	3 oz	109	40

FOOD	PORTION	CALORIES	CHOLESTEROL
raw	3 oz	85	31
raw	1 fillet (7.6 oz)	217	81

SODA
(see also DRINK MIXER)

FOOD	PORTION	CALORIES	CHOLESTEROL
7-Up	1 oz	12	0
7-Up Cherry	1 oz	13	0
7-Up Cherry Diet	1 oz	tr	0
7-Up Diet	1 oz	tr	0
7-Up Gold	1 oz	13	0
7-Up Gold Diet	1 oz	tr	0
Apple Sparkling (Welch's)	12 oz	180	0
Birch Beer Diet (Shasta)	12 oz	4	0
Black Cherry (Shasta)	12 oz	162	0
Cherry Cola (Shasta)	12 oz	140	0
Citrus Mist (Shasta)	12 oz	170	0
Club (Schweppes)	6 oz	0	0
Club Soda (Shasta)	12 oz	0	0
Coca-Cola	6 oz	77	0
Coca-Cola Caffeine-Free	6 oz	77	0
Coca-Cola Cherry	6 oz	76	0
Coca-Cola Classic	6 oz	72	0

FOOD	PORTION	CALORIES	CHOLESTEROL
Cola (Shasta)	8 oz	98	0
Cola (Shasta)	12 oz	147	0
Cola Diet (Shasta)	8 oz	0	0
Collins (Shasta)	12 oz	118	0
Creme (Shasta)	12 oz	154	0
Diet Cherry Coca-Cola	6 oz	tr	0
Diet Coke	6 oz	tr	0
Diet Coke Caffeine-Free	6 oz	tr	0
Diet Minute Maid Lemon-Lime	6 oz	10	0
Diet Minute Maid Orange	6 oz	4	0
Diet Sprite	6 oz	2	0
Dr Pepper	1 oz	13	0
Dr Pepper Diet	1 oz	tr	0
Dr. Diablo (Shasta)	12 oz	140	0
Fanta Ginger Ale	6 oz	63	0
Fanta Grape	6 oz	86	0
Fanta Orange	6 oz	88	0
Fanta Root Beer	6 oz	78	0
Fresca	6 oz	2	0
Fruit Punch (Shasta)	12 oz	173	0
Ginger Ale (Health Valley)	13 oz	153	0

FOOD	PORTION	CALORIES	CHOLESTEROL
Ginger Ale (Schweppes)	6 oz	63	0
Ginger Ale (Shasta)	8 oz	80	0
Ginger Ale (Shasta)	12 oz	120	0
Ginger Ale Diet (Schweppes)	6 oz	tr	0
Ginger Ale Diet (Shasta)	8 oz	0	0
Ginger Beer (Schweppes)	6 oz	68	0
Grape (Schweppes)	6 oz	92	0
Grape (Shasta)	12 oz	177	0
Grape Sparkling (Welch's)	12 oz	180	0
Grapefruit (Schweppes)	6 oz	77	0
Lemon-Lime (Schweppes)	6 oz	71	0
Lemon-Lime (Shasta)	8 oz	97	0
Lemon-Lime (Shasta)	12 oz	146	0
Lemon-Lime Diet (Shasta)	8 oz	0	0
Like Cola	1 oz	13	0
Like Cola Sugar Free	1 oz	tr	0
Mello Yellow	6 oz	87	0

FOOD	PORTION	CALORIES	CHOLESTEROL
Minute Maid Lemon-Lime	6 oz	71	0
Minute Maid Orange	6 oz	87	0
Mr. PIBB	6 oz	71	0
Orange (Shasta)	12 oz	177	0
Orange Sparkling (Welch's)	12 oz	180	0
Orange Sparkling (Schweppes)	6 oz	86	0
Pepper Free	1 oz	12	0
Pepper Free Diet	1 oz	tr	0
Ramblin' Root Beer	6 oz	88	0
Red Berry (Shasta)	12 oz	158	0
Red Pop (Shasta)	12 oz	158	0
Root Beer (Health Valley)	13 oz	120	0
Root Beer (Schweppes)	6 oz	75	0
Root Beer (Shasta)	12 oz	154	0
Sarsaparilla (Health Valley)	13 oz	153	0
Seltzer (Schweppes)	6 oz	0	0
Seltzer Flavored (Schweppes)	6 oz	0	0
Seltzer Light Black Cherry Cider (Crystal Geyser)	6 oz	60	0

FOOD	PORTION	CALORIES	CHOLESTEROL
Seltzer Light Cranberry-Raspberry (Crystal Geyser)	6 oz	60	0
Seltzer Light Kiwi Lemonade (Crystal Geyser)	6 oz	60	0
Seltzer Light Natural Peach (Crystal Geyser)	6 oz	60	0
Seltzer Light Vanilla Creme (Crystal Geyser)	6 oz	60	0
Seltzer No Salt Added No Calories (Manischewitz)	8 oz	0	0
Shasta Free Cola	12 oz	151	0
Sprite	6 oz	71	0
Strawberry (Shasta)	12 oz	147	0
Strawberry, Sparkling (Welch's)	12 oz	180	0
TAB	6 oz	tr	0
TAB Caffeine-Free	6 oz	tr	0
Tonic Water (Shasta)	12 oz	0	0
Wild Berry (Health Valley)	13 oz	142	0
club	12 oz	0	0
cola	12 oz	151	0
cream	12 oz	191	0
ginger ale	12 oz can	124	0
grape	12 oz	161	0
lemon-lime	12 oz	149	0

FOOD	PORTION	CALORIES	CHOLESTEROL
orange	12 oz	177	0
root beer	12 oz	152	0
tonic water	12	125	0

SOLE

FROZEN

Sole a la Monterey (King & Prince)	6 oz	221	11
Sole a la Monterey (King & Prince)	8 oz	295	15

SOUFFLE

HOME RECIPE

cheese	1 cup	308	196
grand marnier	1 cup	109	139
lemon, chilled	1 cup	176	2
raspberry, chilled	1 cup	173	3
spinach souffle	1 cup	218	184

SOUP

CANNED

5 Bean Chunky (Health Valley)	7.5 oz	80	0
Barley w/ Beef; as prep w/ water (Campbell)	1 cup	86	tr
Bean (Health Valley)	4 oz	115	0
Bean w/ Bacon, Special Request (Campbell's)	8 oz	120	5

FOOD	PORTION	CALORIES	CHOLESTEROL
Bean w/ Bacon, Special Request (Campbell's)	8 oz	120	5
Beef Broth (Pritikin Foods)	6⅞ oz	20	<5
Borscht (Gold's)	8 oz	100	0
Borscht Low Calorie (Manischewitz)	8 oz	20	0
Borscht w/ Beets (Manischewitz)	8 oz	80	0
Borscht, Lo-Cal (Gold's)	8 oz	20	0
Chicken Vegetable Soup (Pritikin Foods)	7¼ oz	70	0
Chicken Broth (Health Valley)	4 oz	15	4
Chicken Broth (Pritikin Foods)	6⅞ oz	14	0
Chicken Gumbo (Pritikin Foods)	7⅜ oz	60	5
Chicken Soup w/ Ribbon Pasta (Pritikin Foods)	7¼ oz	60	0
Chicken w/ Rice, Special Request (Campbell's)	8 oz	60	10
Clam Chowder (Health Valley)	4 oz	80	7
Country Vegetable (Lunch Bucket)	1 container (8.25 oz)	90	0
Lentil (Health Valley)	4 oz	90	0

FOOD	PORTION	CALORIES	CHOLESTEROL
Lentil Soup (Pritikin Foods)	7⅜ oz	100	0
Manhattan Clam Chowder (Pritikin Foods)	7⅜ oz	70	2
Minestrone (Health Valley)	7.5 oz	90	0
Minestrone Chunky (Health Valley)	4 oz	70	0
Minestrone Soup (Pritikin Foods)	7⅜ oz	110	0
Mushroom (Health Valley)	4 oz	70	0
Mushroom (Pritikin Foods)	7⅜ oz	60	2
Navy Bean (Pritikin Foods)	7⅜ oz	130	2
New England Chowder (American Original Foods)	4 oz	64	5
New England Clam Chowder (Pritikin Foods)	7⅜ oz	118	2
Potato (Health Valley)	4 oz	70	0
Schav (Gold's)	8 oz	25	15
Split Pea Soup (Pritikin Foods)	7½ oz	130	5
Split Pea Green (Health Valley)	4 oz	70	0
Tomato (Health Valley)	4 oz	60	0
Tomato Soup w/ Tomato Pieces (Pritikin Foods)	7¼ oz	70	0

FOOD	PORTION	CALORIES	CHOLESTEROL
Turkey Vegetable Soup w/ Ribbon Pasta (Pritikin Foods)	7⅜ oz	50	5
Vegetable (Health Valley)	7.5 oz	80	0
Vegetable Beef (Lunch Bucket)	1 container (8.25 oz)	140	15
Vegetable Chicken Chunky (Health Valley)	4 oz	120	12
Vegetable Soup (Pritikin Foods)	7⅜ oz	70	0
asparagus, cream of; as prep w/ milk	1 cup	161	22
asparagus, cream of; as prep w/ water	1 cup	87	5
bean w/ frankfurters; as prep w/ water	1 cup	187	12
bean w/ frankfurters; not prep	1 can (11¼ oz)	454	29
bean black; as prep w/ water	1 cup	116	0
bean black; not prep	1 can (11 oz)	285	0
bean w/ bacon; not prep	1 can (11½ oz)	420	6
bean w/ bacon; as prep w/ water	1 cup	173	3
bean w/ ham, chunky, ready-to-serve	1 can (19¼ oz)	519	49
bean w/ ham, chunky, ready-to-serve	1 cup	231	22
beef broth, ready-to-serve	1 can (14 oz)	27	1

FOOD	PORTION	CALORIES	CHOLESTEROL
beef broth, ready-to-serve	1 cup	16	tr
beef, chunky, ready-to-serve	1 cup	171	14
beef, chunky, ready-to-serve	1 can (19 oz)	383	32
beef noodle; as prep w/ water	1 cup	84	5
beef noodle; not prep	1 can (10¾ oz)	204	12
black bean turtle soup	1 cup	218	0
celery, cream of; as prep w/ milk	1 can (10¾ oz)	400	78
celery, cream of; as prep w/ milk	1 cup	165	32
celery, cream of; as prep w/ water	1 cup	90	15
celery, cream of; not prep	1 can (10¾ oz)	219	34
cheese; as prep w/ milk	1 cup	230	48
cheese; as prep w/ milk	1 can (11 oz)	558	116
cheese; as prep w/ water	1 can (11 oz)	377	72
cheese; as prep w/ water	1 cup	155	30
cheese; not prep	1 can (11 oz)	377	72
chicken vegetable, chunky, ready-to-serve	1 can (19 oz)	374	38
chicken vegetable, chunky, ready-to-serve	1 cup	167	17
chicken vegetable; as prep w/ water	1 cup	74	10

FOOD	PORTION	CALORIES	CHOLESTEROL
chicken vegetable; not prep	1 can (10½ oz)	181	21
chicken & dumplings; as prep w/ water	1 cup	406	34
chicken & dumplings; not prep	1 can (10½ oz)	236	80
chicken broth; as prep w/ water	1 can (10¾ oz)	95	2
chicken broth; as prep w/ water	1 cup	39	1
chicken broth; not prep	1 can (10¾ oz)	94	3
chicken, chunky, ready-to-serve	1 cup	178	30
chicken, chunky, ready-to-serve	1 can (10¾ oz)	216	37
chicken, cream of; as prep w/ milk	1 cup	191	27
chicken, cream of; as prep w/ water	1 can (10¾ oz)	464	66
chicken, cream of; as prep w/ water	1 cup	116	10
chicken, cream of; not prep	1 can (10¾ oz)	283	24
chicken gumbo; as prep w/ water	1 cup	56	5
chicken gumbo; not prep	1 can (10¾ oz)	137	9
chicken noodle w/ meatballs, ready-to-serve	1 cup	99	10
chicken noodle w/ meatballs, ready-to-serve	1 can (20 oz)	227	23

FOOD	PORTION	CALORIES	CHOLESTEROL
chicken noodle; as prep w/ water	1 cup	75	7
chicken noodle; not prep	1 can (10½ oz)	182	15
chicken rice, chunky, ready-to-serve	1 can (19 oz)	286	27
chicken rice, chunky, ready-to-serve	1 cup	127	12
chicken rice; as prep w/ water	1 cup	251	7
chicken rice; not prep	1 can (10½ oz)	146	15
chicken rice; not prep	1 can (10½ oz)	146	15
chili beef; as prep w/ water	1 cup	169	12
chili beef; not prep	1 can (11¼ oz)	411	32
clam chowder, Manhattan, chunky, ready-to-serve	1 cup	133	14
clam chowder, Manhattan, chunky, ready-to-serve	1 can (19 oz)	299	32
clam chowder, Manhattan; as prep w/ water	1 cup	78	2
clam chowder, Manhattan; not prep	1 can (10¾ oz)	187	6
clam chowder, New England; as prep w/ milk	1 cup	163	22
clam chowder, New England; as prep w/ water	1 cup	95	5
clam chowder, New England; not prep	1 can (10¾ oz)	214	12
consomme w/ gelatin; as prep w/ water	1 cup	29	0

FOOD	PORTION	CALORIES	CHOLESTEROL
consomme w/ gelatin; not prep	1 can (10½ oz)	71	0
crab, ready-to-serve	1 cup	76	10
crab, ready-to-serve	1 can (13 oz)	114	10
escarole, ready-to-serve	1 can (19½ oz)	61	6
escarole, ready-to-serve	1 cup	27	2
gazpacho, ready-to-serve	1 cup	57	0
gazpacho, ready-to-serve	1 can (13 oz)	87	0
lentil w/ ham, ready-to-serve	1 can (20 oz)	320	17
lentil w/ ham, ready-to-serve	1 cup	140	7
minestrone, chunky, ready-to-serve	1 cup	127	5
minestrone, chunky, ready-to-serve	1 can (19 oz)	285	11
minestrone; as prep w/ water	1 cup	83	2
minestrone; not prep	1 can (10½ oz)	202	3
mushroom w/ beef stock; as prep w/ water	1 can (10¾ oz)	208	18
mushroom w/ beef stock; as prep w/ water	1 cup	85	7
mushroom w/ beef stock; not prep	1 can (10¾ oz)	208	18
mushroom, cream of; as prep w/ milk	1 can (10¾ oz)	494	48
mushroom, cream of; as prep w/ milk	1 cup	203	20

FOOD	PORTION	CALORIES	CHOLESTEROL
mushroom, cream of; as prep w/ water	1 cup	129	2
mushroom, cream of; not prep	1 can (10¾ oz)	313	3
onion; as prep w/ water	1 cup	57	0
onion; not prep	1 can (10½ oz)	138	0
oyster stew; as prep w/ milk	1 cup	134	32
oyster stew; as prep w/ milk	1 can (10½ oz)	325	77
oyster stew; as prep w/ water	1 cup	59	14
oyster stew; not prep	1 can (10½ oz)	144	33
pea, green; as prep w/ milk	1 can (11¼ oz)	579	43
pea, green; as prep w/ milk	1 cup	239	18
pea, green; as prep w/ water	1 cup	164	0
pea, green; not prep	1 can (11¼ oz)	398	0
pepperpot; as prep w/ water	1 cup	103	10
pepperpot; not prep	1 can (10½ oz)	251	24
potato, cream of; as prep w/ milk	1 can (10¾ oz)	360	54
potato, cream of; as prep w/ milk	1 cup	148	22
potato, cream of; as prep w/ water	1 cup	73	5
potato, cream of; not prep	1 can (10¾ oz)	178	15

FOOD	PORTION	CALORIES	CHOLESTEROL
scotch broth; not prep	1 can (10½ oz)	195	12
scotch broth; as prep w/ water	1 cup	80	5
shrimp, cream of; as prep w/ milk	1 can (10¾ oz)	400	84
shrimp, cream of; as prep w/ milk	1 cup	165	35
shrimp, cream of; as prep w/ water	1 cup	90	17
shrimp, cream of; not prep	1 can (10¾ oz)	219	40
split pea w/ ham, chunky, ready-to-serve	1 cup	184	7
split pea w/ ham, chunky, ready-to-serve	1 can (19 oz)	413	16
split pea w/ ham; as prep w/ water	1 cup	189	8
split pea w/ ham; not prep	1 can (11½ oz)	459	20
stockpot; as prep w/ water	1 cup	100	5
stockpot; not prep	1 can (11 oz)	242	9
tomato beef w/ noodle; as prep w/ water	1 cup	140	5
tomato beef w/ noodle; not prep	1 can (10¾ oz)	341	9
tomato bisque; as prep w/ milk	1 can (11 oz)	481	53
tomato bisque; as prep w/ milk	1 cup	198	22

FOOD	PORTION	CALORIES	CHOLESTEROL
tomato bisque; as prep w/ water	1 cup	123	4
tomato bisque; not prep	1 can (11 oz)	300	11
tomato rice; as prep w/ water	1 cup	120	2
tomato rice; not prep	1 can (11 oz)	291	3
tomato; as prep w/ milk	1 can (10¾ oz)	389	42
tomato; as prep w/ milk	1 cup	160	17
tomato; as prep w/ water	1 cup	86	0
tomato; not prep	1 can (10¾ oz)	208	0
turkey, chunky, ready-to-serve	1 can (18¾ oz)	306	21
turkey, chunky, ready-to-serve	1 cup	136	9
turkey noodle; as prep w/ water	1 cup	69	5
turkey noodle; not prep	1 can (10¾ oz)	168	12
turkey vegetable; as prep w/ water	1 cup	74	2
turkey vegetable; not prep	1 can (10½ oz)	179	3
vegetable, chunky, ready-to-serve	1 cup	122	0
vegetable, chunky, ready-to-serve	1 can (19 oz)	274	0
vegetable w/ beef broth; as prep w/ water	1 cup	81	2

FOOD	PORTION	CALORIES	CHOLESTEROL
vegetable w/ beef broth; not prep	1 can (10½ oz)	197	6
vegetable w/ beef; as prep w/ water	1 cup	79	5
vegetable w/ beef; not prep	1 can (10¾ oz)	192	12
vegetarian vegetable; as prep w/ water	1 cup	72	0
vegetarian vegetable; not prep	1 can (10½ oz)	176	0
vichyssoise	1 cup	148	22
vichyssoise	1 can (10¾ oz)	360	54
DRY			
Beef Flavor Noodle; as prep w/ water (Cup-a-Soup)	6 oz	10	0
Beef Noodle; as prep (Estee)	6 oz	20	1
Beef; as prep (Diamond Crystal)	6 oz	30	tr
Beefy Tomato; as prep w/ water (Cup-a-Soup Trim)	6 oz	10	0
Chicken Vegetable; as prep w/ water (Cup-a-Soup)	8 oz	40	5
Chicken Flavor; as prep w/ water (Cup-a-Soup)	6 oz	25	5
Chicken Flavored; as prep w/ water (Lots-a-Noodles)	7 oz	120	30

FOOD	PORTION	CALORIES	CHOLESTEROL
Chicken Noodle Instant; as prep (Estee)	6 oz	25	4
Chicken Noodle; as prep w/ water (Cup-a-Soup)	6 oz	90	15
Chicken w/ Rice; as prep w/ water (Cup-a-Soup)	6 oz	45	5
Chicken; as prep w/ water (Cup-a-Soup Trim)	6 oz	10	0
Chicken; as prep (Diamond Crystal)	6 oz	30	2
Cream of Mushroom; as prep w/ water (Cup-a-Soup)	6 oz	80	0
Cream of Chicken; as prep w/ water (Cup-a-Soup)	6 oz	80	0
Cream of Chicken; as prep w/ water (Lots-a-Noodles)	7 oz	150	35
Cream; as prep (Diamond Crystal)	6 oz	90	5
French Onion; as prep w/ water (Cup-a-Soup Trim)	6 oz	10	0
Green Pea; as prep w/ water (Cup-a-Soup)	6 oz	120	0
Herb Chicken; as prep w/ water (Cup-a-Soup Trim)	6 oz	10	0
Minestrone Soup Mix; as prep (Manischewitz)	6 oz	50	0

FOOD	PORTION	CALORIES	CHOLESTEROL
Mushroom Instant; as prep (Estee)	6 oz	40	1
Onion Instant; as prep (Estee)	6 oz	25	1
Onion; as prep w/ water (Cup-a-Soup)	6 oz	30	0
Split Pea Soup Mix; as prep (Manischewitz)	6 oz	45	0
Tomato Instant; as prep (Estee)	6 oz	40	0
Tomato; as prep w/ water (Cup-a-Soup)	6 oz	80	0
Tomato; as prep (Diamond Crystal)	6 oz	70	3
asparagus, cream of; as prep w/ water	1 cup	59	tr
asparagus, cream of; not prep	1 pkg (2.2 oz)	234	1
bean w/ bacon; as prep w/ water	1 cup	105	3
bean w/ bacon; not prep	1 pkg (1 oz)	105	3
beef broth cube; as prep w/ water	1 cup	8	tr
beef broth; as prep w/ water	1 cup	19	1
beef broth; as prep w/ water	1 cube	6	tr
beef broth; not prep	1 pkg (.2 oz)	14	1
beef noodle; as prep w/ water	6 oz	30	1
beef noodle; as prep w/ water	1 cup	41	2

FOOD	PORTION	CALORIES	CHOLESTEROL
beef noodle; not prep	1 pkg (.3 oz)	30	1
cauliflower; as prep w/ water	1 cup	68	tr
cauliflower; not prep	1 pkg (.7 oz)	68	tr
celery, cream of; as prep w/ water	1 cup	63	1
celery, cream of; not prep	1 pkg (.6 oz)	62	1
chicken vegetable; as prep w/ water	1 cup	49	3
chicken vegetable; not prep	1 pkg (.4 oz)	37	2
chicken broth cube; as prep w/ water	1 cup	13	1
chicken broth cube; not prep	1 cube	9	1
chicken broth; as prep w/ water	1 cup	21	1
chicken broth; not prep	1 pkg (.2 oz)	16	1
chicken, cream of; as prep w/ water	1 cup	107	3
chicken, cream of; not prep	1 pkg (.6 oz)	80	2
chicken noodle; as prep w/ water	1 cup	53	3
chicken noodle; not prep	1 pkg (2.6 oz)	257	10
chicken rice; as prep w/ water	1 cup	60	3
chicken rice; not prep	1 pkg (.6 oz)	60	3

FOOD	PORTION	CALORIES	CHOLESTEROL
clam chowder, Manhattan; not prep	1 pkg (.7 oz)	65	0
clam chowder, New England; not prep	1 pkg (.8 oz)	95	1
consomme, w/ gelatin; as prep w/ water	1 cup	17	0
consomme, w/ gelatin; not prep	1 pkg (2 oz)	77	0
leek; as prep w/ water	1 cup	71	3
leek; not prep	1 pkg (2.7 oz)	294	9
minestrone; as prep w/ water	1 cup	79	3
minestrone; not prep	1 pkg (2.7 oz)	279	6
mushroom, instant; not prep	1 pkg (.6 oz)	74	0
mushroom; as prep w/ water	1 cup	96	1
mushroom; not prep	1 pkg (2.6 oz)	328	2
onion, French; not prep	1 pkg (1.4 oz)	115	2
onion; as prep w/ water	1 cup	28	0
onion; not prep	1 pkg (1.4 oz)	115	2
oxtail; as prep w/ water	1 cup	71	3
oxtail; not prep	1 pkg (2.6 oz)	280	11
pea, green; as prep w/ water	1 cup	133	3
pea, green; not prep	1 pkg (4 oz)	402	1

FOOD	PORTION	CALORIES	CHOLESTEROL
pea, split; as prep w/ water	1 cup	133	3
pea, split; not prep	1 pkg (4 oz)	402	1
tomato vegetable; as prep w/ water	1 cup	55	tr
tomato vegetable; not prep	1 pkg (1.4 oz)	125	1
tomato; as prep w/ water	1 cup	102	1
tomato; not prep	1 pkg (.7 oz)	77	1
vegetable, beef; as prep w/ water	1 cup	53	1
vegetable, beef; not prep	1 pkg (2.6 oz)	256	6
vegetable, cream of; as prep w/ water	1 cup	105	0
vegetable, cream of; not prep	1 pkg (.62 oz)	79	0

HOME RECIPE

FOOD	PORTION	CALORIES	CHOLESTEROL
black bean turtle soup	1 cup	241	0
corn & cheese chowder	¾ cup	215	66
corn chowder	1 cup	233	75
gazpacho	1 cup	46	0
greek	¾ cup	63	83
hot & sour	1 cup	74	70
lentil	1 cup	175	0
mock turtle	1 cup	256	164
potato	1 cup	201	37

FOOD	PORTION	CALORIES	CHOLESTEROL
seafood chowder	1 cup	170	68
vegetable	1 cup	70	0
vegetable beef	1 cup	320	54
wonton	1 cup	205	89

SOUR CREAM
(*see also* SOUR CREAM SUBSTITUTE)

FOOD	PORTION	CALORIES	CHOLESTEROL
LOWFAT			
Lean Cream (Land O'Lakes)	1 Tbsp	20	4
Lean Cream w/ Chives (Land O'Lakes)	1 Tbsp	20	4
Lite Delite (Friendship)	2 Tbsp	35	8
REGULAR			
Friendship	2 Tbsp	55	42
Sour Cream (Land O'Lakes)	1 Tbsp	32	7
Sour Cream (Land O'Lakes)	1 Tbsp	25	5
half & half	1 Tbsp	20	6
sour cream	1 Tbsp	26	5
sour cream	1 cup	493	102

SOUR CREAM SUBSTITUTE

FOOD	PORTION	CALORIES	CHOLESTEROL
Formagg Sour Sour Cream Style	1 oz	40	0

FOOD	PORTION	CALORIES	CHOLESTEROL
imitation, non-dairy	1 oz	59	0
imitation, non-dairy	1 cup	479	0
sour cream, non-butterfat	1 Tbsp	21	1
sour cream, non-butterfat	1 cup	417	13

SOY

(*see also* ICE CREAM, NON-DAIRY; TEXTURED VEGETABLE PROTEIN; TOFU)

Soo Moo Soybean Milk (Health Valley)	8.5 oz	120	0
Soy Sauce (Kikkoman)	1 Tbsp	10	tr
Soy Sauce Lite (Kikkoman)	1 Tbsp	11	tr
Soy Sauce Mix (Diamond Crystal)	1 tsp	5	0
lecithin	1 Tbsp	120	0
milk	1 cup	79	0
soy sauce	1 Tbsp	7	0
soy sauce, shoyu	1 Tbsp	9	0
soy sauce, tamari	1 Tbsp	11	0
soybean sprouts	½ cup	45	0
soybean, roasted & toasted	1 oz	129	0
soybeans, roasted	½ cup	405	0
soybeans, dry-roasted	½ cup	387	0
soybeans, raw	1 cup	774	0
soybeans; cooked	1 cup	298	0

FOOD	PORTION	CALORIES	CHOLESTEROL

SPAGHETTI
(see PASTA, SPAGHETTI SAUCE)

SPAGHETTI SAUCE
(see also PIZZA, TOMATO)

JARRED

FOOD	PORTION	CALORIES	CHOLESTEROL
Estee Spaghetti Sauce	4 oz	70	0
Pritikin Foods Spaghetti Sauce	4 oz	60	0
Pritikin Foods Spaghetti Sauce w/ Mushrooms	4 oz	60	0
Ragu Chunky Gardenstyle Extra Tomatoes, Garlic & Onions	4 oz	80	0
Ragu Chunky Gardenstyle Extra Tomatoes, Garlic & Onions w/ pasta	4 oz + 5 oz pasta	290	0
Ragu Chunky Gardenstyle Green Peppers & Mushrooms	4 oz	80	0
Ragu Chunky Gardenstyle Green Peppers & Mushrooms w/ pasta	4 oz + 5 oz pasta	290	0
Ragu Chunky Gardenstyle Italian Garden Combination	4 oz	80	0
Ragu Chunky Gardenstyle Italian Garden Combination w/ pasta	4 oz + 5 oz pasta	290	0
Ragu Chunky Gardenstyle Mushrooms & Onions	4 oz	80	0
Ragu Chunky Gardenstyle Mushrooms & Onions w/ pasta	4 oz + 5 oz pasta	290	0

FOOD	PORTION	CALORIES	CHOLESTEROL
Ragu Chunky Gardenstyle Sweet Green & Red Peppers	4 oz	80	0
Ragu Chunky Gardenstyle Sweet Green & Red Peppers w/ pasta	4 oz + 5 oz pasta	290	0
Ragu Extra Thick & Zesty Flavored w/ Meat	4 oz	100	2
Ragu Extra Thick & Zesty Flavored w/ Meat w/ pasta	4 oz + 5 oz pasta	310	2
Ragu Extra Thick & Zesty Plain	4 oz	100	0
Ragu Extra Thick & Zesty Plain w/ pasta	4 oz + 5 oz pasta	310	0
Ragu Extra Thick & Zesty w/ Mushrooms	4 oz	110	0
Ragu Extra Thick & Zesty w/ Mushrooms w/ pasta	4 oz + 5 oz pasta	320	0
Ragu Homestyle Flavored w/ Meat	4 oz	70	2
Ragu Homestyle Flavored w/ Meat w/ pasta	4 oz + 5 oz pasta	280	2
Ragu Homestyle Plain	4 oz	70	0
Ragu Homestyle Plain w/ pasta	4 oz + 5 oz pasta	280	0
Ragu Homestyle w/ Mushrooms	4 oz	70	0
Ragu Homestyle w/ Mushrooms w/ pasta	4 oz + 5 oz pasta	280	0
Ragu Old World Style Flavored w/ Meat	4 oz	80	2
Ragu Old World Style Flavored w/ Meat w/ pasta	4 oz + 5 oz pasta	290	2

FOOD	PORTION	CALORIES	CHOLESTEROL
Ragu Old World Style Marinara Sauce	4 oz	90	0
Ragu Old World Style Marinara Sauce w/ pasta	4 oz + 5 oz pasta	300	0
Ragu Old World Style Plain	4 oz	80	0
Ragu Old World Style Plain w/ pasta	4 oz + 5 oz pasta	290	0
Ragu Old World Style w/ Extra Cheese	4 oz	80	1
Ragu Old World Style w/ Extra Cheese w/ pasta	4 oz + 5 oz pasta	290	1
Ragu Old World Style w/ Extra Garlic	4 oz	80	0
Ragu Old World Style w/ Extra Garlic w/ pasta	4 oz + 5 oz pasta	290	0
Ragu Old World Style w/ Mushrooms	4 oz	80	0
Ragu Old World Style w/ Mushrooms w/ pasta	4 oz + 5 oz pasta	290	0
Ragu Thick & Hearty Flavored w/ Leaner Ground Beef	4 oz	120	2
Ragu Thick & Hearty Flavored w/ Leaner Ground Beef w/ pasta	4 oz + 5 oz pasta	330	2
Ragu Thick & Hearty Marinara	4 oz	110	0
Ragu Thick & Hearty Marinara w/ pasta	4 oz + 5 oz pasta	320	0
Ragu Thick & Hearty Plain	4 oz	110	0
Ragu Thick & Hearty Plain w/ pasta	4 oz + 5 oz pasta	320	0

FOOD	PORTION	CALORIES	CHOLESTEROL
Ragu Thick & Hearty w/ Mushrooms	4 oz	110	0
Ragu Thick & Hearty w/ Mushrooms w/ pasta	4 oz + 5 oz pasta	320	0
marinara sauce	1 cup	171	0
spaghetti sauce	15½ oz jar	479	0
MIX			
spaghetti sauce; not prep	1 pkg 1.5 oz	118	0
w/mushrooms; not prep	1 pkg 1.4 oz	118	11

SPICES
(*see* HERBS/SPICES)

SPINACH

CANNED			
Northwest Premium (S&W)	½ cup	25	0
Spinach (Libby)	½ cup	25	0
Spinach (Seneca)	½ cup	25	0
spinach	½ cup	25	0
FRESH			
cooked	½ cup	21	0
raw; chopped	½ cup	6	0

FOOD	PORTION	CALORIES	CHOLESTEROL
FROZEN			
Chopped (Birds Eye)	⅓ cup	22	0
Chopped; cooked (Health Valley)	7.2 oz	57	0
Creamed (Birds Eye)	⅓ cup	59	tr
Leaf (Birds Eye)	⅓ cup	22	0
Leaf; cooked (Health Valley)	6.7 oz	53	0
Spinach Au Gratin (Budget Gourmet)	6 oz	120	40
frzn; cooked	½ cup	27	0
frzn; not prep	10 oz pkg	68	0

SPORTS DRINKS

thirst quencher	1 cup	60	0

SQUAB

FRESH			
breast, raw	3.5 oz	135	91

SQUASH
(*see also* ZUCCHINI)

CANNED			
crookneck; sliced	½ cup	14	0
FRESH			
acorn; cooked, mashed	½ cup	41	0

FOOD	PORTION	CALORIES	CHOLESTEROL
acorn; cubed, baked	½ cup	57	0
butternut; baked	½ cup	41	0
crookneck, iced; cooked	½ cup	18	0
hubbard; baked	½ cup	51	0
hubbard; cooked, mashed	½ cup	35	0
scallop; cooked	½ cup	14	0
spaghetti; cooked	½ cup	23	0
summer, all varieties, raw; sliced	½ cup	13	0
summer; sliced, cooked	½ cup	18	0
winter, all varieties, raw; cubed	½ cup	21	0
winter; cubed, cooked	½ cup	39	0
FROZEN Butternut (Southland)	4 oz	45	0
Winter Cooked (Birds Eye)	⅓ cup	45	0
butternut; cooked, mashed	½ cup	47	0
crookneck; sliced, cooked	½ cup	24	0
SEEDS seeds, dried	1 oz	154	0
seeds, whole, roasted	1 oz	127	0

SQUID

FRESH fried	3 oz	149	221
raw	3 oz	78	198

FOOD	PORTION	CALORIES	CHOLESTEROL

STRAWBERRY

FRESH

| strawberries | 1 cup | 45 | 0 |

FROZEN

Strawberries Halved Quick Thaw (Birds Eye)	½ cup	119	0
Strawberries Halved in Lite Syrup (Birds Eye)	½ cup	87	0
Strawberries Whole in Lite Syrup (Birds Eye)	½ cup	81	0
strawberries, sweetened	1 cup	200	0
strawberries, unsweetened	1 cup	52	0

JUICE

| Strawberry (Smucker's) | 8 oz | 130 | 0 |

STUFFING/DRESSING

Beef (Stove Top)	½ cup	165	19
Chicken (Stove Top)	½ cup	181	22
Chicken Flexible Serve (Stove Top)	½ cup	180	17
Chicken w/ Rice (Stove Top)	½ cup	184	22
Cornbread (Stove Top)	½ cup	163	19

FOOD	PORTION	CALORIES	CHOLESTEROL
Cornbread Flexible Serve (Stove Top)	½ cup	180	17
Herb Homestyle Flexible Serve (Stove Top)	½ cup	180	17
Long Grain & Wild Rice (Stove Top)	½ cup	184	22
Pork (Stove Top)	½ cup	179	21
San Francisco Style Americana (Stove Top)	½ cup	162	19
Savory Herbs (Stove Top)	½ cup	180	22
Select Chicken Florentine (Stove Top)	½ cup	203	31
Select Garden Herb (Stove Top)	½ cup	219	34
Select Vegetable & Almond (Stove Top)	½ cup	227	34
Select Wild Rice & Mushroom (Stove Top)	½ cup	172	21
Turkey (Stove Top)	½ cup	179	21
HOME RECIPE			
bread; as prep w/ water & fat	½ cup	251	tr
bread; as prep w/ water, egg & fat	½ cup	107	75
sausage	½ cup	292	12

FOOD	PORTION	CALORIES	CHOLESTEROL

SUCKER

FRESH

white, raw	3 oz	79	35
white, raw	1 fillet (5.6 oz)	147	66

SUGAR
(see also FRUCTOSE, SUGAR SUBSTITUTE, SYRUP*)*

brown	1 cup	836	0
cube	1 cube	27	0
powdered	1 cup	493	0
white	1 cup	770	0

SUGAR SUBSTITUTE
(see also FRUCTOSE*)*

Adolph's	1 tsp	0	0
Diamond	1 tsp	tr	0
Spoon for Spoon	1 tsp	2	0
Sucaryl	1 tsp	0	0
Sugar Twin	1 tsp	tr	0
Sweet'n Low Brown Sugar Substitute	1/10 tsp	2	0
Sweet'n Low Granulated	1 pkg (1 g)	4	0
Sweet'n Low Liquid	10 drops	0	0
Sweet'n Low	1 tsp	12	0
Sweet'n It (Estee)	6 drops	0	0

FOOD	PORTION	CALORIES	CHOLESTEROL

SUNDAE TOPPINGS
(*see* ICE CREAM TOPPINGS)

SUNFISH

FRESH
| pumpkinseed, raw | 3 oz | 76 | 57 |

SUNFLOWER SEEDS

Sunflower (Planters)	1 oz	160	0
Sunflower Nuts, Oil Roasted (Planters)	1 oz	170	0
Sunflower Nuts, Dry Roasted (Planters)	1 oz	160	0
Sunflower Nuts, Dry Roasted, Unsalted (Planters)	1 oz	170	0
dried	1 oz	162	0
dry roasted	1 oz	165	0
oil roasted	1 oz	175	0
sunflower butter	1 Tbsp	93	0
toasted	1 oz	176	0

SWEET POTATO
(*see also* YAM)

CANNED
Surf (American Original Foods)	4 oz	100	20
Surf (American Original Foods)	4 oz	90	40
in syrup pack	½ cup	106	0

FOOD	PORTION	CALORIES	CHOLESTEROL
mashed	½ cup	233	0
pieces	1 cup	183	0
FRESH			
baked in skin	1 (3½ oz)	118	0
mashed	½ cup	172	0
raw	1 (4.6 oz)	136	0
FROZEN			
frzn; baked	½ cup	88	0

SWISS CHARD

FRESH			
cooked	½ cup	18	0
raw; chopped	½ cup	3	0

SWORDFISH

FRESH			
cooked	1 piece (3.7 oz)	164	53
cooked	3 oz	132	43
raw	3 oz	103	33
raw	1 piece (4.8 oz)	164	54

SYRUP
(*see also* ICE CREAM TOPPINGS, PANCAKE/WAFFLE SYRUP)

All Flavors Fruit Syrup (Smucker's)	2 Tbsp	100	0
Blueberry (Estee)	1 Tbsp	4	0

FOOD	PORTION	CALORIES	CHOLESTEROL
Corn Syrup Light (Karo)	1 Tbsp	60	0
Corn Syrup Light (Karo)	1 cup	960	0
Corn Syrup Dark (Karo)	1 Tbsp	60	0
Corn Syrup Dark (Karo)	1 cup	975	0
Fruit Flavored, All Varieties (Smucker's)	1 Tbsp	50	0
Maple Rich (Home Brands)	1 oz	110	0

TAHINI
(*see* SESAME)

TAMARIND

FRESH			
tamarind	1	5	0

TANGERINE

FRESH			
tangerine	1	37	0
JUICE			
Mandarin Tangerine (Dole)	6 oz	97	0
frzn, sweetened; as prep	1 cup	110	0
frzn; not prep	6 oz can	344	0
sweetened	1 cup	125	0

FOOD	PORTION	CALORIES	CHOLESTEROL

TAPIOCA

| Minute Tapioca (General Foods) | 1 Tbsp | 35 | 0 |

TEA/HERBAL TEA

HERBAL

Almond Orange (Bigelow)	5 oz	tr	0
Almond Sunset (Celestial Seasonings)	1 cup	3	0
Apple Orchard (Bigelow)	1 cup	5	0
Apple Spice (Bigelow)	5 oz	tr	0
Chamomile (Bigelow)	5 oz	tr	0
Chamomile (Celestial Seasonings)	1 cup	2	0
Chamomile Mint (Bigelow)	5 oz	tr	0
Cinnamon Apple Spice (Celestial Seasonings)	1 cup	3	0
Cinnamon Orange (Bigelow)	5 oz	tr	0
Cinnamon Rose (Celestial Seasonings)	1 cup	2	0
Country Peach Spice (Celestial Seasonings)	1 cup	3	0
Cranberry Cove (Celestial Seasonings)	1 cup	3	0
Early Riser (Bigelow)	1 cup	3	0

FOOD	PORTION	CALORIES	CHOLESTEROL
Emperor's Choice (Celestial Seasonings)	1 cup	4	0
Feeling Free (Bigelow)	1 cup	1	0
Fruit & Almond (Bigelow)	1 cup	1	0
Ginseng Plus (Celestial Seasonings)	1 cup	3	0
Grandma's Tummy Mints (Celestial Seasonings)	1 cup	2	0
Hibiscus & Rose Hips (Bigelow)	5 oz	1	0
I Love Lemon (Bigelow)	1 cup	1	0
Lemon & C (Bigelow)	5 oz	tr	0
Lemon Mist (Celestial Seasonings)	1 cup	2	0
Lemon Zinger (Celestial Seasonings)	1 cup	4	0
Looking Good (Bigelow)	1 cup	1	0
Mandarin Orange Spice (Celestial Seasonings)	1 cup	5	0
Mellow Mint (Celestial Seasonings)	1 cup	2	0
Mint Blend (Bigelow)	5 oz	tr	0
Mint Magic (Celestial Seasonings)	1 cup	1	0
Mint Medley (Bigelow)	1 cup	1	0

FOOD	PORTION	CALORIES	CHOLESTEROL
Mo's 24 (Celestial Seasonings)	1 cup	2	0
Nice Over Ice (Bigelow)	1 cup	1	0
Orange & C (Bigelow)	5 oz	tr	0
Orange & Spice (Bigelow)	1 cup	1	0
Orange Zinger (Celestial Seasonings)	1 cup	5	0
Peppermint (Bigelow)	5 oz	tr	0
Peppermint (Celestial Seasonings)	1 cup	2	0
Raspberry Patch (Celestial Seasonings)	1 cup	4	0
Red Zinger (Celestial Seasonings)	1 cup	4	0
Roastaroma (Celestial Seasonings)	1 cup	11	0
Roasted Grain & Carob (Bigelow)	5 oz	3	0
Sleepytime (Celestial Seasonings)	1 cup	5	0
Spearmint (Bigelow)	5 oz	tr	0
Spearmint (Celestial Seasonings)	1 cup	5	0
Strawberry Fields (Celestial Seasonings)	1 cup	4	0
Sunburst C (Celestial Seasonings)	1 cup	3	0

FOOD	PORTION	CALORIES	CHOLESTEROL
Sweet Dreams (Bigelow)	1 cup	1	0
Take-A-Break (Bigelow)	1 cup	3	0
Wild Forest Blueberry (Celestial Seasonings)	1 cup	2	0
REGULAR Amaretto Nights (Celestial Seasonings)	1 cup	3	0
Apple Spice and Tea (Celestial Seasonings)	1 cup	tr	0
Bavarian Chocolate Orange (Celestial Seasonings)	1 cup	7	0
Caffeine-Free (Celestial Seasonings)	1 cup	4	0
Chinese Fortune (Bigelow)	1 cup	1	0
Cinnamon Stick (Bigelow)	1 cup	1	0
Cinnamon Vienna (Celestial Seasonings)	1 cup	2	0
Classic English Breakfast (Celestial Seasonings)	1 cup	3	0
Constant Comment (Bigelow)	1 cup	1	0
Darjeeling Gardens (Celestial Seasonings)	1 cup	3	0
Darjeeling Blend (Bigelow)	1 cup	1	0
Earl Grey (Bigelow)	1 cup	1	0

FOOD	PORTION	CALORIES	CHOLESTEROL
English Teatime (Bigelow)	1 cup	1	0
Extraordinary Earl Grey (Celestial Seasonings)	1 cup	3	0
Fruit Tea Fruit Cooler; as prep (Lipton)	8 oz	87	0
Iced Berry Tea; as prep (Crystal Light)	8 oz	3	0
Iced Tea (SIPPS)	8.45 oz	100	0
Iced Tea (Shasta)	12 oz	124	0
Irish Cream Mist (Celestial Seasonings)	1 cup	3	0
Lemon Lift (Bigelow)	1 cup	1	0
Lemons and Tea (Celestial Seasonings)	1 cup	tr	0
Morning Thunder (Celestial Seasonings)	1 cup	3	0
Orange Pekoe (Bigelow)	1 cup	1	0
Orange Spice and Tea (Celestial Seasonings)	1 cup	tr	0
Peppermint Stick (Bigelow)	1 cup	1	0
Plantation Mint (Bigelow)	1 cup	1	0
Raspberries and Tea (Celestial Seasonings)	1 cup	2	0
Raspberry Royale (Bigelow)	1 cup	1	0

FOOD	PORTION	CALORIES	CHOLESTEROL
Swiss Mint (Celestial Seasonings)	1 cup	tr	0
instant, sugar sweetened, lemon flavor powder; as prep w/ water	9 oz	87	0
instant, unsweetened powder; as prep w/ water	8 oz	2	0
instant, unsweetened, lemon flavor powder; as prep w/ water	8 oz	4	0
tea	6 oz	2	0

TEMPEH

FOOD	PORTION	CALORIES	CHOLESTEROL
tempeh	½ cup	165	0

TEXTURED VEGETABLE PROTEIN
(*see also* MEAT SUBSTITUTE, SOY)

FOOD	PORTION	CALORIES	CHOLESTEROL
simulated meat products	1 oz	88	0

TOFU
(*see also* ICE CREAM, NON-DAIRY)

FOOD	PORTION	CALORIES	CHOLESTEROL
fried	1 piece (½ oz)	35	0
fuyu, salted & fermented	1 block (⅓ oz)	13	0
koyadofu, dried, frozen	1 piece (½ oz)	82	0
raw, firm	¼ block (3 oz)	118	0
raw, regular	¼ block (4 oz)	88	0

FOOD	PORTION	CALORIES	CHOLESTEROL

TOFUTTI
(see ICE CREAM, NON-DAIRY)

TOMATO
(see also PIZZA, SPAGHETTI SAUCE)

CANNED

FOOD	PORTION	CALORIES	CHOLESTEROL
Aspic Supreme (S&W)	½ cup	60	0
California Sliced (Contadina)	½ cup	40	0
Crushed Tomatoes in Tomato Puree (Contadina)	½ cup	30	0
Diced Tomatoes in Rich Puree (S&W)	½ cup	35	0
Italian Paste (Contadina)	2 oz	65	tr
Italian Stewed (S&W)	½ cup	35	0
Italian Style (Contadina)	½ cup	25	0
Italian Style Stewed (Cantadina)	½ cup	35	0
Italian Style w/ Basil (S&W)	½ cup	25	0
Kosher Tomatoes (Claussen)	1	9	0
Paste (Contadina)	2 oz	50	0
Paste (S&W)	6 oz	150	0

FOOD	PORTION	CALORIES	CHOLESTEROL
Peeled Ready Cut (S&W)	½ cup	25	0
Puree (Contadina)	½ cup	40	0
Puree (S&W)	½ cup	60	0
Sauce (S&W)	½ cup	40	0
Sauce, Thick & Zesty (Contadina)	½ cup	40	0
Stewed (Contadina)	½ cup	35	0
Stewed Tomatoes (S&W)	½ cup	35	0
Stewed Tomatoes 50% Salt Reduced (S&W)	½ cup	35	0
Tomato Sauce (Health Valley)	4 oz	30	0
Tomato Sauce No Salt Added (Health Valley)	4 oz	30	0
Whole Peeled (Contadina)	½ cup	25	0
Whole Peeled (S&W)	½ cup	25	0
red, whole	1 cup	47	0
sauce, spanish style	½ cup	40	0
stewed	1 cup	68	0
tomato paste	½ cup	110	0
tomato puree	1 cup	102	0

FOOD	PORTION	CALORIES	CHOLESTEROL
tomato sauce	1 cup	74	0
tomato sauce w/ mushrooms	1 cup	85	0
tomato sauce w/ onion	½ cup	50	0
tomato sauce w/ tomato tidbits	½ cup	39	0
wedges in tomato juice	1 cup	67	0
FRESH			
green	1	30	0
red	1	24	0
scalloped	½ cup	88	8
stewed	1 cup	59	0
JUICE			
California (S&W)	5½ oz	35	0
tomato juice	6 fl oz	32	0

TONGUE

beef, raw	4 oz	252	98
beef; simmered	3 oz	241	91
pork, raw	4 oz	254	114
pork; braised	3 oz	230	124

TOPPINGS
(*see* ICE CREAM TOPPINGS)

TORTILLA CHIPS
(*see* CHIPS)

FOOD	PORTION	CALORIES	CHOLESTEROL

TROUT

FRESH

FOOD	PORTION	CALORIES	CHOLESTEROL
rainbow, raw	3 oz	100	48
rainbow, raw	1 fillet (2.8 oz)	93	45
rainbow, cooked	1 fillet (2.1 oz)	94	45
rainbow, cooked	3 oz	129	62
seatrout, raw	1 fillet (8.4 oz)	248	198
seatrout, raw	3 oz	88	71

TUNA
(see also TUNA DISHES)

CANNED

FOOD	PORTION	CALORIES	CHOLESTEROL
Chunk Light in Oil (Bumble Bee)	3 oz	200	30
Chunk Light in Water (Bumble Bee)	3 oz	90	30
Chunk White in Oil (Bumble Bee)	3 oz	200	30
Chunk White in Water (Bumble Bee)	3 oz	90	30
Solid White in Oil (Bumble Bee)	3 oz	190	30
Solid White in Water (Bumble Bee)	3 oz	90	30
Tuna (Health Valley)	6.5 oz	180	30
Tuna Diet No Salt (Health Valley)	6.5 oz	200	30

FOOD	PORTION	CALORIES	CHOLESTEROL
Tuna Salad (The Spreadables)	¼ can	90	13
light in oil	3 oz	169	15
light in oil	1 can (6 oz)	399	30
white in oil	3 oz	158	26
white in oil	1 can (6.2 oz)	331	55
white in water	1 can (6 oz)	234	72
white in water	3 oz	116	35
FRESH bluefin, raw	3 oz	122	32
bluefin; cooked	3 oz	157	42
skipjack, raw	3 oz	88	40
skipjack, raw	½ fillet (6.9 oz)	204	93
yellowfin, raw	3 oz	92	38
READY-TO-USE Salad (Wampler Longacre)	1 oz	61	7
tuna salad	3 oz	159	11
tuna salad	1 cup	383	27

TUNA DISHES

FOOD	PORTION	CALORIES	CHOLESTEROL
Tuna Sandwich (Micrwave Chefwich)	1 (5 oz)	380	28
HOME RECIPE pattie	1 (3 oz)	228	69

OOD	PORTION	CALORIES	CHOLESTEROL
stuffed green pepper	1 (9.9 oz)	261	59
una casserole	¾ cup	299	56

TURKEY

(*see also* DINNER, HOT DOG, TURKEY DISHES, TURKEY SUBSTITUTE)

CANNED

Turkey Salad (The Spreadables)	¼ can	100	20

FRESH

Breast (Land O'Lakes)	3 oz	100	50
Breast Boneless Roast, Fresh Young; cooked (Perdue)	3 oz	162	63
Breast, Fresh Young, meat only; cooked	3 oz	162	63
Breast Half, Fresh Young, meat only; cooked (Perdue)	3 oz	162	63
Breast Hen w/ Wing; cooked (Louis Rich)	1 oz	53	16
Breast Hen w/o Back; cooked (Louis Rich)	1 oz	47	17
Breast Hen w/o Wing; cooked (Louis Rich)	1 oz	53	11
Breast Roast; cooked (Louis Rich)	1 oz	41	18
Breast Slices; cooked (Louis Rich)	1 oz	44	13
Breast Steak Fresh Young; cooked (Perdue)	3 oz	115	71

FOOD	PORTION	CALORIES	CHOLESTEROL
Breast Steaks; cooked (Louis Rich)	1 oz	40	19
Breast Tender-loins, Fresh Young; cooked (Perdue)	3 oz	115	71
Breast Tender-loins; cooked (Louis Rich)	1 oz	41	11
Breast; cooked (Louis Rich)	1 oz	50	12
Drumsticks, Fresh Young, meat only; cooked (Perdue)	3 oz	173	73
Drumsticks; cooked (Louis Rich)	1 oz	55	33
Ground Lean 90% Fat Free; cooked (Louis Rich)	3.5 oz	183	85
Ground Lean 90% Fat Free; cooked (Louis Rich)	1 oz	51	24
Ground Turkey (Bil Mar Foods)	3 oz	163	60
Ground; cooked (Louis Rich)	1 oz	61	24
Ground; cooked (Louis Rich)	3.5 oz	217	87
Thighs Boneless, Fresh Young; cooked (Perdue)	3 oz	153	70
Thighs, Fresh Young, meat only; cooked (Perdue)	3 oz	211	73
Thighs; cooked (Louis Rich)	1 oz	65	28

FOOD	PORTION	CALORIES	CHOLESTEROL
Whole, Fresh Young, meat only; cooked (Perdue)	3 oz	178	70
Whole; cooked (Louis Rich)	3.5 oz	200	18
Whole; cooked (Louis Rich)	1 oz	56	18
Wing Drumettes; cooked (Louis Rich)	1 oz	52	20
Wings, Fresh Young, meat only; cooked (Perdue)	3 oz	196	69
Wings Drummettes, Fresh Young, meat only; cooked (Perdue)	3 oz	196	69
Wing Portions, Fresh Young, meat only; cooked (Perdue)	3 oz	196	69
Wings; cooked (Louis Rich)	1 oz	54	26
Young Whole (Land O'Lakes)	3 oz	130	65
Young, Whole, Butter Basted (Land O'Lakes)	3 oz	140	85
Young, Whole, Self-Basting (Land O'Lakes)	3 oz	120	77
back, meat & skin, raw	½ back (1.1 lbs)	940	416
back, meat & skin, raw	1.6 oz	81	36
back, meat & skin; roasted	½ back (13.3 oz)	903	358
breast, meat & skin, raw	½ breast (3.9 lbs)	2700	1195

FOOD	PORTION	CALORIES	CHOLESTEROL
breast, meat & skin, raw	5.4 oz	234	103
breast, meat & skin; roasted	4 oz	217	87
breast, meat & skin; roasted	½ breast (2.9 lbs)	2510	1002
dark meat w/ skin, raw	5.3 oz	232	117
dark meat w/ skin, raw	½ turkey (3.9 lbs)	2681	1355
dark meat w/ skin; roasted	½ turkey (2.6 lbs)	2553	1081
dark meat w/ skin; roasted	3.6 oz	222	94
dark meat w/o skin, raw	4.7 oz	163	99
dark meat w/o skin, raw	½ turkey (3.4 lbs)	1879	1142
dark meat w/o skin; roasted	1 cup	260	123
dark meat w/o skin; roasted	3.2 oz	167	79
flesh & skin, raw	½ turkey (8.5 lbs)	6013	2796
flesh & skin, raw	11.9 oz	522	243
flesh & skin; roasted	½ turkey (6 lbs)	5545	2265
flesh & skin; roasted	8.4 oz	482	197
flesh, raw	½ turkey (7.2 lbs)	3867	2240
flesh, raw	10 oz	335	194
flesh; roasted	7.2 oz	345	159
flesh; roasted	1 cup	235	108
leg, meat & skin, raw	2.7 lbs	1736	939
leg, meat & skin, raw	3.8 oz	150	81
leg, meat & skin; roasted	2.5 oz	144	63

FOOD	PORTION	CALORIES	CHOLESTEROL
leg, meat & skin; roasted	1.8 lbs	1660	727
light meat w/ skin, raw	6.5 oz	288	125
light meat w/ skin, raw	½ turkey (4.7 lbs)	3331	1439
light meat w/ skin; roasted	½ turkey (3.4 lbs)	2992	1182
light meat w/ skin; roasted	4.8 oz	260	103
light meat w/o skin, raw	5.4 oz	176	95
light meat w/o skin, raw	½ turkey (3.9 lbs)	2023	1097
light meat w/o skin; roasted	1 cup	2153	97
light meat w/o skin; roasted	4.1 oz	180	81
neck, meat, raw	1 neck (6.3 oz)	243	142
neck, meat; simmered	1 neck (5.3 oz)	274	186
skin, raw	½ turkey (1.3 lbs)	2180	564
skin, raw	1.8 oz	188	49
skin; roasted	½ turkey (13.1 oz)	1578	436
skin; roasted	1 oz	135	37
whole, flesh, skin, giblets & neck, raw	18.4 lbs	12799	6826
whole, flesh, skin, giblets & neck; roasted	13.1 lbs	11873	5745
whole, flesh, skin, giblets & neck; roasted	10 oz	514	249
wing, meat & skin, raw	1 oz	57	22

FOOD	PORTION	CALORIES	CHOLESTEROL
wing, meat & skin, raw	12.2 oz	656	250
wing, meat & skin, roasted	8.3 oz	524	192
roast, boneless, seasoned, light & dark meat, raw	10 oz	340	
FROZEN PREPARED Kibun Turkey Pasta Salad w/ dressing	½ pkg	250	15
Kibun Turkey Pasta Salad w/o dressing	½ pkg	140	10
READY-TO-USE Baked Ham (Wampler Longacre)	1 oz	38	22
Baked Ham w/ 12% water (Wampler Longacre)	1 oz	33	19
Baked Ham w/ 20% water (Wampler Longacre)	1 oz	39	16
Bologna (Louis Rich)	1 slice (28 g)	59	20
Bologna (Wampler Longacre)	1 oz	56	22
Bologna Mild (Louis Rich)	1 slice (28 g)	61	13
Bologna Red Rind (Mr. Turkey)	1 oz	63	20
Bologna Sliced (Wampler Longacre)	1 oz	57	21
Breast Barbecued (Louis Rich)	1 oz	36	11
Breast & White Turkey Deli Chef (Wampler Longacre)	1 oz	35	12

FOOD	PORTION	CALORIES	CHOLESTEROL
Breast & White Turkey No Skin Covering (Wampler Longacre)	1 oz	39	11
Breast BBQ Quarter (Mr. Turkey)	1 oz	34	11
Breast Fillets w/ Cheese (Land O'Lakes)	5 oz	300	35
Breast Gourmet (Wampler Longacre)	1 oz	31	10
Breast Gourmet Browned & Roasted (Wampler Longacre)	1 oz	35	16
Breast Gourmet Browned & Glazed (Wampler Longacre)	1 oz	28	11
Breast Gourmet Skinless (Wampler Longacre)	1 oz	28	10
Breast Hickory Smoked (Louis Rich)	1 oz	31	12
Breast Honey Roasted (Louis Rich)	1 slice (28 g)	29	11
Breast Mini Gourmet (Wampler Longacre)	1 oz	35	15
Breast Oven Roasted (Louis Rich)	1 slice (28 g)	31	11
Breast Oven Roasted (Louis Rich)	1 oz	30	11
Breast Oven Roasted Oven Lite (Wampler Longacre)	1 oz	35	14
Breast Oven Roasted Quarter (Mr. Turkey)	1 oz	34	12

FOOD	PORTION	CALORIES	CHOLESTEROL
Breast Premium (Wampler Longacre)	1 oz	29	11
Breast Premium Browned & Glazed (Wampler Longacre)	1 oz	29	11
Breast Premium Skinless (Wampler Longacre)	1 oz	26	8
Breast Premium Skinless Browned & Roasted (Wampler Longacre)	1 oz	26	8
Breast Roll Sliced (Wampler Longacre)	1 oz	37	10
Breast Salt Watchers (Wampler Longacre)	1 oz	35	19
Breast Skinless Gourmet High Yield (Wampler Longacre)	1 oz	28	10
Breast Smoked (Bil Mar Foods)	1 oz	31	10
Breast Smoked Chunk (Louis Rich)	1 oz	34	11
Breast Smoked Gourmet (Wampler Longacre)	1 oz	37	15
Breast Smoked Lean-Lite (Wampler Longacre)	1 oz	38	16
Breast Smoked Mini Gourmet (Wampler Longacre)	1 oz	37	15
Breast Smoked Quarter (Mr. Turkey)	1 oz	35	10
Breast Smoked Sliced (Louis Rich)	1 slice (21 g)	21	7
Breast Smoked Sliced (Wampler Longacre)	1 oz	27	9

FOOD	PORTION	CALORIES	CHOLESTEROL
Breasts, Bronze Label (Land O'Lakes)	3 oz	100	50
Breasts, Gold Label, Browned (Land O'Lakes)	3 oz	120	55
Breasts, Gold Label, Skin On (Land O'Lakes)	3 oz	120	55
Breasts, Gold Label, Skinless (Land O'Lakes)	3 oz.	90	50
Breasts, Silver Label (Land O'Lakes)	3 oz	100	50
Cheese Patties (Bil Mar Foods)	3 oz	213	37
Chunk Ham w/ 12% water (Wampler Longacre)	1 oz	36	20
Chunk Ham w/ 20% water (Wampler Longacre)	1 oz	39	16
Chunk Pastrami (Wampler Longacre)	1 oz	35	24
Cotto Salami (Louis Rich)	1 slice (28 g)	52	22
Cotto Salami (Mr. Turkey)	1 oz	45	16
Dark Smoked Cured (Wampler Longacre)	1 oz	45	21
Diced Combination Roll (Wampler Longacre)	1 oz	43	14
Diced Ham w/ 20% water (Wampler Longacre)	1 oz	39	16
Diced White Roll (Wampler Longacre)	1 oz	43	12
Diced, White/Dark Mixed (Land O'Lakes)	3 oz	120	35

FOOD	PORTION	CALORIES	CHOLESTEROL
Ham (Land O'Lakes)	3 oz	100	55
Ham Chopped (Louis Rich)	1 slice (28 g)	42	17
Ham Cured Thigh Meat (Louis Rich)	1 slice (28 g)	34	19
Ham Cured Thigh Meat Square (Louis Rich)	1 slice (21 g)	24	12
Ham Cured Thigh Meat Water Added (Louis Rich)	1 slice (28 g)	34	18
Ham Honey Cured (Louis Rich)	1 slice (21 g)	25	15
Ham Lean-Lite (Wampler Longacre)	1 oz	36	6
Ham Sliced (Wampler Longacre)	1 oz	37	17
Ham Smoked Breakfast (Mr. Turkey)	1 oz	33	16
Ham Smoked Buffet Style (Bil Mar Foods)	1 oz	32	17
Luncheon Loaf (Louis Rich)	1 slice (28 g)	43	14
Luncheon Loaf Square Spiced (Bil Mar Foods)	1 slice (1 oz)	51	11
Nuggets (Mr. Turkey)	1 nugget	33	6
Nuggets White Breaded Fully Cooked (Wampler Longacre)	1 oz	87	13

FOOD	PORTION	CALORIES	CHOLESTEROL
Oscar Mayer Breast Oven Roasted	1 slice (21 g)	22	9
Oscar Mayer Breast Smoked	1 slice (21 g)	20	9
Pastrami (Bil Mar Foods)	1 slice (1 oz)	28	17
Pastrami (Louis Rich)	1 slice (28 g)	33	14
Pastrami (Wampler Longacre)	1 oz	35	24
Pastrami Sliced (Wampler Longacre)	1 oz	34	20
Pastrami Square (Louis Rich)	1 slice (23 g)	23	13
Patties (Land O'Lakes)	2¼ oz	170	30
Patties (Mr. Turkey)	3 oz	195	36
Roast White w/ Gravy (Land O'Lakes)	3 oz	110	20
Roast White/Dark w/ Gravy (Land O'Lakes)	3 oz	120	20
Roasted Thighs (Wampler Longacre)	1 oz	38	18
Roll Breast & White Turkey (Deli Chef)	1 oz	39	10
Roll Combination Turkey (Wampler Longacre)	1 oz	43	14
Roll White Turkey (Wampler Longacre)	1 oz	43	12

FOOD	PORTION	CALORIES	CHOLESTEROL
Roll, Blue Label, Mixed (Land O'Lakes)	3 oz	120	50
Roll, Blue Label, White (Land O'Lakes)	3 oz	110	50
Roll, Red Label, Mixed (Land O'Lakes)	3 oz	110	50
Roll, Red Label, White (Land O'Lakes)	3 oz	110	50
Salad (Wampler Longacre)	1 oz	71	15
Salami (Louis Rich)	1 slice (28 g)	52	20
Salami (Wampler Longacre)	1 oz	45	21
Salami Sliced (Wampler Longacre)	1 oz	46	25
Smoked (Louis Rich)	1 slice (28 g)	33	12
Sticks (Mr. Turkey)	1 stick	65	12
Summer Sausage (Louis Rich)	1 slice (28 g)	52	22
Turkey (Carl Buddig)	1 oz	50	6
Turkey Bologna (Mr. Turkey)	1 oz	63	20
Turkey Breakfast Sausage; cooked (Louis Rich)	1 (1 oz)	59	22
Turkey Breast (Bil Mar Foods)	1 slice (1 oz)	31	10

FOOD	PORTION	CALORIES	CHOLESTEROL
Turkey Breast Smoked Sliced (Bil Mar Foods)	1 oz	31	10
Turkey Ham (Carl Buddig)	1 oz	40	19
Turkey Ham Smoked (Bil Mar Foods)	1 oz	32	18
Turkey Ham Square Chopped (Bil Mar Foods)	1 slice (1 oz)	37	17
Turkey Ham w/ 20% Water (Wampler Longacre)	1 oz	39	16
Turkey Salami (Carl Buddig)	1 oz	40	19
Turkey Smoked Sausage w/ Cheese; cooked (Louis Rich)	1 (1 oz)	58	19
Turkey Smoked Sausage; cooked (Louis Rich)	1 (1 oz)	55	19
Turkey Sticks (Land O'Lakes)	2 (1 oz each)	150	25
White Meat, Diced (Mr. Turkey)	2 oz	84	32
Whole Smoked (Wampler Longacre)	1 oz	40	16
bologna, turkey	1 slice (28 g)	57	28
breast	1 slice (21 g)	23	9
breast	1 oz	47	17

FOOD	PORTION	CALORIES	CHOLESTEROL
poultry salad sandwich spread	1 Tbsp	109	4
poultry salad sandwich spread	1 oz	238	9
prebasted breast, meat & skin; roasted	3.8 lbs	2175	718
prebasted breast, meat & skin; roasted	½ breast (1.9 lbs)	1087	359
prebasted thigh, meat & skin; roasted	11 oz	494	194
prebasted thigh, meat & skin; roasted	2 thighs (1.4 lbs)	990	389
roll, light & dark meat	1 slice (28 g)	42	16
roll, light meat	1 slice (28 g)	42	12
salami, cooked	1 pkg (8 oz)	446	186
salami, cooked	1 slice (28 g)	56	23
turkey loaf, breast meat	2 slices (1.5 oz)	47	17
turkey loaf, breast meat	1 pkg (6 oz)	187	69

TURKEY DISHES
(*see also* DINNER, TURKEY SUBSTITUTE)

HOME RECIPE

| stew | ¾ cup | 336 | 138 |

FOOD	PORTION	CALORIES	CHOLESTEROL
turkey loaf	1 slice (4.7 oz)	263	138

TURKEY SUBSTITUTE

Meatless Turkey (Loma Linda)	2 slices (2 oz)	95	0
Smoked Turkey, frzn (Worthington)	3.5 oz	239	2

TURNIP

CANNED greens	½ cup	17	0
FRESH greens, raw; chopped	½ cup	7	0
greens; chopped, cooked	½ cup	15	0
raw; cubed	½ cup	18	0
FROZEN frzn; not prep	10 oz pkg	44	0
greens & turnips; not prep	10 oz pkg	59	0
greens; cooked	½ cup	24	0
greens; not prep	10 oz pkg	62	0

VANILLA EXTRACT

Pure Vanilla Extract (Virginia Dare)	1 tsp	10	0

FOOD	PORTION	CALORIES	CHOLESTEROL

VEAL
(*see also* BEEF, VEAL DISHES)

FRESH

FOOD	PORTION	CALORIES	CHOLESTEROL
cutlet, w/ bone, lean & fat; cooked	3 oz	184	86
loin chop, w/ bone, lean & fat; cooked	1 sm (2.9 oz)	190	82
loin chop, w/ bone, lean & fat; cooked	1 med (3.9 oz)	257	111
loin chop, w/ bone, lean only; cooked	1 sm (2.4 oz)	143	68
loin chop, w/ bone, lean only; cooked	1 med (3.3 oz)	194	93
loin roast, w/ bone, lean & fat; roasted	3 oz	199	86
loin roast, w/ bone, lean only; roasted	3 oz	130	84
rib chop, w/bone, lean & fat; cooked	1 med (3.5 oz)	269	99
round, lean & fat; chopped, cooked	½ cup	151	71
round, lean & fat; ground, cooked	½ cup	119	56
round, patty; cooked	3 oz	184	86
shoulder arm roast, w/o bone, lean & fat; braised	3 oz	200	86
shoulder arm roast, w/o bone, lean only; braised	3 oz	170	84
shoulder arm steak, w/ bone, lean only; cooked	3.5 oz	196	97

FOOD	PORTION	CALORIES	CHOLESTEROL

VEAL DISHES

HOME RECIPE

| parmigiana | 4.2 oz | 279 | 136 |
| veal loaf | 1 slice (4.7 oz) | 270 | 135 |

VEGETABLES, MIXED
(see also individual vegetables)

CANNED

Beets Pickled w/ Onions (Libby)	½ cup	80	0
Beets Pickled w/ Onions (Seneca)	½ cup	80	0
Garden Salad Marinated (S&W)	½ cup	60	0
Green Beans & Wax Beans (S&W)	½ cup	20	0
Mixed Vegetables (Hanover)	½ cup	110	0
Mixed Vegetables (Libby)	½ cup	40	0
Mixed Vegetables (Seneca)	½ cup	40	0
Mixed Vegetables Old Fashioned Harvest Time (S&W)	½ cup	35	0
Okra Creole Gumbo (Trappey's)	½ cup	25	0
Okra Cut & Tomatoes (Trappey's)	½ cup	25	0

FOOD	PORTION	CALORIES	CHOLESTEROL
Okra Cut, Tomatoes & Corn (Trappey's)	½ cup	25	0
Peas & Carrots (Libby)	½ cup	50	0
Peas & Carrots (Seneca)	½ cup	50	0
Succotash (Libby)	½ cup	80	0
Succotash (Seneca)	½ cup	80	0
Succotash Country Style (S&W)	½ cup	80	0
Sweet Peas & Diced Carrots (S&W)	½ cup	50	0
Sweet Peas w/ Tiny Pearl Onions (S&W)	½ cup	60	0
Vegetable Salad (Hanover)	½ cup	90	0
corn w/ red & green peppers	½ cup	86	0
mixed vegetables	½ cup	44	0
peas and carrots	½ cup	48	0
peas and onions	½ cup	30	0
succotash	½ cup	102	0
FROZEN			
Broccoli Cut & Cauliflower Cut (Hanover)	½ cup	20	0
Broccoli, Carrots & Pasta Twists in Lightly Seasoned Sauce (Birds Eye)	⅔ cup	87	0

FOOD	PORTION	CALORIES	CHOLESTEROL
Broccoli, Cauliflower & Carrots Farm Fresh Mixtures (Birds Eye)	¾ cup	33	0
Broccoli, Cauliflower w/ Creamy Italian Cheese Sauce (Birds Eye)	½ cup	89	14
Broccoli, Cauliflower, Carrots w/ Cheese Sauce (Birds Eye)	½ cup	99	4
Broccoli, Baby Carrots & Water Chestnuts Farm Fresh Mixtures (Birds Eye)	¾ cup	45	0
Broccoli, Corn & Red Peppers Farm Fresh Mixtures (Birds Eye)	⅔ cup	60	tr
Brussels Sprouts, Cauliflower & Carrots Farm Fresh Mixtures (Birds Eye)	¾ cup	40	0
Caribbean Blend (Hanover)	½ cup	20	0
Carrots, Baby Whole Sweet Peas & Onions Deluxe Vegetable (Birds Eye)	½ cup	48	0
Cauliflower, Baby Whole Carrots & Snow Peas Farm Fresh Mixtures (Birds Eye)	⅔ cup	38	0
Chinese Style International Recipe (Birds Eye)	½ cup	68	tr

FOOD	PORTION	CALORIES	CHOLESTEROL
Chinese Style Stir Fry Vegetable (Birds Eye)	½ cup	36	0
Chow Mein Style International Recipe (Birds Eye)	½ cup	89	tr
Corn, Green Beans & Pasta Curls in Light Cream Sauce (Birds Eye)	½ cup	107	1
Garden Medley (Hanover)	½ cup	20	0
Green Peas & Pearl Onions (Birds Eye)	½ cup	71	0
Italian Style International Recipe (Birds Eye)	½ cup	101	0
Japanese Style International Recipe (Birds Eye)	½ cup	88	tr
Japanese Style Stir Fry Vegetable (Birds Eye)	½ cup	29	0
Mandarin Style International Recipe (Birds Eye)	½ cup	86	tr
Medley Vegetable Crisp (Ore Ida)	3 oz	160	5
Mixed Vegetables (Birds Eye)	½ cup	58	tr
Mixed Vegetables (Hanover)	½ cup	50	0

FOOD	PORTION	CALORIES	CHOLESTEROL
Mixed Vegetables w/ Onion Sauce (Birds Eye)	⅓ cup	97	tr
New England Style International Recipe (Birds Eye)	½ cup	124	tr
Oriental Blend (Hanover)	½ cup	25	0
Pasta Primavera Style International Recipe (Birds Eye)	½ cup	121	3
Peas & Cauliflower in Cream Sauce (Budget Gourmet)	5.75 oz	170	20
Peas & Pearl Onions w/ Cream Sauce (Birds Eye)	½ cup	137	4
Peas & Potatoes w/ Cream Sauce (Birds Eye)	½ cup	126	1
Peas & Water Chestnuts Oriental (Budget Gourmet)	5 oz	120	5
Peppers & Onions (Southland)	2 oz	15	0
Rutabaga & Yellow Turnips (Southland)	4 oz	50	0
San Francisco Style International Recipe (Birds Eye)	½ cup	90	tr
Soup Mix Vegetables (Southland)	3.2 oz	50	0

FOOD	PORTION	CALORIES	CHOLESTEROL
Spring Vegetables in Cheese Sauce (Budget Gourmet)	5 oz	90	20
Stew Vegetables (Ore Ida)	3 oz	60	0
Stew Vegetables (Southland)	4 oz	60	0
Succotash (Hanover)	½ cup	80	0
Summer Vegetables (Hanover)	½ cup	35	0
Vegetables for Soup (Hanover)	½ cup	60	0
Vegetables New England Recipe (Budget Gourmet)	5.5 oz	210	20
mixed; cooked	½ cup	54	0
mixed; not prep	10 oz pkg	201	0
peas & carrots; cooked	½ cup	38	0
peas & carrots; not prep	½ cup	37	0
peas & onions; not prep	½ cup	48	0
peas and onions; cooked	½ cup	40	0
succotash	10 oz pkg	265	0
succotash; cooked	½ cup	79	0
HOME RECIPE			
caponata	¼ cup	28	0
succotash	½ cup	111	0
JUICE			
Beefamato (Mott's)	6 oz	80	0

FOOD	PORTION	CALORIES	CHOLESTEROL
Clamato (Mott's)	6 oz	96	0
vegetable cocktail	6 fl oz	34	0

VINEGAR

FOOD	PORTION	CALORIES	CHOLESTEROL
Apple Cider (White House)	2 Tbsp	4	0
White Distilled (White House)	2 Tbsp	4	0

WAFFLES

FOOD	PORTION	CALORIES	CHOLESTEROL
FROZEN READY-TO-USE Raisins, Bran & Whole Grain, Nutri-Grain (Eggo)	1	130	0
HOME RECIPE waffle	7" diam	282	70
waffle	9" sq	602	150
MIX mix; as prep w/ egg & milk	1 waffle (2.6 oz)	210	0

WALNUTS

FOOD	PORTION	CALORIES	CHOLESTEROL
Black Walnuts (Planters)	1 oz	190	0
English Walnuts, Whole, Halves or Pieces (Planters)	1 oz	190	0

FOOD	PORTION	CALORIES	CHOLESTEROL
Walnut Topping (Kraft)	1 Tbsp	90	0
black, dried	1 oz	172	0
black, dried; chopped	1 cup	759	0
English, dried	1 oz	182	0
English, dried; chopped	1 cup	770	0

WATERCHESTNUTS

CANNED Chinese; sliced	½ cup	35	0

WATERCRESS
(*see also* CRESS)

FRESH raw; chopped	½ cup	2	0

WATERMELON

seeds, dried	1 oz	158	0
watermelon; diced	1 cup	50	0

WAX BEANS

CANNED Cut Wax Beans (Owatonna)	½ cup	20	0
Golden Cut Premium (S&W)	½ cup	20	0
Wax Beans (Libby)	½ cup	20	0
Wax Beans (Seneca)	½ cup	20	0

FOOD	PORTION	CALORIES	CHOLESTEROL

WHALE

FRESH
raw	3.5 oz	156	15

WHELK (SNAIL)

FRESH
cooked	3 oz	233	110
raw	3 oz	117	55

WHIPPED TOPPINGS
(*see also* CREAM)

Cool Whip (Non-Dairy)	1 Tbsp	11	tr
Cool Whip Extra Creamy Dairy	1 Tbsp	16	tr
D-Zerta w/ NutraSweet; as prep	1 Tbsp	7	tr
D-Zerta; as prep	¼ cup	47	tr
Dream Whip; as prep	1 Tbsp	9	tr
Real Cream Topping (Kraft)	¼ cup	25	10
Whipped Topping (Kraft)	¼ cup	35	0
Whipped Topping; as prep (Estee)	1 Tbsp	4	0
cream, pressurized	1 Tbsp	8	2
cream, pressurized	1 cup	154	46
frzn, non-dairy	¼ cup	60	0

FOOD	PORTION	CALORIES	CHOLESTEROL
frzn, non-dairy	1 Tbsp	13	0
non-dairy, powdered	1 Tbsp	8	tr
non-dairy, pressurized	1 Tbsp	11	0
pressurized, non-dairy	¼ cup	46	0

WHITE BEANS

FOOD	PORTION	CALORIES	CHOLESTEROL
CANNED			
white	1 cup	306	0
DRIED			
cooked	1 cup	249	0
raw	1 cup	674	0
small white, raw	1 cup	723	0
small white, cooked	1 cup	253	0

WHITEFISH

FOOD	PORTION	CALORIES	CHOLESTEROL
FRESH			
raw	3 oz	114	51
raw	1 fillet (6.9 oz)	266	119
SMOKED			
whitefish	1 oz	39	9
whitefish	3 oz	92	28

WHITING

FOOD	PORTION	CALORIES	CHOLESTEROL
FRESH			
cooked	1 fillet (2.5 oz)	83	60

FOOD	PORTION	CALORIES	CHOLESTEROL
cooked	3 oz	98	71
raw	3 oz	77	57
raw	1 fillet (3.2 oz)	83	61

WINE
(*see also* WINE COOLERS)

FOOD	PORTION	CALORIES	CHOLESTEROL
dessert	2 oz	90	0
red	3.5 oz	74	0
rose	3.5 oz	73	0
sherry	2 oz	84	0
vermouth, dry	3.5 oz	105	0
vermouth, sweet	3.5 oz	167	0
white	3.5 oz	70	0

WINE COOLERS

FOOD	PORTION	CALORIES	CHOLESTEROL
Bartles & Jaymes	12 oz	192	0

WINGED BEANS

DRIED
FOOD	PORTION	CALORIES	CHOLESTEROL
cooked	1 cup	252	0
raw	1 cup	745	0

WOLFFISH

FRESH
FOOD	PORTION	CALORIES	CHOLESTEROL
Atlantic, raw	3 oz	82	39
Atlantic, raw	½ fillet (5.4 oz)	147	70

FOOD	PORTION	CALORIES	CHOLESTEROL
YAM			
(*see also* SWEET POTATO)			
CANNED			
Candied (S&W)	½ cup	180	0
Yams Golden Cut in Syrup (Sugary Sam)	½ cup	110	0
Yams Golden Whole in Heavy Syrup (Trappey's)	½ cup	130	0
Yams Southern Whole in Extra Heavy Syrup (S&W)	½ cup	139	0
FRESH			
mountain yam, Hawaii, raw; cubed	½ cup	46	0
mountain yam, Hawaii; cooked	½ cup	59	0
yam; cubed, cooked	½ cup	79	0
YARDLONG BEANS			
DRIED			
cooked	1 cup	202	0
raw	1 cup	580	0
YEAST			
baker's dry active	1 pkg (7 g)	20	0
brewer's dry	1 Tbsp	25	0

FOOD	PORTION	CALORIES	CHOLESTEROL

YELLOW BEANS

DRIED

cooked	1 cup	254	0
raw	1 cup	676	0

YOGURT

(*see also* YOGURT DRINKS; YOGURT, FROZEN)

Yoplait yogurt made in and/or distributed from California will have a slightly different fat content to comply with California law.

All Flavors (TCBY)	5 oz	160	11-15
Amaretto Almond Yo Creme (Yoplait)	5 oz	240	30
Apple Cinnamon Breakfast Yogurt (Yoplait)	6 oz	220	10
Apple Original (Yoplait)	4 oz	120	5
Apple Original (Yoplait)	6 oz	190	10
Banana Strawberry Non-Fat Lite (Colombo)	8 oz	190	5
Banana Custard Style (Yoplait)	6 oz	190	20
Banana Fruit-on-the-Bottom (Dannon)	8 oz	240	10
Bavarian Chocolate Yo Creme (Yoplait)	5 oz	270	30

FOOD	PORTION	CALORIES	CHOLESTEROL
Berries Breakfast Yogurt (Yoplait)	6 oz	230	10
Black Cherry (Breyers)	8 oz	270	15
Black Cherry Lowfat (Light N'Lively)	6 oz	180	5
Blueberry (Breyers)	8 oz	260	15
Blueberry (Dannon)	8 oz	200	10
Blueberry (Yoplait 150)	6 oz	150	5
Blueberry Custard Style (Yoplait)	6 oz	190	20
Blueberry Fruit-on-the-Bottom (Dannon)	8 oz	240	10
Blueberry Fruit-on-the-Bottom (Dannon)	4.4 oz	130	5
Blueberry Lowfat (Light N'Lively)	6 oz	180	5
Blueberry Non-Fat Lite (Colombo)	8 oz	160	5
Blueberry Original (Yoplait)	4 oz	120	5
Blueberry Original (Yoplait)	6 oz	190	10
Boysenberry Fruit-on-the-Bottom (Dannon)	8 oz	240	10
Boysenberry Original (Yoplait)	4 oz	120	5

FOOD	PORTION	CALORIES	CHOLESTEROL
Cherries Jubilee (Yoplait)	5 oz	220	30
Cherry (Yoplait 150)	6 oz	150	5
Cherry Custard Style (Yoplait)	6 oz	180	20
Cherry Fruit-on-the-Bottom (Dannon)	8 oz	240	10
Cherry Fruit-on-the-Bottom (Dannon)	4.4 oz	130	5
Cherry Original (Yoplait)	4 oz	120	5
Cherry w/ Almonds Breakfast Yogurt (Yoplait)	6 oz	210	10
Coffee (Dannon)	8 oz	200	10
Coffee/Lowfat (Friendship)	8 oz	210	14
Dutch Apple Fruit-on-the-Bottom (Dannon)	8 oz	240	10
Exotic Fruit Fruit-on-the-Bottom (Dannon)	8 oz	240	10
Fruit Cocktail Non-Fat Lite (Colombo)	8 oz	160	5
Lemon (Dannon)	8 oz	200	10
Lemon Custard Style (Yoplait)	6 oz	190	20

FOOD	PORTION	CALORIES	CHOLESTEROL
Lemon Original (Yoplait)	4 oz	120	5
Mixed Berries Extra Smooth (Dannon)	4.4 oz	130	10
Mixed Berries Fruit-on-the-Bottom (Dannon)	8 oz	240	10
Mixed Berries Fruit-on-the-Bottom (Dannon)	4.4 oz	130	5
Mixed Berries Hearty Nuts & Raisins (Dannon)	8 oz	260	10
Mixed Berry (Breyers)	8 oz	270	15
Mixed Berry Custard Style (Yoplait)	6 oz	180	20
Mixed Berry Original (Yoplait)	4 oz	120	5
Orange Original (Yoplait)	4 oz	120	5
Orchard Fruit Hearty Nuts & Raisins (Dannon)	8 oz	260	10
Peach (Breyers)	8 oz	270	15
Peach (Yoplait 150)	6 oz	150	5
Peach Lowfat (Light N'Lively)	6 oz	180	5
Peach Non-Fat Lite (Colombo)	8 oz	190	5

FOOD	PORTION	CALORIES	CHOLESTEROL
Peach Original (Yoplait)	4 oz	120	5
Peach Fruit-on-the-Bottom (Dannon)	8 oz	240	10
Pina Colada Fruit-on-the-Bottom (Dannon)	8 oz	240	10
Pina Colada Original (Yoplait)	4 oz	120	5
Pina Colada Original (Yoplait)	4 oz	120	5
Pineapple (Breyers)	8 oz	270	15
Pineapple Lowfat (Light N'Lively)	6 oz	180	5
Pineapple Original (Yoplait)	4 oz	120	5
Plain (Breyers)	8 oz	190	20
Plain (Friendship)	8 oz	170	30
Plain (Yoplait)	4 oz	80	10
Plain (Yoplait)	6 oz	120	15
Plain Lowfat (Dannon)	8 oz	140	15
Plain Non-Fat (Dannon)	8 oz	110	<5
Raspberries & Cream (Yoplait)	5 oz	230	30

FOOD	PORTION	CALORIES	CHOLESTEROL
Raspberry (Dannon)	8 oz	200	10
Raspberry (Yoplait 150)	6 oz	150	5
Raspberry Custard Style (Yoplait)	6 oz	190	20
Raspberry Original (Yoplait)	4 oz	120	5
Raspberry Original (Yoplait)	4 oz	120	5
Raspberry Extra Smooth (Dannon)	4.4 oz	130	10
Raspberry Fruit-on-the-Bottom (Dannon)	8 oz	240	10
Raspberry Fruit-on-the-Bottom (Dannon)	4.4 oz	130	5
Red Raspberry (Breyers)	8 oz	260	15
Red Raspberry Lowfat (Light N'Lively)	6 oz	170	5
Strawberries Romanoff (Yoplait)	5 oz	220	30
Strawberry (Breyers)	8 oz	270	15
Strawberry (Dannon)	8 oz	200	10
Strawberry (Yoplait 150)	6 oz	150	5
Strawberry Banana (Breyers)	8 oz	280	15

FOOD	PORTION	CALORIES	CHOLESTEROL
Strawberry Banana (Dannon)	8 oz	200	10
Strawberry Banana Breakfast Yogurt (Yoplait)	6 oz	240	10
Strawberry Banana Fruit-on-the-Bottom (Dannon)	4.4 oz	130	5
Strawberry Banana Lowfat (Light N'Lively)	6 oz	200	5
Strawberry Custard Style (Yoplait)	6 oz	190	20
Strawberry Extra Smooth (Dannon)	4.4 oz	130	10
Strawberry Fruit-on-the-Bottom (Dannon)	8 oz	240	10
Strawberry Fruit-on-the-Bottom (Dannon)	4.4 oz	130	5
Strawberry Lowfat (Light N'Lively)	6 oz	180	5
Strawberry Non-Fat Lite (Colombo)	8 oz	190	5
Strawberry Original (Yoplait)	4 oz	120	5
Strawberry w/ Almonds Breakfast Yogurt (Yoplait)	6 oz	210	10
Strawberry-Banana (Yoplait 150)	6 oz	150	5

FOOD	PORTION	CALORIES	CHOLESTEROL
Strawberry-Banana Original (Yoplait)	4 oz	120	5
Strawberry-Rhubarb Original (Yoplait)	4 oz	120	5
Sunrise Peach Breakfast Yogurt (Yoplait)	6 oz	230	10
Tropical Fruits Breakfast Yogurt (Yoplait)	6 oz	230	10
Vanilla (Dannon)	8 oz	200	10
Vanilla (Dannon)	4.4 oz	110	5
Vanilla Bean (Breyers)	8 oz	230	7
Vanilla Custard Style (Yoplait)	6 oz	180	20
Vanilla Hearty Nuts & Raisins (Dannon)	8 oz	270	10
Vanilla Lowfat (Friendship)	8 oz	210	14
With Fruit Lowfat (Friendship)	8 oz	230	14
coffee, lowfat	1 cup	193	11
coffee, lowfat	4 oz	97	6
coffee, lowfat	8 oz	194	11
fruit, all flavors, lowfat	1 cup	232	9
fruit, lowfat	4 oz	113	5
fruit, lowfat	8 oz	225	10
plain	4 oz	70	14

FOOD	PORTION	CALORIES	CHOLESTEROL
plain	8 oz	139	29
plain lowfat	1 cup	143	14
plain lowfat	4 oz	72	7
plain lowfat	8 oz	144	14
plain skim milk	1 cup	127	5
plain skim milk	4 oz	63	2
plain skim milk	8 oz	127	4
plain whole milk	1 cup	138	30
vanilla lowfat	8 oz	194	11
vanilla lowfat	4 oz	97	6
vanilla lowfat	1 cup	193	11

YOGURT DRINKS

FOOD	PORTION	CALORIES	CHOLESTEROL
Exotic Fruit Dan'up (Dannon)	8 oz	190	10
Mixed Berry Dan'up (Dannon)	8 oz	190	10
Raspberry Dan'up (Dannon)	8 oz	190	10
Strawberry Banana Dan'up (Dannon)	8 oz	190	10
Strawberry Dan'up (Dannon)	8 oz	190	10

YOGURT, FROZEN

FOOD	PORTION	CALORIES	CHOLESTEROL
Black Cherry (Sealtest)	½ cup	100	5
Peach (Sealtest)	½ cup	100	5

FOOD	PORTION	CALORIES	CHOLESTEROL
Red Raspberry (Sealtest)	½ cup	100	5
Strawberry (Sealtest)	½ cup	100	5
Vanilla (Colombo)	4 oz	99	7

YORKSHIRE PUDDING

Yorkshire pudding (home recipe)	3" sq	171	86

ZABAGLIONE
(*see* CUSTARD)

ZABAIONE
(*see* CUSTARD)

ZUCCHINI

CANNED			
Italian Style (S&W)	½ cup	45	0
Italian style	½ cup	33	0
FRESH			
cooked; sliced	½ cup	14	0
raw, sliced	½ cup	9	0
FROZEN			
Zucchini Vegetable Crisp (Ore Ida)	3 oz	150	5

FOOD	PORTION	CALORIES	CHOLESTEROL
Zucchini Sliced (Southland)	3.2 oz	15	0
cooked	½ cup	19	0
HOME RECIPE			
croquettes	½ cup	118	75
sticks	½ cup	81	18

Food	Value	Calories		
Zucchini sliced (not fried)	3.7 oz	18		0
cooked		16 oz	18	0
HOME RECIPE prepared		16 oz		
store		4 oz	81	79

PART II

Restaurant, Take-Out and Fast-Food Chains

FOOD	PORTION	CALORIES	CHOLESTEROL

ARBY'S

FOOD	PORTION	CALORIES	CHOLESTEROL
Bac'n Cheddar Deluxe	1	561	78
Beef'n Cheddar	1	490	51
Chicken Breast Sandwich	1	595	57
Chicken Club Sandwich	1	621	108
Chicken Roasted Breast	1	254	200
Chicken Roasted Leg	1	319	214
Chicken Salad Sandwich	1	386	30
Chicken Salad & Croissant	1	472	12
Chicken Salad w/ Tomato & Lettuce	1	515	12
French Fries	1 reg	211	6
Hot Ham 'n Cheese	1 reg	353	50
Potato Superstuffed Broccoli & Cheese	1	541	24
Potato Superstuffed Deluxe	1	648	72
Potato Superstuffed Mushroom & Cheese	1	506	21
Potato Superstuffed Taco	1	619	145
Potato Baked Plain	1	290	0
Potato Cakes	1	201	1
Roast Beef	1	350	39
Roast Beef Deluxe	1	486	59
Roast Beef Jr	1	218	20
Roast Beef King	1	467	49
Roast Beef Super	1	501	40
Shake, Chocolate	1	384	32

FOOD	PORTION	CALORIES	CHOLESTEROL
Shake, Jamocha	1	424	31
Shake, Vanilla	1	295	30
Tossed Salad, Plain	1	44	0
Tossed Salad w/ 20 Calorie Italian Dressing	1	57	0
Turkey Deluxe	1	375	39

BASKIN-ROBBINS

FOOD	PORTION	CALORIES	CHOLESTEROL
Chocolate Ice Cream	1 scoop	270	37
Jamoca Almond Fudge Ice Cream	1 scoop	270	32
Low, Lite 'N Luscious Chunky Banana	4 oz	100	3
Low, Lite 'N Luscious Jamoca Chip	4 oz	110	3
Low, Lite 'N Luscious Pineapple Coconut	4 oz	110	3
Pralines 'N Cream Ice Cream	1 scoop	280	36
Vanilla Frozen Yogurt	4 oz	124	8
Vanilla Ice Cream	1 scoop	240	52

BRAZIER
(*see* DAIRY QUEEN)

BURGER KING

FOOD	PORTION	CALORIES	CHOLESTEROL
7-UP	1 reg	144	0
Apple Pie	1	305	4
Bacon Double Cheeseburger	1	510	104
Breakfast Croissan'wich w/ Bacon	1	355	249

FOOD	PORTION	CALORIES	CHOLESTEROL
Breakfast Croissan'wich w/ Ham	1	335	262
Breakfast Croissan'wich w/ Sausage	1	538	293
Cheeseburger	1	317	48
Chicken Specialty Sandwich	1	688	82
Chicken Tenders	6 pieces	204	47
Coffee, black	6 oz	2	0
Diet Pepsi	1 reg	1	0
French Fries	1 reg	227	14
French Toast Sticks	1 serving	499	74
Great Danish	1	500	6
Ham & Cheese Specialty Sandwich	1	471	70
Hamburger	1	275	37
Milk, 2%	8 oz	121	18
Milk, Whole	8 oz	157	35
Onion Rings	1 reg	274	0
Orange Juice	6 oz	80	0
Pepsi-Cola	1 reg	159	0
Salad Dressing, 1000 Island	3 Tbsp	117	17
Salad Dressing, Bleu Cheese	3 Tbsp	156	22
Salad Dressing, House	3 Tbsp	130	11
Salad Dressing, Italian, Reduced Calorie	3 Tbsp	14	0
Salad w/o Dressing	1 reg	28	0
Scrambled Egg Platter	1	468	370

FOOD	PORTION	CALORIES	CHOLESTEROL
Scrambled Egg Platter w/ Bacon	1	536	378
Scrambled Egg Platter w/ Sausage	1	702	420
Whaler Fish Sandwich	1	488	77
Whopper Double Beef	1	863	168
Whopper Double Beef w/ Cheese	1	946	191
Whopper Jr. Sandwich	1	322	41
Whopper Jr. Sandwich w/ Cheese	1	364	52
Whopper Sandwich	1	628	90
Whopper Sandwich w/ Cheese	1	711	113

CARL'S JR.

FOOD	PORTION	CALORIES	CHOLESTEROL
BAKERY SELECTIONS			
Chocolate Cake	1 piece	380	70
Chocolate Chip Cookies	2.5 oz	353	15
Danish	1	300	0
Muffin, Blueberry	1	256	34
Muffin, Bran	1	220	50
BEVERAGES			
Iced Tea	1 reg	2	0
Milk, 2%	10 oz	175	0
Orange Juice	1 sm	94	0
Shake	1 reg	353	17
Soda	1 reg	243	0
Soda, Diet	1 reg	2	0

FOOD	PORTION	CALORIES	CHOLESTEROL
BREAKFAST ITEMS			
Bacon	2 strips	50	8
English Muffin w/ Margarine	1	180	0
French Toast Dips w/o syrup	1 serving	480	54
Hash Brown Nuggets	1 serving	170	10
Hot Cakes w/ Margarine w/o Syrup	1 serving	360	15
Sausage	1 patty	190	25
Scrambled Eggs	1 serving	120	245
Sunrise Sandwich w/ Bacon	1	370	120
Sunrise Sandwich w/ Sausage	1	500	165
REGULAR MENU SELECTIONS			
American Cheese	½ oz	63	16
California Roast Beef 'n Swiss	1	360	130
Cheeseburger Double Western Bacon	1	890	145
Cheeseburger Western Bacon	1	630	105
Chicken Club Sandwich Charbroiler	1	510	85
Chicken Sandwich Charbroiler BBQ	1	320	50
Country Fried Steak Sandwich	1	610	45
Filet of Fish Sandwich	1	550	90
French Fries	1 reg	360	15
Hamburger, Famous Star	1	590	45
Hamburger, Happy Star	1	220	45
Hamburger, Old Time Star	1	400	80
Hamburger, Super Star	1	770	125

FOOD	PORTION	CALORIES	CHOLESTEROL
Onion Rings	1 serving	310	10
Potato w/ Bacon & Cheese	1	650	45
Potato w/ Broccoli & Cheese	1	470	10
Potato Fiesta	1	550	40
Potato Lite	1	250	0
Potato w/ Sour Cream & Chives	1	350	10
Potato w/ Cheese	1	550	40
Swiss Cheese	½ oz	57	16
Zucchini	1 serving	300	10
SALADS AND DRESSINGS			
Dressing, Blue Cheese	1 oz	151	18
Dressing, French, Reduced Calorie	1 oz	38	0
Dressing, House	1 oz	110	10
Dressing, Italian	1 oz	120	0
Dressing, 1000 Island	1 oz	110	5
Salad-to-Go, Chef	1	180	63
Salad-to-Go, Chicken	1	206	83
Salad-to-Go, Garden	1	46	7
Salad-to-Go, Taco	1	356	99
SOUPS			
Boston Clam Chowder	7 oz	140	22
Cream of Broccoli	7 oz	140	22
Lumber Jack Mix Vegetable	7 oz	70	3
Old Fashioned Chicken Noodle	7 oz	80	14

FOOD	PORTION	CALORIES	CHOLESTEROL
CHICK-FIL-A			
Carrot-Raisin Salad	2.7 oz	116	6
Carrot-Raisin Salad	13 oz	570	30
Chick-fil-A Nuggets	8 pack	287	62
Chick-fil-A Nuggets	12 pack	430	92
Chick-fil-A Sandwich	1	426	66
Chick-fil-A, no bun	3.6 oz	219	42
Chicken Salad Cup	3.4 oz	309	21
Chicken Salad Plate	1	475	97
Chicken Salad Sandwich (Wheat)	1	449	50
Coleslaw	4 oz	175	13
Coleslaw	15 oz	718	52
Fudge Brownie w/ Nuts	1	369	0
Hearty Breast of Chicken Soup	8.5 oz	152	46
Ice Cream	4.5 oz	134	24
Iced Tea, Unsweetened	9 oz	3	0
Lemon Pie	1 slice	329	7
Lemonade	10 oz	124	tr
Orange Juice	6 oz	82	0
Potato Salad	4 oz	198	6
Potato Salad	16 oz	850	23
Waffle Potato Fries	1 reg	270	8
DAIRY QUEEN/BRAZIER			
FOOD SELECTION All White Chicken Nuggets	1 serving	276	39

FOOD	PORTION	CALORIES	CHOLESTEROL
Chicken Breast Fillet	1	608	78
Chicken Breast Fillet w/ Cheese	1	661	87
DQ Hounder	1	480	80
DQ Hounder w/ Cheese	1	533	89
DQ Hounder w/ Chili	1	575	89
Double Hamburger	1	530	85
Double Hamburger w/ Cheese	1	650	95
Fish Fillet	1	430	40
Fish Fillet w/ Cheese	1	483	49
French Fries	1 reg	200	10
French Fries	1 lg	320	15
Hot Dog	1	280	45
Hot Dog w/ Cheese	1	330	55
Hot Dog w/ Chili	1	320	55
Onion Rings	1 reg	280	15
Single Hamburger	1	360	45
Single Hamburger w/ Cheese	1	410	50
Super Hot Dog	1	520	80
Super Hot Dog w/ Cheese	1	580	100
Super Hot Dog w/ Chili	1	570	100
Triple Hamburger	1	710	135
Triple Hamburger w/ Cheese	1	820	145
ICE CREAM			
Banana Split	1	540	30
Buster Bar	1	460	10

FOOD	PORTION	CALORIES	CHOLESTEROL
Chipper Sandwich	1	318	13
Cone	1 sm	140	10
Cone	1 reg	240	15
Cone	1 lg	340	25
DQ Sandwich	1	140	5
Dilly Bar	1	210	10
Dipped Cone	1 sm	190	10
Dipped Cone	1 reg	340	20
Dipped Cone	1 lg	510	30
Double Delight	1	490	25
Float	1	410	20
Freeze	1	500	30
Fudge Nut Bar	1	406	10
Heath Blizzard	1	800	65
Hot Fudge Brownie Delight	1	600	20
Malt	1 sm	406	10
Malt	1 reg	520	35
Malt	1 lg	760	50
Mr. Misty	1 sm	190	0
Mr. Misty	1 reg	250	0
Mr. Misty	1 lg	340	0
Mr. Misty Float	1	390	20
Mr. Misty Freeze	1	500	30
Mr. Misty Kiss	1	70	0
Parfait	1	430	30
Peanut Buster Parfait	1	740	30

FOOD	PORTION	CALORIES	CHOLESTEROL
Shake	1 sm (10 oz)	490	35
Shake	1 reg (15 oz)	710	50
Shake	1 lg (17 oz)	831	60
Shake	1 xlg (21 oz)	990	70
Strawberry Shortcake	1	540	30
Sundae	1 sm	190	10
Sundae	1 reg	310	20

DOMINO'S PIZZA
(*see also* PIZZA, SHAKEY'S)

10" PIZZA

FOOD	PORTION	CALORIES	CHOLESTEROL
Double Cheese	2 slices	284	24
Double Cheese, Pepperoni	2 slices	331	35
Ground Beef	2 slices	250	21
Ground Beef, Pepperoni	2 slices	297	32
Mushroom, Sausage	2 slices	248	18
Pepperoni	2 slices	265	23
Pepperoni, Mushroom	2 slices	267	23
Pepperoni, Sausage	2 slices	293	29
Plain Cheese	2 slices	218	12
Sausage	2 slices	246	18

14" PIZZA

FOOD	PORTION	CALORIES	CHOLESTEROL
Double Cheese	2 slices	365	31
Double Cheese, Pepperoni	2 slices	427	45

FOOD	PORTION	CALORIES	CHOLESTEROL
Ground Beef	2 slices	321	26
Ground Beef, Pepperoni	2 slices	382	40
Mushroom, Sausage	2 slices	322	24
Pepperoni	2 slices	343	29
Pepperoni, Mushroom	2 slices	346	29
Pepperoni, Sausage	2 slices	380	38
Plain Cheese	2 slices	281	15
Sausage	2 slices	318	24
LARGE PIZZA Double Cheese	2 slices	700	42
Double Cheese, Pepperoni	2 slices	778	60
Ground Beef	2 slices	527	34
Ground Beef, Pepperoni	2 slices	605	52
Mushroom, Sausage	2 slices	532	33
Pepperoni	2 slices	556	39
Pepperoni, Mushroom	2 slices	550	39
Pepperoni, Sausage	2 slices	606	51
Plain Cheese	2 slices	478	21
Sausage	2 slices	528	33
SMALL PIZZA Double Cheese	2 slices	480	35
Double Cheese, Pepperoni	2 slices	453	46
Ground Beef	2 slices	361	30
Ground Beef, Pepperoni	2 slices	431	46
Mushroom, Sausage	2 slices	365	28
Pepperoni	2 slices	384	34
Pepperoni, Mushroom	2 slices	388	34

FOOD	PORTION	CALORIES	CHOLESTEROL
Pepperoni, Sausage	2 slices	431	44
Plain Cheese	2 slices	314	17
Sausage	2 slices	360	35

DRUTHER'S INTERNATIONAL

FOOD	PORTION	CALORIES	CHOLESTEROL
Bacon and Egg Biscuit	1	258	253
Bacon and Egg Plate; fried	1	721	500
Bacon and Egg Plate; scrambled	1	742	501
Biscuits and Gravy	1 serving	331	3
Cheeseburger	1	380	69
Chicken Snack, Thigh, Drumstick	1 snack	925	77
Chicken Snack, Wing, Breast	1 snack	970	159
Deluxe Quarter Hamburger	1	660	127
Double Cheeseburger	1	500	105
Eight Piece Chicken Dinner	1	3664	601
Fish and Chips	1 dinner	729	112
Fish Dinner	1	770	117
Fish Sandwich	1	349	56
Ham and Egg Biscuit	1	217	256
Ham and Egg Plate	1	681	511
Ham and Egg Plate; scrambled	1	703	511
Hamburger	1	327	55
Sausage and Egg Biscuit	1	246	257
Sausage and Egg Plate; fried	1	741	515
Sausage and Egg Plate; scrambled	1	762	515

FOOD	PORTION	CALORIES	CHOLESTEROL
Three Piece Chicken Dinner, Thigh, Breast, Wing	1	1309	271
Three Piece Chicken Dinner, Thigh, Breat, Drumstick	1	1281	273
Twelve Piece Chicken Dinner	1	5496	982
Two Piece Chicken Dinner	1	925	157
Two Piece Chicken Dinner, Breast, Wing	1	970	159
Two Sausages/Two Biscuits	1 meal	358	34

DUNKIN' DONUTS
(see also DOUGHNUT)

CROISSANT

Almond	1	435	2
Chocolate	1	502	2
Plain	1	291	2

DOUGHNUT

Apple Filled w/ Cinnamon Sugar	1	219	1
Bavarian Creme Filled	1	226	2
Bavarian Filled w/ Chocolate Frosting	1	231	1
Blueberry Filled	1	196	1
Chocolate Frosted Yeast Ring	1	246	1
Chocolate Cake Ring w/ Glaze	1	324	2
Coconut Coated Cake Ring	1	417	2
French Cruller w/ Glaze	1	201	16
Honey Dipped Coffee Roll	1	348	1
Honey Dipped Cruller	1	370	2

FOOD	PORTION	CALORIES	CHOLESTEROL
Honey Dipped Yeast Ring	1	208	2
Jelly Filled	1	274	2
Lemon Filled	1	221	1
Munchkin Cake w/ Powdered Sugar	1	69	tr
Munchkin Chocolate w/ Glaze	1	88	1
Munchkin Yeast w/ Glaze	1	43	tr
Plain Cake Ring	1	319	2
Sugared Jelly Stick	1	332	2
MISCELLANEOUS			
Biscuit	1	332	tr
Brownie	1	280	20
Chocolate Chip Cookie	1	129	6
Macaroon	1	351	3
MUFFIN			
Apple Spice	1	327	26
Banana Nut	1	327	23
Blueberry	1	263	21
Bran	1	353	12
Cherry	1	317	31
Corn	1	347	25

HARDEE'S

FOOD	PORTION	CALORIES	CHOLESTEROL
American Cheese	½ oz	47	12
Apple Turnover	1	282	tr
Bacon Cheeseburger	1	556	60
Big Cookie	1	278	9

FOOD	PORTION	CALORIES	CHOLESTEROL
Big Country Breakfast Ham Platter	1	665	369
Big Country Breakfast Platter	1	716	350
Big Country Breakfast Sausage Platter	1	940	442
Big Deluxe	1	503	50
Biscuit	1	257	0
Biscuit Gravy	4 oz	144	21
Biscuit w/ Bacon & Egg	1	405	369
Biscuit w/ Cheese	1	304	12
Biscuit w/ Cinnamon 'N' Raisin	1	276	tr
Biscuit w/ Country Ham	1	328	12
Biscuit w/ Egg	1	334	160
Biscuit w/ Sausage	1	426	17
Biscuit w/ Sausage & Egg	1	503	177
Biscuit w/ Steak	1	491	16
Biscuit w/ Sugar Cured Ham	1	299	17
Canadian Sunrise	1	489	253
Cheeseburger	1	309	28
Cheeseburger, ¼ lb	1	511	77
Chicken Fillet	1	510	57
Egg	1 oz	77	160
Fisherman's Fillet	1	469	80
French Fries	1 reg	239	tr
French Fries	1 lg	406	tr
Hamburger	1	276	22
Hash Rounds	1	200	10

FOOD	PORTION	CALORIES	CHOLESTEROL
Hot Ham 'N' Cheese	1	376	59
Jelly	1 Tbsp	49	0
Milkshake	11 oz	391	tr
Mushroom 'N' Swiss	1	512	86
Roast Beef Sandwich	1	312	68
Roast Beef Sandwich, Big	1	440	86
Salad Chef	1	277	179
Salad Side	1	21	tr
Turkey Club	1	426	45

JACK-IN-THE-BOX

Bacon Cheeseburger	1	705	85
Breakfast Jack	1	307	203
Cheeseburger	1	325	41
Cheesecake	1	309	63
Chicken Strips	4 pieces	349	68
Chicken Strips	6 pieces	523	103
Chicken Supreme	1	524	82
Club Pita (no sauce)	1	277	43
Coca-Cola Classic	12 oz	144	0
Coffee, black	8 oz	2	0
Crescent, Canadian	1	452	226
Crescent, Sausage	1	584	187
Crescent, Supreme	1	547	178
Diet Coke	12 oz	8	0
Dinner, Chicken Strip (no sauce)	1	689	100

FOOD	PORTION	CALORIES	CHOLESTEROL
Dinner, Shrimp (no sauce)	1	731	157
Dinner, Sirloin Steak (no sauce)	1	699	75
Dr Pepper	12 oz	144	0
Dressing, Buttermilk House	1 pkg	181	10
Dressing, Reduced Calorie French	1 pkg	80	0
Dressing, Thousand Island	1 pkg	156	11
Dressing, Bleu Cheese	1 pkg	131	9
Egg Rolls	3 pieces	405	30
Egg Rolls	5 pieces	675	50
Fajita Pita	1	278	30
Fish Supreme	1	554	66
French Fries	1 reg	221	8
French Fries	1 lg	353	13
French Fries	1 jumbo	442	16
Grape Jelly	1 pkg	38	0
Guacamole	1 oz	55	0
Ham & Swiss Burger	1	754	106
Hamburger	1	288	26
Hash Brown	1	116	3
Hot Apple Turnover	1	410	15
Hot Club Supreme	1	524	82
Iced Tea	12 oz	3	0
Jumbo Jack	1	584	73
Jumbo Jack w/ Cheese	1	677	102
Lowfat Milk	8 oz	122	18

FOOD	PORTION	CALORIES	CHOLESTEROL
Milk Shake, Chocolate	1 reg	330	25
Milk Shake, Vanilla	1 reg	320	25
Moby Jack	1	444	47
Monterey Burger	1	865	152
Mushroom Burger	1	470	64
Nachos, Cheese	1 serving	571	37
Nachos, Supreme	1 serving	787	59
Onion Rings	1 serving	383	27
Orange Juice	6 oz	80	0
Pancake Platter	1	612	99
Pancake Syrup	1 pkg	121	0
Pizza Pocket	1	497	32
Ramblin' Root Beer	12 oz	176	0
Salad, Chef	1	295	107
Salad, Pasta & Seafood	1	394	48
Salad, Side	1	51	tr
Salad, Taco	1	377	102
Salsa	1 oz	8	0
Sauce, A-1 Steak	1 pkg	35	0
Sauce, BBQ	1 pkg	39	tr
Sauce, Mayo-Mustard	1 pkg	124	10
Sauce, Mayo-Onion	1 pkg	143	20
Sauce, Seafood Cocktail	1 pkg	57	0
Sauce, Sweet & Sour	1 pkg	39	0
Scrambled Egg Platter	1	662	354
Shrimp	10 pieces	270	84

FOOD	PORTION	CALORIES	CHOLESTEROL
Shrimp	15 pieces	404	126
Sprite	12 oz	144	0
Swiss & Bacon Burger	1	678	127
Taco	1	191	21
Taco, Super	1	288	37
Ultimate Cheeseburger	1	942	127

KENTUCKY FRIED CHICKEN

CHICKEN DISHES			
Extra Crispy Center Breast	1	353	93
Extra Crispy Drumstick	1	173	65
Extra Crispy Side Breast	1	354	66
Extra Crispy Thigh	1	371	121
Extra Crispy Wing	1	218	63
Kentucky Nugget Sauce, Barbecue	1 oz	35	1
Kentucky Nugget Sauce, Honey	1 oz	49	1
Kentucky Nugget Sauce, Mustard	1 oz	36	1
Kentucky Nugget Sauce, Sweet & Sour	1 oz	58	1
Kentucky Nuggets	1 nugget	46	12
Original Center Breast	1	257	93
Original Drumstick	1	147	81
Original Side Breast	1	276	96
Original Thigh	1	278	122
Original Wing	1	181	67

FOOD	PORTION	CALORIES	CHOLESTEROL
SIDE DISHES			
Baked Beans	1 portion	105	1
Buttermilk Biscuit	1	269	1
Chicken Gravy	1 serving	59	2
Coleslaw	1 serving	103	4
Corn on the Cob	1 ear	176	1
Kentucky Fries	1 reg	268	2
Mashed Potatoes	1 serving	59	1
Mashed Potatoes w/ Gravy	1 serving	62	1
Potato Salad	1 serving	141	11

LONG JOHN SILVER'S

FOOD	PORTION	CALORIES	CHOLESTEROL
2 Piece Fish & Fryes	1	651	75
2 Piece Kitchen Breaded Fish Dinner	1	818	76
3 Piece Fish Dinner	1	1180	119
3 Piece Fish & Fryes	1	853	106
3 Piece Kitchen Breaded Fish Dinner	1	940	101
3 Piece Chicken Planks Dinner	1	885	25
4 Piece Chicken Planks Dinner	1	1037	25
6 Piece Chicken Nuggets Dinner	1	699	25
Batter Fried Fish	1	202	31
Batter Fried Shrimp	1	47	17
Batter Fried Shrimp Dinner	1	711	127
Clam Chowder	1	128	17

FOOD	PORTION	CALORIES	CHOLESTEROL
Clam Dinner	1	955	27
Coleslaw	1	182	12
Fish & Chicken	1	935	56
Fish & More	1	978	88
Fish Sandwich Platter	1	835	75
Fryes	1 reg	247	13
Hush Puppies	1	145	1
Kitchen Breaded Fish	1	122	25
Ocean Chef Salad	1	229	64
Oyster Dinner	1	789	55
Scallop Dinner	1	747	37
Seafood Platter	1	976	95
Seafood Salad	1	426	113

McDONALD'S

BEVERAGES

Coca-Cola Classic	16 oz	190	0
Diet Coke	16 oz	1	0
Grapefruit Juice	6 oz	80	0
Milk, 2%	8 oz	121	18
Milk Shake, Chocolate	10 oz	388	41
Milk Shake, Strawberry	10 oz	384	41
Milk Shake, Vanilla	10 oz	354	41
Orange Drink	16 oz	177	0
Orange Juice	6 oz	80	0
Sprite	16 oz	190	0

FOOD	PORTION	CALORIES	CHOLESTEROL
BREAKFAST ITEMS			
Biscuit w/ Bacon, Egg & Cheese	1	449	336
Biscuit w/ Biscuit Spread	1	260	1
Biscuit w/ Sausage	1	440	49
Biscuit w/ Sausage & Egg	1	529	358
Egg McMuffin	1	293	299
English Muffin w/ Butter	1	169	9
Hashbrown Potatoes	1	131	9
Hotcakes w/ Butter & Syrup	1 portion	413	21
Pork Sausage	1.7 oz	180	48
Sausage McMuffin	1	372	64
Sausage McMuffin w/ Egg	1	451	336
Scrambled Eggs	1 portion	157	545
DESSERTS			
Apple Pie	1	262	6
Cone, Soft Serve	1	144	16
Cookies, Chocolate Chip	1 pkg	325	4
Cookies, McDonaldland	1 pkg	288	0
Danish, Apple	1	389	25
Danish, Cinnamon Raisin	1	445	34
Danish, Iced Cheese	1	395	47
Danish, Raspberry	1	414	26
Sundae, Hot Caramel	1	343	35
Sundae, Hot Fudge	1	313	28
Sundae, Strawberry	1	283	27

FOOD	PORTION	CALORIES	CHOLESTEROL
MAIN MENU SELECTIONS			
Big Mac	1	562	103
Cheeseburger	1	308	53
Chicken McNuggets	1 portion	288	65
Filet-O-Fish	1	442	50
French Fries	1 reg	220	9
French Fries	1 lg	312	12
Hamburger	1	257	37
McD.L.T.	1	674	112
McNuggets Sauce, Barbeque	1 oz	53	0
McNuggets Sauce, Honey	1 oz	46	0
McNuggets Sauce, Hot Mustard	1 oz	66	5
McNuggets Sauce, Sweet & Sour	1 oz	57	0
Quarter Pounder	1	517	118
SALADS AND DRESSINGS			
1000 Island Dressing	½ oz	78	8
Bacon Bits	.1 oz	16	0
Bleu Cheese Dressing	½ oz	69	6
Chef Salad	1	231	152
Chicken Salad Oriental	1	141	78
Chow Mein Noodles	.3 oz	45	2
Croutons	.4 oz	52	0
French Dressing	½ oz	58	0
Lite Vinaigrette Dressing	½ oz	15	0
Oriental Dressing	½ oz	24	0
Ranch Dressing	½ oz	83	5

FOOD	PORTION	CALORIES	CHOLESTEROL
Shrimp Salad	1	104	193
Side Salad	1	57	53

RAX

MEXICAN BAR

FOOD	PORTION	CALORIES	CHOLESTEROL
Banana Pepper Rings	1 Tbsp	2	tr
Cheese Sauce, Nacho	3.5 oz	470	11
Cheese Sauce, Regular	3.5 oz	420	11
Green Onions	¼ cup	10	0
Japapeno Peppers	1 oz	6	0
Olives	3.5 oz	110	0
Refried Beans	3 oz	120	2
Sour Topping	3.5 oz	130	tr
Spanish Rice	3.5 oz	90	tr
Spicy Meat Sauce	3.5 oz	80	12
Taco Sauce	3.5 oz	30	tr
Taco Shell	1	40	tr
Tomatoes	1 oz	6	0
Tortilla Chips	1 oz	140	tr
Tortillas	1	110	tr

MISCELLANEOUS

FOOD	PORTION	CALORIES	CHOLESTEROL
Cherry Coke	10 oz	120	0
Chocolate Chip Cookie	1	130	tr
Coca-Cola	10 oz	120	0
Coffee, decafe, black	6 oz	2	0
Coffee, regular, black	6 oz	2	0
Creamer, Non-Dairy	⅜ oz	14	0

FOOD	PORTION	CALORIES	CHOLESTEROL
Diet Coke	10 oz	tr	0
Drive-Thru Salad, Chef Salad w/o dressing	1	230	322
Drive-Thru Salad, Garden w/o dressing	1	160	273
Fanta Root Beer	10 oz	120	0
Hot Cocoa Mix	10 oz	110	tr
Hot Tea	6 oz	tr	0
Iced Tea	6 oz	tr	0
Milk, 2%	8 oz	110	20
Milk, Whole	8 oz	150	30
Milk Shake, Chocolate	1	560	63
Milk Shake, Strawberry	1	560	62
Milk Shake, Vanilla	1	500	58
Sprite	10 oz	110	0
Whipped Topping	1 dip	50	2
PASTA BAR			
Alfredo Sauce	3.5 oz	80	10
Chicken Noodle Soup	3.5 oz	40	10
Creme of Broccoli Soup	3.5 oz	50	tr
Parmesan Cheese Substitute	1 oz	80	tr
Pasta Shells	3.5 oz	170	0
Pasta/Vegetable Blend	3.5 oz	100	0
Rainbow Rotine	3.5 oz	180	2
Spaghetti	3.5 oz	140	0
Spaghetti Sauce	3.5 oz	80	tr
Spaghetti Sauce w/ Meat	3.5 oz	150	tr

FOOD	PORTION	CALORIES	CHOLESTEROL
POTATOES			
BBQ Potato	1	730	18
Cheese & Bacon Potato	1	780	23
Cheese & Broccoli Potato	1	760	11
Chili & Cheese Potato	1	700	25
French Fries, salted or unsalted	1 reg	260	4
French Fries, salted or unsalted	1 lg	390	6
Plain	1	270	0
Plain w/ margarine	1	370	0
Sour Topping Potato	1	400	tr
SALAD BAR			
Alfalfa Sprouts	1 oz	8	0
Applesauce	1 cup	100	0
Bacon Bits	.5 oz	40	12
Banana Chips	1 oz	100	0
Beets	1 cup	60	0
Blue Cheese Dressing	1 Tbsp	50	8
Broccoli	½ cup	16	0
Cabbage	1 cup	16	0
Cantaloupe	2 pieces	16	0
Carrots	¼ cup	8	0
Cauliflower	½ cup	16	0
Celery	1 Tbsp	14	0
Cheddar Cheese Tidbits	1 oz	160	tr
Cherry Peppers	1 Tbsp	6	0
Chow Mein Noddles	1 oz	140	tr

FOOD	PORTION	CALORIES	CHOLESTEROL
Coconut	1 oz	160	0
Coleslaw	3.5 oz	70	tr
Cottage Cheese	1 cup	250	47
Crackers (Saltines)	2	16	tr
Croutons	.5 oz	50	tr
Cucumbers	4 slices	2	0
Eggs	1.5 oz	70	267
French Dressing	1 Tbsp	60	tr
Garbanzo Beans	½ cup	360	0
Gelatin, Lime	½ cup	90	0
Gelatin, Strawberry	½ cup	90	0
Grapefruit Sections	1 cup	80	0
Grapes	1 cup	100	0
Green Peppers	¼ cup	8	0
Honeydew Melons	2 pieces	25	0
Italian Dressing	1 Tbsp	50	0
Kale	1 oz	16	0
Kidney Beans	1 cup	220	0
Lettuce	1 leaf	2	0
Lite Blue Cheese Dressing	1 Tbsp	35	3
Lite French Dressing	1 Tbsp	40	tr
Lite Italian Dressing	1 Tbsp	30	5
Lite Thousand Island Dressing	1 Tbsp	40	5
Macaroni Salad	3.5 oz	160	tr
Mushrooms	¼ cup	4	0
Oil	1 Tbsp	130	0

FOOD	PORTION	CALORIES	CHOLESTEROL
Onions	¼ cup	12	0
Pasta Salad	3.5 oz	80	tr
Peaches	2 slices	16	0
Peas	1 oz	25	0
Pickle Spear	1	8	0
Pineapple, canned	3.5 oz	100	0
Pineapple, fresh	1 slice	45	0
Poppy Seed Dressing	1 Tbsp	60	6
Potato Salad	1 cup	260	7
Pudding, Butterscotch	3.5 oz	140	2
Pudding, Chocolate	3.5 oz	140	2
Pudding, Vanilla	3.5 oz	140	2
Radishes	.5 oz	2	0
Ranch Dressing	1 Tbsp	45	5
Red Cabbage	¼ cup	4	0
Sesame Sticks	1 oz	150	0
Shredded Imitation Cheddar Cheese	1 oz	90	6
Soynuts	1 oz	120	0
Strawberries	2 oz	18	0
Sunflower Seeds w/ Raisins	1 oz	130	0
Thousand Island Dressing	1 Tbsp	70	8
Three Bean Salad	½ cup	100	0
Tomatoes	1 oz	6	0
Turkey Bits	2 oz	70	49
Vinegar	1 Tbsp	2	0
Watermelon	2 pieces	18	0

FOOD	PORTION	CALORIES	CHOLESTEROL
SANDWICHES AND INGREDIENTS			
American Slices	1 slice	60	15
BBC	1	720	137
BBC Sauce	.75 oz	140	41
BBQ Meat Topping	3.25 oz	140	24
BBQ Sandwich	1	420	24
Bacon	1 slice	80	30
Banana Pepper Rings	1 Tbsp	2	tr
Bun	1 sm	180	tr
Double Works Burger	1	440	50
Fish	3.5 oz	230	tr
Fish Sandwich	1	460	tr
Ham	2.5 oz	70	24
Ham & Swiss Sandwich	1	430	37
Hamburger	1	130	25
Hamburger Seasoning Salt	1 sprinkle	tr	tr
Horseradish Sauce	.75 oz	10	tr
Kaiser Bun	4"	180	tr
Kaiser Bun	6"	280	tr
Ketchup	1 Tbsp	6	tr
Mayonnaise	.75 oz	150	tr
Mustard	1 Tbsp	4	tr
Onions	3 rings	4	0
Onions, Diced	¼ cup	18	0
Philly Vegetables	2 oz	30	tr
Philly Beef & Cheese Sandwich	1	470	49

FOOD	PORTION	CALORIES	CHOLESTEROL
Pickle Slices	4 slices	2	0
Pickle Spears	1	8	0
Regular BBQ Sauce	1 oz	40	tr
Roast Beef	2.8 oz	140	36
Roast Beef Sandwich	1 lg	570	36
Roast Beef Sandwich	1 reg	320	36
Roast Beef Sandwich (Uncle Al)	1 sm	260	19
Shredded Lettuce	¼ cup	2	0
Smokey BBQ Sauce	1 oz	40	tr
Sweet Pickle Relish	1 Tbsp	20	tr
Swiss	1 slice	30	13
Tartar Sauce	.5 oz	50	tr
Tomato	1 slice	2	0
Turkey	2.5 oz	80	27
Turkey & Bacon Club	1	470	87
Works Burger	1	310	25

RED LOBSTER

All of the following are for a cooked portion unless otherwise noted.

FOOD	PORTION	CALORIES	CHOLESTEROL
Atlantic Cod	1 lunch serving	100	70
Atlantic Ocean Perch	1 lunch serving	130	75
Blacktip Shark	1 lunch serving	150	60
Calamari; breaded & fried	1 lunch serving	360	140

FOOD	PORTION	CALORIES	CHOLESTEROL
Calico Scallops	1 lunch serving	180	115
Catfish	1 lunch serving	170	85
Cherrystone Clams	1 lunch serving	130	80
Chicken Breast	4 oz before cooking	120	65
Deep Sea Scallops	1 lunch serving	130	50
Flounder	1 lunch serving	100	70
Grouper	1 lunch serving	110	65
Haddock	1 lunch serving	110	85
Halibut	1 lunch serving	110	60
Hamburger	5 oz before cooking	320	105
King Crab Legs	1 lb	170	100
Langostino	1 lunch serving	120	210
Lemon Sole	1 lunch serving	120	65
Mackerel	1 lunch serving	190	100
Maine Lobster	1¼ lb	240	310
Mako Shark	1 lunch serving	140	100

FOOD	PORTION	CALORIES	CHOLESTEROL
Monkfish	1 lunch serving	110	80
Mussels	3 oz	70	50
Norwegian Salmon	1 lunch serving	230	80
Oysters, raw	6	110	60
Pollack	1 lunch serving	120	90
Porterhouse Steak	18 oz before cooking	1420	290
Rainbow Trout	1 lunch serving	170	90
Red Rockfish	1 lunch serving	90	85
Red Snapper	1 lunch serving	110	70
Rock Lobster	1 tail	230	200
Shrimp	8–12 pieces	120	230
Sirloin Steak	7 oz before cooking	570	140
Snow Crab Legs	1 lb	150	130
Sockeye Salmon	1 lunch serving	160	50
Strip Steak	7 oz before cooking	690	140
Swordfish	1 lunch serving	100	100

FOOD	PORTION	CALORIES	CHOLESTEROL
Tilefish	1 lunch serving	100	80
Yellowfin Tuna	1 lunch serving	180	70

ROY ROGERS

FOOD	PORTION	CALORIES	CHOLESTEROL
Bacon Cheeseburger	1	581	103
Biscuit	1	231	5
Breakfast Crescent Sandwich	1	401	148
Breakfast Crescent Sandwich w/ Bacon	1	431	156
Breakfast Crescent Sandwich w/ Ham	1	442	305
Breakfast Crescent Sandwich w/ Sausage	1 reg	449	168
Breakfast Crescent Sandwich w/ Sausage	1 lg	608	94
Brownie	1	264	10
Cheeseburger	1	563	95
Chicken Breast	4.8 oz	412	118
Chicken Breast & Wing	6.5 oz	604	165
Chicken Leg	1.8 oz	140	40
Chicken Nuggets	6 nuggets	267	51
Chicken Thigh	3.2 oz	296	85
Chicken Thigh & Leg	5 oz	436	125
Chicken Wing	1.7 oz	192	47
Coffee, black	1 reg	0	0

FOOD	PORTION	CALORIES	CHOLESTEROL
Coke	12 oz	145	0
Coleslaw	1 reg	110	5
Danish, Apple	1	249	15
Danish, Cheese	1	254	11
Danish, Cherry	1	271	11
Diet Coke	12 oz	1	0
French Fries	1 reg	268	42
French Fries	1 lg	357	56
Hamburger	1	456	73
Hot Chocolate	6 oz	123	35
Hot Topped Potato w/ Bacon 'n Cheese	1	397	34
Hot Topped Potato w/ Broccoli 'n Cheese	1	376	19
Hot Topped Potato w/ Oleo	1	274	0
Hot Topped Potato w/ Sour Cream 'n Chives	1	408	31
Hot Topped Potato w/ Taco Beef 'n Cheese	1	463	37
Hot Topped Potato, Plain	1	211	0
Ice Tea	1 reg	0	0
Large Roast Beef Sandwich	1	360	73
Large Roast Beef Sandwich w/ Cheese	1	467	95
Macaroni Salad	1 reg	186	5
Milk, Whole	8 oz	150	33
Orange Juice	7 oz	99	0
Orange Juice	10 oz	136	0

FOOD	PORTION	CALORIES	CHOLESTEROL
Pancake Platter w/ Syrup, Butter	1	452	53
Pancake Platter w/ Syrup, Butter, Bacon	1	493	63
Pancake Platter w/ Syrup, Butter, Ham	1	506	73
Pancake Platter w/ Syrup, Butter, Sausage	1	608	94
Potato Salad	1 reg	107	5
RR Bar Burger	1	611	115
Roast Beef Sandwich	1	317	55
Roast Beef Sandwich w/ Cheese	1	424	77
Shake, Chocolate	1	358	37
Shake, Strawberry	1	315	37
Shake, Vanilla	1	306	40
Strawberry Shortcake	1	447	28
Sundae, Caramel	1	293	23
Sundae, Hot Fudge	1	337	23
Sundae, Strawberry	1	216	23
SALAD BAR			
Beets, Sliced	¼ cup	16	0
Broccoli	½ cup	20	0
Carrots, Shredded	¼ cup	42	0
Croutons	2 Tbsp	70	0
Cucumbers	5–6 slices	4	0
Green Peas	¼ cup	7	0

FOOD	PORTION	CALORIES	CHOLESTEROL
Green Peppers	2 Tbsp	4	0
Lettuce	1 cup	10	0
Mushrooms	¼ cup	5	0
Sunflower Seeds	2 Tbsp	157	0
Tomatoes	3 slices	20	0

SHAKEY'S
(*see also* PIZZA, DOMINO'S PIZZA)

All servings are based on 1 slice from a 12" pie cut into 10 slices.

PIZZA			
Homestyle Shakey's Special	1 slice	384	29
Homestyle Cheese	1 slice	303	21
Homestyle w/ Onion, Green Peppers, Olives, Mushrooms	1 slice	320	21
Homestyle w/ Pepperoni	1 slice	343	27
Homestyle w/ Sausage, Mushrooms	1 slice	343	24
Homestyle w/ Sausage, Pepperoni	1 slice	374	24
Thick Crust, Cheese Only	1 slice	170	13
Thick Crust, Shakey's Special	1 slice	208	18
Thick Crust w/ Pepperoni	1 slice	185	17
Thick Crust w/ Sausage, Mushrooms	1 slice	179	15
Thick Crust w/ Sausage, Pepperoni	1 slice	177	19
Thick Crust w/ Green Pepper, Black Olives, Mushrooms	1 slice	162	13
Thin Crust, Cheese Only	1 slice	133	14

FOOD	PORTION	CALORIES	CHOLESTEROL
Thin Crust, Shakey's Special	1 slice	171	16
Thin Crust w/ Pepperoni	1 slice	148	14
Thin Crust w/ Sausage, Mushroom	1 slice	141	13
Thin Crust w/ Sausage, Pepperoni	1 slice	166	17
Thin Crust w/ Onion, Green Pepper, Black Olives, Mushroom	1 slice	125	11

TACO BELL

FOOD	PORTION	CALORIES	CHOLESTEROL
Bellbeefer	1	312	39
Bellbeefer, Green	1	306	39
Burrito, Double Beef Supreme, Green	1	459	59
Burrito Supreme Platter	1	774	79
Burrito Supreme Platter, Green	1	762	79
Burrito, Bean	1	360	14
Burrito, Bean, Green	1	354	14
Burrito, Beef	1	402	59
Burrito, Beef, Green	1	396	59
Burrito, Combo	1	381	36
Burrito, Combo, Green	1	375	36
Burrito, Double Beef Supreme	1	464	59
Burrito Supreme	1	422	35
Burrito Supreme, Green	1	416	35
Cinnamon Crispas	1	266	2

FOOD	PORTION	CALORIES	CHOLESTEROL
Enchirito	1	382	56
Enchirito, Green	1	370	56
Fabulous Steak Fajita	1	235	14
Fabulous Steak Fajita w/ Guacamole	1	269	14
Fabulous Steak Fajita w/ Sour Cream	1	281	14
Mexican Pizza	1	714	81
Nachos	1	356	9
Nachos Bellgrande	1	719	43
Pico De Gallo	1	8	tr
Pintos & Cheese	1	194	19
Pintos & Cheese, Green	1	189	19
Ranch Dressing	2½ oz	236	35
Salsa	3 oz.	18	0
Seafood Salad w/o Dressing	1	648	82
Seafood Salad w/o Dressing & Shell	1	216	81
Seafood Salad w/ Ranch Dressing	1	884	117
Taco	1	184	32
Taco Bellgrande	1	351	55
Taco Bellgrande Platter	1	1002	80
Taco Bellgrande Platter, Green	1	990	80
Taco Light	1	411	57
Taco Light Platter	1	1062	82
Taco Light Platter, Green	1	1051	82
Taco Salad w/ Ranch Dressing	1	1167	121

FOOD	PORTION	CALORIES	CHOLESTEROL
Taco Salad w/ Salsa	1	949	85
Taco Salad w/o Beans	1	822	80
Taco Salad w/o Salsa	1	931	85
Taco Salad w/o Shell	1	524	82
Taco Sauce	1 pkg	2	0
Taco Sauce, Hot	1 pkg	3	0
Taco, Soft	1	228	32
Tostada	1	243	18
Tostada, Beefy	1	322	40
Tostada, Beefy, Green	1	316	40
Tostada, Green	1	238	18

WENDY'S

SANDWICH TOPPINGS

All Wendy's sandwiches are custom-made. The following list of sandwich toppings allows you to calculate the cholesterol and calories in any sandwich you order.

FOOD	PORTION	CALORIES	CHOLESTEROL
Single Hamburger Patty, no bun	1 (4 oz)	210	75
Bacon	1 strip	30	5
Big Classic	1	470	80
Biscuit, Buttermilk	1	320	tr
Breakfast Potatoes	1	360	20
Breakfast Sandwich	1	370	200
Bun, Kaiser	1	180	5
Bun, Multi-Grain	1	140	tr
Bun, White	1	140	tr
Chicken Breast Fillet	1	200	60

FOOD	PORTION	CALORIES	CHOLESTEROL
Chicken Fried Steak	1	580	95
Chili	1 reg	240	25
Chocolate Chip Cookie	1	320	5
Coca-Cola	8 oz	100	0
Coffee, Decaffeinated, black	6 oz	2	0
Coffee, black	6 oz	2	0
Creamer, Non- Dairy	⅜ oz	14	0
Crispy Chicken Nuggets; cooked in animal/ vegetable oil	6 pieces	290	55
Crispy Chicken Nuggets; cooked in vegetable oil	6 pieces	310	50
Diet Coke	8 oz	0	0
Diet Pepsi	8 oz	0	0
Dr Pepper	8 oz	100	0
Egg, Fried	1 egg	90	230
Eggs, Scrambled	2 eggs	190	450
Fish Fillet	1	210	45
French Fries; cooked in vegetable oil	1 reg	300	5
French Fries; cooked in animal /vegetable oil	1 reg	310	15
French Toast	2 slices	400	115
French Toast, Apple Topping	1 pkg	130	0
French Toast, Blueberry Topping	1 pkg	60	0
French Toast, Syrup	1 pkg	140	0
Frosty Dairy Dessert	1 sm	400	50
Grape Jelly	1 pkg	40	0

FOOD	PORTION	CALORIES	CHOLESTEROL
Half & Half	⅜ oz	14	5
Hot Chocolate	6 oz	110	tr
Kid's Meal Hamburger	1	200	35
Lemonade	12 oz	160	0
Milk, 2%	8 oz	110	20
Milk, Chocolate	8 oz	190	25
Milk, Whole	8 oz	140	30
Mountain Dew	8 oz	110	0
Nuggets Sauce, Barbecue	1 pkg	50	0
Nuggets Sauce, Honey	1 pkg	45	0
Nuggets Sauce, Sweet & Sour	1 pkg	45	0
Nuggets Sauce, Sweet Mustard	1 pkg	50	0
Omelet #1	1	290	355
Omelet #2	1	250	450
Omelet #3	1	280	525
Omelet #4	1	210	460
Orange Juice	6 oz	80	0
Pepsi-Cola	8 oz	110	0
Sausage Gravy	6 oz	440	85
Sausage Patty	1	200	45
Slice, Lemon-Lime	8 oz	100	0
Slice, Mandarin Orange	8 oz	110	0
Taco Salad	1	430	45
Taco Sauce	1 pkg	10	0
Tea, Hot or Iced	6 oz hot 12 oz iced	0	0

FOOD	PORTION	CALORIES	CHOLESTEROL
Toast, Wheat w/ Margarine	2 slices	190	5
Toast, White	2 slices	250	20
GARDEN SPOT SALAD BAR			
Alfalfa Sprouts	1 oz	8	0
American Cheese	1 oz	90	5
Bacon Bits	1 tsp	10	tr
Blueberries	1 Tbsp	6	0
Breadsticks	2	35	tr
Broccoli	½ cup	12	0
Cabbage, Red	¼ cup	4	0
Cantaloupe	2 pieces (2 oz)	18	0
Carrots	¼ cup	10	0
Cauliflower	½ cup	12	0
Celery	1 Tbsp	tr	0
Cheddar Cheese (imitation)	1 oz	80	tr
Cherry Tomatoes, Pickled	1 Tbsp	14	0
Coleslaw	¼ cup	80	40
Cottage Cheese	½ cup	110	20
Cucumbers	4 slices	2	0
Eggs; hard cooked, chopped	1 Tbsp	30	90
Grapefruit	2 oz	10	0
Grapes	¼ cup	30	0
Green Peas	1 oz	25	0
Green Peppers	¼ cup	8	0
Honeydew Melon	2 pieces (2 oz)	20	0
Jalapeno Peppers	1 Tbsp	9	0

FOOD	PORTION	CALORIES	CHOLESTEROL
Lettuce	1 cup	8	0
Mozzarella Cheese (imitation)	1 oz	90	tr
Mushrooms	¼ cup	4	0
Oranges	2 oz	25	0
Parmesan, Grated	1 oz	130	20
Pasta Salad	¼ cup	130	5
Peaches	2 pieces	17	0
Pepper Rings, Pickled	1 Tbsp	2	0
Pineapple Chunks	½ cup	70	0
Provolone Cheese	1 oz	90	tr
Radishes	½ oz	2	0
Red Onions	3 rings	2	0
Salad Dressing, Blue Cheese	1 Tbsp	60	10
Salad Dressing, Celery Seed	1 Tbsp	70	5
Salad Dressing, French Style	1 Tbsp	70	0
Salad Dressing, Golden Italian	1 Tbsp	50	0
Salad Dressing, Oil	1 Tbsp	120	0
Salad Dressing, Ranch	1 Tbsp	50	5
Salad Dressing, Reduced Calorie Bacon/Tomato	1 Tbsp	45	tr
Salad Dressing, Reduced Calorie Creamy Cucumber	1 Tbsp	50	tr
Salad Dressing, Reduced Calorie Italian	1 Tbsp	25	0
Salad Dressing, Reduced Calorie Thousand Island	1 Tbsp	54	5
Salad Dressing, Thousand Island	1 Tbsp	70	10

FOOD	PORTION	CALORIES	CHOLESTEROL
Salad Dressing, Wine Vinegar	1 Tbsp	2	0
Strawberries	2 oz	18	0
Sunflower Seeds & Raisins	1 oz	140	0
Swiss Cheese (imitation)	1 oz	90	5
Tomatoes	1 oz	6	0
Watermelon	2 pieces (2 oz)	18	0

HOT STUFFED BAKED POTATOES

FOOD	PORTION	CALORIES	CHOLESTEROL
Bacon & Cheese	1	570	22
Broccoli & Cheese	1	500	23
Cheese	1	590	22
Chili & Cheese	1	510	22
Plain	1	250	0
Sour Cream & Chives	1	460	15

SANDWICH TOPPINGS

FOOD	PORTION	CALORIES	CHOLESTEROL
American Cheese	1 slice	60	15
Bacon	1 strip	30	5
Ketchup	1 tsp	6	0
Lettuce	1 leaf	2	0
Mayonnaise	1 Tbsp	90	10
Mustard	1 tsp	4	0
Onion	3 rings	2	0
Pickles, Dill	4 slices	2	0
Tomatoes	1 slice	2	0

ZANTIGO

FOOD	PORTION	CALORIES	CHOLESTEROL
Beef Enchilada	1	315	49

FOOD	PORTION	CALORIES	CHOLESTEROL
Cheese Enchilada	1	390	63
Hot Chilito	1	329	32
Mild Chilito	1	330	26
Taco	1	198	31
Taco Burrito	1	415	44

APPENDIX
Baby Foods

BABY FOODS

Strained foods packed for infant feeding are often used to feed adults when they cannot chew regular foods. It is for this reason that we include the following products. It is neither necessary nor desirable to limit cholesterol intake in infant and toddler diets.

FOOD	PORTION	CALORIES	CHOLESTEROL
CEREAL			
Baby Cereal (Health Valley)	1 oz	60	0
Baby Cereal Brown Rice (Health Valley)	1 oz	60	0
BAKED GOODS			
Animal Shaped Cookies (Gerber)	2	60	tr
Arrowroot Cookies (Gerber)	2	50	tr
Pretzels (Gerber)	2	50	0
Toddler Biter Biscuits (Gerber)	1	50	tr
Zwieback Toast (Gerber)	2	60	tr
CHUNKY FOODS			
Homestyle Noodles & Beef (Gerber)	6 oz	150	14
Macaroni Alphabets w/ Beef & Tomato Sauce (Gerber)	6.25 oz	130	13

FOOD	PORTION	CALORIES	CHOLESTEROL
Noodles & Chicken w/ Carrots & Peas (Gerber)	6 oz	100	20
Rice w/ Beef & Tomato Sauce (Gerber)	6.25 oz	150	12
Saucy Rice w/ Chicken (Gerber)	6 oz	150	18
Spaghetti Tomato Sauce & Beef (Gerber)	6.25 oz	160	10
Vegetables & Beef (Gerber)	6.25 oz	140	10
Vegetables & Chicken (Gerber)	6.25 oz	140	16
Vegetables & Ham (Gerber)	6.25 oz	120	10
Vegetables & Turkey (Gerber)	6.25 oz	110	20

JUNIOR AND TODDLER MEATS

FOOD	PORTION	CALORIES	CHOLESTEROL
Beef (Gerber)	3.5 oz	110	27
Chicken (Gerber)	3.5 oz	140	58
Chicken Sticks (Gerber)	2.5 oz	120	65
Ham (Gerber)	3.5 oz	120	29
Meat Sticks (Gerber)	2.5 oz	110	33
Turkey (Gerber)	3.5 oz	130	53

FOOD	PORTION	CALORIES	CHOLESTEROL
Turkey Sticks (Gerber)	2.5 oz	120	61
Veal (Gerber)	3.5 oz	100	27
JUNIOR DESSERTS			
Dutch Apple (Gerber)	6 oz	128	7
Fruit Dessert (Gerber)	6 oz	128	0
Hawaiian Delight (Gerber)	6 oz	105	3
Peach Cobbler (Gerber)	6 oz	128	0
Vanilla Custard Pudding (Gerber)	6 oz	128	23
JUNIOR DINNERS			
Beef Egg Noodle Dinner (Gerber)	7.5 oz	140	12
Beef w/ Vegetables (Gerber)	4.5 oz	130	13
Chicken Noodle Dinner (Gerber)	7.5 oz	120	18
Chicken w/ Vegetables (Gerber)	4.5 oz	130	21
Ham w/ Vegetables (Gerber)	4.5 oz	110	13
Macaroni Tomato Beef Dinner (Gerber)	7.5 oz	130	8
Spaghetti Tomato Sauce Beef Dinner (Gerber)	7.5 oz	140	9

FOOD	PORTION	CALORIES	CHOLESTEROL
Split Peas w/ Ham Dinner (Gerber)	7.5 oz	150	5
Turkey Rice Dinner (Gerber)	7.5 oz	120	24
Turkey w/ Vegetables (Gerber)	4.5 oz	140	15
Vegetable Bacon Dinner (Gerber)	7.5 oz	180	7
Vegetable Beef Dinner (Gerber)	7.5 oz	140	9
Vegetable Chicken Dinner (Gerber)	7.5 oz	120	17
Vegetable Ham Dinner (Gerber)	7.5 oz	140	9
Vegetable Lamb Dinner (Gerber)	7.5 oz	140	6
Vegetable Turkey Dinner (Gerber)	7.5 oz	120	24
STRAINED DESSERTS			
Banana Apple (Gerber)	4.5 oz	90	0
Cherry Vanilla Pudding (Gerber)	4.5 oz	90	3
Chocolate Custard Pudding (Gerber)	4.5 oz	110	14
Dutch Apple (Gerber)	4.5 oz	100	4
Fruit Dessert (Gerber)	4.5 oz	100	0
Hawaiian Dessert (Gerber)	4.5 oz	120	2

FOOD	PORTION	CALORIES	CHOLESTEROL
Orange Pudding (Gerber)	4.5 oz	110	11
Peach Cobbler (Gerber)	4.5 oz	100	0
Vanilla Custard Pudding (Gerber)	4.5 oz	100	15

STRAINED DINNERS

FOOD	PORTION	CALORIES	CHOLESTEROL
Beef Egg Noodle Dinner (Gerber)	4.5 oz	90	6
Beef w/ Vegetables (Gerber)	4.5 oz	120	11
Chicken Noodle Dinner (Gerber)	4.5 oz	80	10
Chicken w/ Vegetables (Gerber)	4.5 oz	140	18
Ham w/ Vegetables (Gerber)	4.5 oz	100	12
Macaroni Cheese Dinner (Gerber)	4.5 oz	90	3
Macaroni Tomato Beef Dinner (Gerber)	4.5 oz	90	3
Turkey Rice Dinner (Gerber)	4.5 oz	80	15
Turkey w/ Vegetables (Gerber)	4.5 oz	130	17
Vegetable Bacon Dinner (Gerber)	4.5 oz	100	4
Vegetable Beef Dinner (Gerber)	4.5 oz	80	5
Vegetable Chicken Dinner (Gerber)	4.5 oz	80	7

FOOD	PORTION	CALORIES	CHOLESTEROL
Vegetable Ham Dinner (Gerber)	4.5 oz	80	4
Vegetable Lamb Dinner (Gerber)	4.5 oz	90	3
Vegetable Liver Dinner (Gerber)	4.5 oz	60	29
Vegetable Turkey Dinner (Gerber)	4.5 oz	70	12

STRAINED MEATS AND EGG YOLKS

FOOD	PORTION	CALORIES	CHOLESTEROL
Beef (Gerber)	3.5 oz	100	29
Chicken (Gerber)	3.5 oz	100	61
Egg Yolks (Gerber)	2.25 oz	128	398
Ham (Gerber)	3.5 oz	110	24
Lamb (Gerber)	3.5 oz	100	38
Pork (Gerber)	3.5 oz	110	35
Turkey (Gerber)	3.5 oz	130	58
Veal (Gerber)	3.5 oz	100	25